eHealth Research Theory and Development

This is the first book to provide a comprehensive overview of the multidisciplinary domain of eHealth – one of the most important recent developments in healthcare. It provides an overview of the possibilities of eHealth for different healthcare sectors, an outline of theoretical underpinnings and effectiveness, and key models, frameworks and methods for its development, implementation, and evaluation. This fully revised second edition brings together up-to-date knowledge on eHealth and includes several new chapters and sections on important topics such as implementation, human-centred design, healthcare systems, and evaluation methods.

The first part of this book is focused on the underpinnings of eHealth, and consists of chapters on behaviour change, the possibilities of technology for healthcare systems, and the current state of affairs of eHealth for mental and public health. In the second part, chapters on development, implementation, and evaluation of eHealth are provided, presenting methods, theories and frameworks from disciplines such as human-centred design, engineering, psychology, business modelling, and implementation science. By drawing together expertise from different disciplines, the book offers a holistic approach to the use of technology to support health and wellbeing, giving readers an insight into how eHealth can offer multiple solutions for the major challenges with which our healthcare system is faced.

Case studies, learning objectives, end of chapter summaries, and a list of key terms, make this accessible book very suitable for students, as well as researchers and healthcare professionals. Due to its multidisciplinary nature, it can be used by readers from a broad range of fields, such as psychology, health sciences, and human-centred design.

Hanneke Kip works as an assistant professor at the Centre for eHealth and Wellbeing Research of the University of Twente and as a researcher at Transfore – a forensic psychiatric organization in the Netherlands.

Nienke Beerlage-de Jong is an assistant professor at the section of Health Technology and Services Research at TechMed Centre of the University of Twente, the Netherlands.

Lisette (J.E.W.C.) van Gemert-Pijnen is a full professor of persuasive health technology at the University of Twente, the Netherlands.

Robbert Sanderman is emeritus professor and previously full professor and head of the Health Psychology group at the Faculty of Medicine at the University Medical Centre Groningen.

Saskia M. Kelders is an associate professor of engaging eHealth technologies at the Department of Psychology, Health and Technology at the University of Twente, Enschede, the Netherlands.

eHealth Research Theory and Development

A Multidisciplinary Approach

Second Edition

Edited by
Hanneke Kip, Nienke Beerlage-de Jong,
Lisette (J.E.W.C.) van Gemert-Pijnen,
Robbert Sanderman, and Saskia M. Kelders

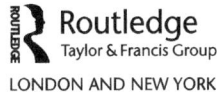

LONDON AND NEW YORK

Designed cover image: © Esther Scheide

Second edition published 2024
by Routledge
4 Park Square, Milton Park, Abingdon, Oxon OX14 4RN

and by Routledge
605 Third Avenue, New York, NY 10158

Routledge is an imprint of the Taylor & Francis Group, an informa business

First edition published by Routledge 2018

Trademark notice: Product or corporate names may be trademarks or registered trademarks, and are used only for identification and explanation without intent to infringe.

British Library Cataloguing-in-Publication Data
A catalogue record for this book is available from the British Library

Library of Congress Cataloging-in-Publication Data
Names: Kip, Hanneke, editor. | Beerlage de Jong, Nienke, editor. |
Gemert-Pijnen, Lisette van, editor. | Sanderman, R. (Robbert), editor. |
Kelders, Saskia M., editor.
Title: EHealth research theory and development : a multidisciplinary
approach / edited by Hanneke Kip, Nienke Beerlage-de Jong,
Lisette van Gemert-Pijnen, Robbert Sanderman & Saskia Kelders.
Description: 2nd edition. | Abingdon, Oxon ; New York, NY : Routledge, 2024. |
Includes bibliographical references and index.
Identifiers: LCCN 2023053869 (print) | LCCN 2023053870 (ebook) |
ISBN 9781032295367 (hardback) | ISBN 9781032295237 (paperback) |
ISBN 9781003302049 (ebook)
Subjects: LCSH: Medical telematics. | Telecommunication in medicine. |
Medical technology. | Medical informatics.
Classification: LCC R119.95 .E37 2024 (print) |
LCC R119.95 (ebook) | DDC 610.1/4–dc23/eng/20240208
LC record available at https://lccn.loc.gov/2023053869
LC ebook record available at https://lccn.loc.gov/2023053870

ISBN: 9781032295367 (hbk)
ISBN: 9781032295237 (pbk)
ISBN: 9781003302049 (ebk)

DOI: 10.4324/9781003302049

Typeset in Times New Roman
by Newgen Publishing UK

Contents

Contributors

Editors

Hanneke Kip works as an assistant professor at the Centre for eHealth and Wellbeing Research of the University of Twente and as a researcher at Transfore – a forensic psychiatric organization. She aims to understand how technologies such as virtual reality, mobile apps, and wearables can be of added value for mental healthcare for people with severe mental illness. She is specifically interested in the working mechanisms and interdisciplinary development, implementation, and evaluation of these technologies.

Nienke Beerlage-de Jong is assistant professor at the section of Health Technology and Services Research at TechMed Centre of the University of Twente, the Netherlands. She also holds a guest appointment at University Medical Centre Groningen, the Netherlands. Her work focuses on eHealth technologies aiming to foster behaviour change in the face of complex healthcare challenges. Her research primarily revolves around planetary- and one-health; fostering multidisciplinary, intersectoral, and cross-national collaborations.

Lisette (J.E.W.C.) van Gemert-Pijnen is a professor of persuasive health technology at the University of Twente. Her research focuses on persuasive designs to increase trust and adherence to technologies and to develop methods for implementation in practice. She founded the first Center for eHealth Research that produced the CeHRes Roadmap. She is involved in a university-wide strategic research programme to accelerate the uptake and implementation of health technologies.

Robbert Sanderman was trained as a clinical psychologist and got his PhD in 1988. In 1999 he became a full professor and head of the Health Psychology group at the Faculty of Medicine of the University Medical Centre Groningen until his retirement in 2020. From 2013 to 2020, he has also been a full Professor of Health Psychology & Head of the Health Psychology Department at the University of Twente. His research is focused on psychological and social adaptive processes in patients diagnosed with a chronic somatic disease (e.g., cancer, diabetes, heart failure, and COPD) and eHealth interventions. He supervised 70 PhD projects, co-edited several handbooks on chronic disease, and co-authored over 450 publications (articles, book chapters, and books).

Saskia M. Kelders is an associate professor at the Department of Psychology, Health and Technology at the University of Twente, Enschede, the Netherlands and extraordinary professor at Optentia Research Focus Area, North-West University, Vaal Triangle Campus. She chairs the 'engaging eHealth Technology lab' at the University of Twente which focuses on improving development, evaluation, and implementation of digital health interventions. Her work combines technological and psychological perspectives and is multidisciplinary in nature. Currently she works on her ERC Starting Grant on engagement as a mechanism of impact for Digital Mental Health Interventions.

Contributing Authors

Christina Bode is associate professor for Health Psychology & Technology at the University of Twente and Programme Director Psychology. Her research and teaching is dedicated to the question of how people with somatic chronic diseases can live a vital life and how this aim can be facilitated with innovative monitoring and behaviour change interventions. She studies explicit reflective and implicit BCTs and Virtual Reality environments in different application fields.

Annemarie Braakman-Jansen, PhD is assistant professor at the department of Psychology Health and Technology at the University of Twente. She is trained as a Health Scientist and obtained her PhD on the epidemiological project 'Prognosis in Early Arthritis' (2003). Her research focus is on design and implementation of sensing and supportive eHealth communication technology within the field of infection prevention and healthy aging for both elderly and (in)formal caregivers.

Catherine Burns is a Professor in Systems Design Engineering at the University of Waterloo, Canada, where she directs the Advanced Interface Design Lab. She holds a Tier 1 Canada Research Chair in Human Factors in Healthcare Systems. Catherine's research is in human factors engineering where she is well known for her work in Cognitive Work Analysis, Ecological Interface Design, and the development of decision support systems. In this area she has contributed over 300 publications and is the co-author of seven books. She is a Fellow of the Human Factors and Ergonomics Society. At the University of Waterloo, Catherine is also Associate Vice President, Health Initiatives where she leads the University of Waterloo's Health Futures strategy.

Rory Coyne is a PhD student in the School of Psychology at University of Galway. He completed the MSc in Health Psychology at the University of Galway in 2021. His PhD research is concentrated on measuring drivers' physiological responses to automated driving systems. He is also a member of the mHealth Research Group at the University of Galway, directed by Professor Jane Walsh.

Rik Crutzen is Professor of Behaviour Change and Technology at Maastricht University's Care and Public Health Research Institute (CAPHRI), where he also chairs the Department of Health Promotion. Besides expertise on behaviour change in general, his work has a specific focus on if and how we can use technological innovations to improve both reach and efficacy of behaviour change interventions to improve health and quality of life.

Roberto R. Cruz Martinez, PhD is a psychologist with a background in sport psychology and health psychology. His main research interest is the study of support strategies via digital technologies for self-regulatory behaviours, in both healthy and ill individuals. Roberto currently works as an information specialist and as open-access specialist at the University of Twente, in the Netherlands.

Tessa Dekkers, PhD is a researcher in digital health and technology, currently an Assistant Professor at the Department of Psychology, Health & Technology of the University of Twente. Her expertise lies in participatory human-centered design, with a focus on enhancing digital health interventions' accessibility and inclusivity, especially for marginalized groups facing health disparities.

Andrea W.M. Evers is professor of Health Psychology at Leiden University, the Netherlands. She is also affiliated to the Technical University Delft and Erasmus University Rotterdam as

Medical Delta Professor Healthy Society. Andrea W.M. Evers uniquely combines fundamental and applied science in her interdisciplinary research, by focusing both on basic research and translational behavioral research in the area of prevention, screening, and innovative interventions (e.g., eHealth tools).

Trish Greenhalgh is a medical doctor and Professor of Primary Care Health Sciences at the University of Oxford, UK. As co-Director of the Interdisciplinary Research In Health Sciences (IRIHS) unit, Trish leads a programme of research at the interface between social sciences and medicine, with strong emphasis on the organisation and delivery of health services.

Christiane Grünloh, PhD is a senior researcher at Roessingh Research and Development (The Netherlands). She has a medical background with several years of experience as a medical assistant (GP, Urology), holds degrees in Media Informatics (BSc, MSc), and a PhD in Human-Computer interaction. Christiane is involved in (inter)national research projects on personalized health technology, adopting different participatory research approaches (e.g., action research, citizen science, human-centered and value sensitive design).

Wim H. van Harten is CEO of Rijnstate Hospital in Arnhem, full professor in Quality Management and Health care Technology and Research group leader in the Netherlands Cancer Institute in Amsterdam. He is President Emeritus of the European Organisation of Cancer Institutes, chair of the OECI working group on cancer economics, and regular chair of Accreditation & Designation site visits of major cancer centers in Europe.

Julia Keizer received her PhD at the University of Twente in 2022. Her research focused on supporting healthcare workers in limiting antibiotic resistance and infections in hospitals. Her research interests include complex healthcare related issues in which cooperation with healthcare workers and bridging theory and practice are crucial. She now works as a policy advisor at the Hospital Group Twente.

Lisa Klein Haneveld works as a researcher at Stichting Transfore, a forensic psychiatric healthcare institution in The Netherlands. She works on projects related to evaluation and implementation of technology, such as VR and biofeedback, to support healthcare professionals and their patients in reaching their treatment goals.

Iris ten Klooster has a background in Human Factors and Engineering Psychology. Currently, she is doing her PhD at the department Psychology, Health and Technology at the University of Twente. Her research focuses on exploring the diverse methods of utilizing data to personalize eHealth technologies.

Laura Kooij is Manager Innovation and Care Transformation in Rijnstate, a large teaching hospital in the Netherlands. She obtained her PhD on digital transformation in hospital care from the University of Twente, with research aimed at implementation and evaluation of eHealth in clinical practice. Her experience in different hospitals is in the field of digital transformation, especially development and implementation of digital health in clinical practice.

Eimear Morrissey, PhD is a postdoctoral researcher at the School of Psychology and School of Medicine at University of Galway. She completed her PhD in Health Psychology in 2018. Her research centres on the self-management of long-term conditions, with a strong focus on Public and Patient Involvement.

Bart (L.J.M.) Nieuwenhuis is (retired) professor at the Department of High-tech Business and Entrepreneurship at the University of Twente. He is owner of the consultancy firm Knowledge for Business (K4B). He combined working for telecom companies and consultancy firms and lecturing and researching while being full professor at various universities in the Netherlands. Bart Nieuwenhuis graduated (cum laude) in Electrical Engineering and received a PhD in Computer Science.

Harri Oinas-Kukkonen is full professor of information systems at the University of Oulu, Finland. He has been listed among the 100 most influential ICT experts in the country and a key person to whom companies should talk to when developing their strategies for ICT services. He is the creator of the Persuasive Systems Design (PSD) model for developing ICT interventions that influence human behaviours. His research focuses on health behaviour change.

Chrysanthi Papoutsi is leading research on the social study of digital health, with a particular interest in the use of qualitative methods to examine how sociotechnical innovations are co-produced, implemented, and used in complex health and care settings.

Olga Perski is a Marie Skłodowska-Curie Postdoctoral Research Fellow at the University of California, San Diego, and Tampere University (Finland). Her research is focused on the development, optimization, and evaluation of interventions for smoking cessation and alcohol reduction delivered via smartphone apps, wearables, chatbots, and virtual reality. She is interested in the technology-enabled, real-time assessment and dynamic modelling of within-person processes, and the development of 'just-in-time adaptive interventions'.

Marcel Pieterse is associate professor at the Department of Psychology, Health and Technology at the University of Twente. He obtained his PhD in 1999 on the design and implementation of a brief smoking cessation intervention for Dutch general practitioners. He has been involved in numerous implementation projects since then. His research interests are treatment and prevention of addictions, healthcare interior design supporting recovery, and automatic processes in health behaviour.

Jacob Pitkow received his Bachelor of Arts in Government from Wesleyan University and completed the Post-Baccalaureate Program in Psychological Science at the University of California, Irvine. He has an interest in integrating psychology, sociology, policy, and technology. In his professional roles he has worked as a Data Scientist at Apple.

Leona Ryan is a Psychologist and Science Foundation Ireland (d-real) PhD scholar. Leona is part of the mHealth Research Group in the University of Galway under the direction of Professor Jane Walsh where behavioural science is leveraged to increase the uptake of innovate digital health interventions across healthcare settings. Leona's research integrates health psychology principles with immersive technologies to support the design of novel education and training interventions for healthcare practitioners.

Stephen M. Schueller, PhD is an Associate Professor of Psychological Science and Informatics at UC Irvine. He received his bachelor's degree in psychology from the University of California, Riverside, his PhD in clinical psychology from the University of Pennsylvania, and completed his clinical internship and postdoctoral fellowship at the University of California, San Francisco. Dr. Schueller's work focuses on increasing access to and accessibility of mental health services through technology.

Rosalie van der Vaart, PhD has ample experience in the development, implementation, and evaluation of digital health interventions, particularly tailored for individuals with chronic somatic conditions. She places great emphasis on co-creation involving all stakeholders, with special attention to the requirements and skills/abilities of end-users and the operational workflows within which the technology is applied.

Lex van Velsen has been involved in the design of numerous eHealth services for chronic disease management, geriatrics, mental health, rehabilitation care, etc. His main focus here is aligning end-user needs, a technology push, and economic viability. Lex holds a PhD in technical communication. Currently, he is Head of Mobile at Nedap Healthcare.

Jane Walsh is the Director of the Mobile Technology and Health (mHealth) Research Group where she leads a programme of research of €20+ million euro funded by Horizon Europe, HRB, and SFI. She was appointed to the Royal Irish Academy Social Sciences Committee and is former Chair of the Psychological Society of Ireland, Division of Health Psychology. Jane was awarded the University of Galway President's Award for Research Excellence (2020).

Jobke Wentzel is a researcher/lecturer at Windesheim University of Applied Sciences, and specializes in eHealth, health care innovation, nursing care, nurse eHealth skills, and technology-related health care worker competences.

Preface

Aim of the Book

In both research and practice, an increasing amount of attention is paid to eHealth – the use of technology to support health, healthcare, and wellbeing. Since the publication of the first edition of this book in 2018, many new studies were conducted, new technologies were introduced, new models and theories were introduced, and existing ones were updated. Furthermore, the challenges that healthcare is faced with have not decreased since then; if anything, problems related to staff shortages, limited budgets, and patients with more complex (chronic) diseases have grown even further. Consequently, due to the rapid pace of technological change and the accompanying new developments in research and practice, a second edition of this book was comprised. In this second edition, we aim to provide an even broader and more in-depth overview of the complex, rapidly developing, and most of all interesting multidisciplinary domain of eHealth.

While eHealth technologies such as Internet-based interventions, mobile apps, and virtual reality have much potential to improve the efficiency and effectiveness of healthcare, their impact on practice is often lagging behind on expectations. One reason for this is that there is no good fit between the technology, the people involved, and their context. To address this multifaceted, complex problem, different perspectives need to be combined to shape the development, implementation, and evaluation processes in which people, technology, and context are accounted for. This book contributes to such a holistic, multidisciplinary approach by bringing together chapters on the development, implementation, and evaluation of eHealth; using methods, frameworks, and theories from disciplines, such as psychology, human-centred design, implementation science, engineering, and business modelling. In this way, this book aims to provide a comprehensive overview of the eHealth domain.

What's New in this Second Edition

In this second edition of the book, we provide an updated overview of the current state of affairs, possibilities, and limitations of eHealth for different healthcare settings. Some lessons learned from the first edition remain as relevant as ever, but other aspects of eHealth development, implementation, and evaluation have evolved and new insights have arisen. Consequently, all chapters have been rewritten and updated with new or updated theories and frameworks, examples from practice, and insights from research. More specifically, chapters have been thoroughly revised, and new chapters were added. The chapter on healthcare (Chapter 4) is entirely rewritten to provide a more comprehensive overview of different healthcare systems and the main challenges of healthcare. More attention is paid to specific frameworks and models that are relevant for healthcare in general. Because of the many new insights on eHealth development, implementation, and evaluation, the CeHRes Roadmap was updated to even better reflect research practice, resulting in a rewritten chapter on this framework (Chapter 7). Moreover, as it remains important, but challenging, to align eHealth interventions to the values of stakeholders, a new chapter on this topic was added (Chapter 9). Furthermore, because of the importance of implementation, a new chapter on models and frameworks for guiding this complex process was written (Chapter 13). In line with this, the chapter with examples and challenges from practice was thoroughly updated (Chapter 14). The chapter on engagement is rewritten, based on new, groundbreaking research on this topic (Chapter 15). Chapter 16 on evaluation is thoroughly revised as well, with more attention for overarching frameworks that can be used to guide evaluation processes. Finally, the chapter on the future of eHealth that was part of the first edition has been removed, because future directions and ethics are now intertwined throughout all chapters.

Target Groups of the Book

This book has multiple target groups. First, it is suited for students of studies (BSc and MSc) related to mental and somatic health and healthcare. Some examples are psychology, health sciences, mental health promotion, and health informatics. Second, as this book covers main principles and theories, more depth can be added, making it well-suited for e.g. PhD students or senior researchers exploring the field of eHealth. Third, the book's focus on the practical application of theoretical principles, methods, and cases derived from practice ensures that it is of added value for professionals working in practice, such as designers, policy makers, or healthcare professionals working with eHealth technologies. Finally, it is important to stress that since the book is not focused on local healthcare settings or on specific cases, but on underlying concepts and authors from multiple countries are involved, it can be used internationally.

In other words: This book is suitable for anyone who wants to look outside of their own discipline and wants to learn more about the new, exciting multidisciplinary domain of eHealth!

Organization of the Book

Structure

This edited, multidisciplinary book is focused on the theoretical underpinnings, development, implementation, and evaluation of eHealth. Chapters are written by experts in their domain, but are all embedded in the book's main structure and are aligned with its main principles. Following this, the book is divided in two sections. The first one is focused on the theoretical underpinnings and practical application of eHealth. The second part centres around the development, implementation, and evaluation. An overview of chapters and their authors is provided in the table below.

Part 1	Underpinnings Of eHealth	
Chapter 1	Introducing eHealth	Lisette (J.E.W.C.) van Gemert-Pijnen, Hanneke Kip, Saskia M. Kelders, Robbert Sanderman, & Nienke Beerlage-de Jong
Chapter 2	Psychological Principles and Health Behaviour Change	Jane Walsh, Eimear Morrissey, Rory Coyne, & Leona Ryan
Chapter 3	Opportunities of Technology to Promote Health and Wellbeing	Saskia M. Kelders
Chapter 4	Healthcare and Digital Transformation	Laura Kooij & Wim H. van Harten
Chapter 5	Mental Health and eHealth Technology	Jacob Pitkow & Stephen Schueller

How to Read this Book

Every chapter starts with a brief introduction of its main topic, followed by learning objectives that provide the main topics of the chapter. These learning objectives pinpoint what the author(s) find(s) most important and assist in distinguishing main matters from side matters. Key terms and their definitions can be found in the glossary at the end of this book. Furthermore, cases derived from practice are provided in boxes or sometimes plain text to illustrate abstract concepts. All chapters also contain references to other chapters when matters are discussed that are explained more elaborately elsewhere. Each chapter ends with several take-home messages that summarize the most important lessons learned from the chapter. Finally, key references are provided for learners that want to know more about the content matter of the chapter.

What to Expect from the Chapters

To provide an oversight of the main topics of each chapter, the learning objectives per chapter are provided below.

Chapter 1 – Introducing eHealth

After completing this chapter, you will be able to:

- Explain the relationship between technology, psychology, and health, and connect them to eHealth;
- State several application areas of eHealth and provide accompanying examples;
- Name several benefits and barriers of eHealth related to its development, implementation, evaluation, and use in practice;
- Explain what a holistic vision of eHealth entails and why it is required to overcome the barriers and achieve the benefits of eHealth;
- Name and explain the importance of interdisciplinary development, implementation, and evaluation of eHealth.

Chapter 2 – Psychological Principles and Health Behaviour Change

After completing this chapter, you will be able to:

- Provide definitions of psychology in general and its subdomains health psychology and positive psychology, and explain how they relate to health, well-being, and technology;
- Explain how self-management and health behaviours impact health and how and why technology can support these behaviours;
- Provide an overview of the science of health behaviour change with an emphasis on the Behaviour Change Technique Taxonomy and explain its relation to eHealth;
- Discuss developments in eHealth technologies for health behaviour change – both the development and evaluation of health behaviour change models and their application to real-world settings;
- Discuss the challenges associated with the use of eHealth technology to change behaviour.

Chapter 3 – Opportunities of Technology to Promote Health and Wellbeing

After completing this chapter, you will be able to:

- Discuss the evolution of technology, in particular technologies relating to supporting health, healthcare, and well-being;
- Provide different examples of technologies for health and discuss their advantages and limitations;
- Discuss important ethical issues concerning the use of technology, and in particular artificial intelligence (AI), in health;
- Explain the basics of common concepts in technology for health, and AI in particular;
- Name and explain different software design models and explain why they are important for eHealth.

Chapter 4 – Healthcare and Digital Transformation

After completing this chapter, you will be able to:

- Understand and explain the basics of healthcare systems from different countries;
- Explain the main challenges facing healthcare;

- Explain the relevant developments in healthcare in terms of healthcare transformation and eHealth technology;
- Explain the need for digital transformation and name important factors that affect this digital transformation;
- Explain and describe relevant theoretical models to explain technology acceptance and implementation of digital health technology in healthcare practice.

Chapter 5 – Mental Health and eHealth Technology

After completing this chapter, you will be able to:

- Describe the predominant models of care incorporating eMental health interventions;
- Reflect on the efficacy, limits, and ethical implications of eMental health interventions;
- Explain the differences between unsupported, supported, and virtual care models of eMental health interventions;
- Explain the potential for eMental health interventions to overcome barriers to traditional treatments;
- Discuss deficits in eMental health intervention research and practice.

Chapter 6 – Public Health, Behavioural Medicine, and eHealth Technology

After completing this chapter, you will be able to:

- Explain what public health and behavioural medicine are;
- Connect the challenges of the fields of public health and behavioural medicine to the possibilities of eHealth;
- State the effectiveness of the use of eHealth to stimulate healthy lifestyle behaviours and psychological adjustment;
- Provide examples of the application of eHealth within the fields of public health (focusing on primary and secondary prevention) and behavioural medicine;
- Discuss the specific possibilities and challenges within the fields of public health and behavioural medicine with regard to the use of eHealth.

Chapter 7 – The CeHRes Roadmap

After completing this chapter, you will be able to:

- Explain the need for a holistic, iterative, and interdisciplinary development, implementation, and evaluation approach for eHealth technology;
- Describe and explain the pillars that underpin holistic eHealth development, implementation, and evaluation;
- Describe and define the six main phases of the CeHRes Roadmap, state their main objectives, and explain the rationale behind each phase;
- Explain how the phases of the CeHRes Roadmap are interrelated and why an iterative, agile development approach is important;
- List several suitable models and methods for eHealth development, implementation, and evaluation and explain the added value of a multi-method, interdisciplinary approach for each phase.

Chapter 8 – The Contextual Inquiry

After completing this chapter, you will be able to:

- Explain why and in what way the contextual inquiry is an essential part of eHealth development;
- Provide concrete examples from practice to illustrate the relevance of conducting a contextual inquiry for the development of suitable eHealth technologies;
- Name and explain goals, benefits, and barriers of multiple research methods that can be used in the contextual inquiry;
- Explain the identification, analysis, and added value of stakeholders during the contextual inquiry and connect this to the entire process of eHealth development, implementation, and evaluation;
- Explain the role of the contextual inquiry within the entire process of developing, implementing, and evaluating eHealth.

Chapter 9 – Activities for Value Sensitive eHealth Design

After completing this chapter, you will be able to:

- Explain the goal, nature, and importance of multiple design activities (personas, scenarios, value propositions, service models, and requirements);
- Explain the interrelationship of multiple design activities and connect this to the fit of an eHealth technology with its context and its user;
- Create a value proposition for your eHealth service;
- Translate the findings from your contextual inquiry into service and technology design of eHealth via multiple design activities.
- Create a design document, including personas, scenarios, and requirements.

Chapter 10 – Business Modelling

After completing this chapter, you will be able to:

- Understand the basics of business modelling and explain its importance for eHealth implementation;
- Understand and apply the business model canvas and the value proposition canvas;
- Explain how to analyze the business impact of eHealth implementation;
- Identify the most relevant quantitative variables for eHealth implementation;
- Perform an indicative quantitative analysis for eHealth implementation.

Chapter 11 – Human-Centred Design

After completing this chapter, you will be able to:

- Explain the basic principles and rationale behind Human-Centred Design and understand their relevance for eHealth design;
- Name and explain several methods and approaches that are suitable for the different phases of HCD and connect them to eHealth design;

- Describe different types of prototypes and connect them to iterative design and the different phases of HCD;
- Explain the relevance of evaluation for HCD and compare the goals of several common evaluation techniques for different design stages;
- Name and explain different methods for remote, online HCD and understand their advantages and disadvantages.

Chapter 12 – Persuasive Health Technology

After completing this chapter, you will be able to:

- Explain what persuasive technology is, and in what way domains such as persuasive communication, health promotion, social marketing, technology acceptance, and human-media interaction are its underlying foundations;
- Analyze the added value of persuasive technology in the context of improving health and explain its relation to behaviour change (techniques);
- Explain the PSD model, name the four categories, and provide examples of accompanying persuasive features;
- Explain in what way persuasive technology can be used to develop and evaluate eHealth technologies;
- Provide examples of how persuasive features can be integrated into an eHealth technology.

Chapter 13 – Innovation, Improvement, and Implementation – Conceptual Frameworks for Thinking through Complex Change

After completing this chapter, you will be able to:

- Explain in broad terms why eHealth technologies, research findings, and other innovations often fail to get taken up to their full potential;
- Distinguish between innovation, improvement, and implementation;
- Define complexity and explain why complex phenomena are different from complicated ones;
- Explain different frameworks (such as DOI, CFIR, or NASSS) to a real initiative to implement an eHealth innovation or achieve an improvement in services;
- Provide examples of how the NASSS framework can be applied to implementation of technology in healthcare.

Chapter 14 – Sustainable eHealth Implementation: A Practical Perspective

After completing this chapter, you will be able to:

- Explain the complexity of eHealth implementation in practice;
- Understand and explain implementation factors that play a role in integrating eHealth in practice and upscaling to the market;
- Identify potential barriers for sustained implementation, in particular related to stakeholder engagement, financing, business modelling, and law and regulations;
- Identify points for improvement of implementation in practice and market.

Chapter 15 – Engagement

After completing this chapter, you will be able to:

- Provide a definition and explain the importance of three key concepts for eHealth: Acceptance, adoption, and adherence;
- Explain the concept, components, and conceptual framework of engagement;
- Name and explain ways of measuring and evaluating engagement;
- Provide examples of how engagement can be used to increase the effectiveness of eHealth technologies;
- Provide an overview of unexplored avenues and future directions for research on engagement with eHealth.

Chapter 16 – Evaluating eHealth

After completing this chapter, you will be able to:

- Provide several reasons for the importance of multi-method, iterative eHealth evaluation processes;
- Explain why eHealth can be seen as a black box and what the pitfalls of only conducting an RCT are;
- Explain how holistic, multi-method evaluations can contribute to opening the black box of eHealth;
- Explain the goals and phases of different types of evaluation frameworks: MOST-design, realist evaluation, and process evaluation;
- Name and explain several methods for the evaluation of effectiveness, efficiency, and adherence and engagement: RCTs, fractional factorial designs, Single Case Experimental Designs (SCEDs), log data analysis, mixed-methods research, and Health Technology Assessment (HTA).

Part 1

Underpinnings Of eHealth

1 Introducing eHealth

Lisette (J.E.W.C.) van Gemert-Pijnen, Hanneke Kip,
Saskia M. Kelders, Robbert Sanderman, &
Nienke Beerlage-de Jong

Introduction

eHealth, the use of technology to improve health, well-being, and healthcare is increasing rapidly. The rapid development of technologies such as VR, mobile apps, and wearables has instigated their application to healthcare. In this chapter, you will read that eHealth can have many advantages, like cost-effectiveness, process optimization, and an increased reach and impact. It has the potential to improve the quality of care, for example, by enabling healthcare professionals to better adhere to guidelines or by increasing patient satisfaction. The COVID-19 pandemic accelerated the use of some technologies, like video-consultation and telemonitoring, and ensured a change in prior regulations regarding the use of technology in healthcare. However, eHealth has not reached its full potential yet. Many eHealth technologies are not used as much or as intended, the goals on efficiency and effectiveness have not been achieved, and problems with financing the technology have been encountered. From this it becomes clear that there is room for improvement in the development, implementation, and evaluation of eHealth.

In this chapter, we introduce eHealth and describe its emergence, describe how eHealth can be used to improve health and well-being, and its possibilities to make healthcare more efficient and effective. We describe how eHealth is used in practice and what the added value of eHealth can be, including observed benefits and barriers. The chapter ends with an outline of the book. After completing this chapter, you will be able to:

- Explain the relationship between technology, psychology, and health, and connect them to eHealth;
- State several areas of application for eHealth and provide accompanying examples;
- Name several benefits and barriers of eHealth related to its development, implementation, evaluation, and use in practice;
- Explain what a holistic vision of eHealth entails and why it is required to overcome the barriers and achieve the benefits of eHealth;
- Name and explain the importance of interdisciplinary development, implementation, and evaluation of eHealth.

DOI: 10.4324/9781003302049-2

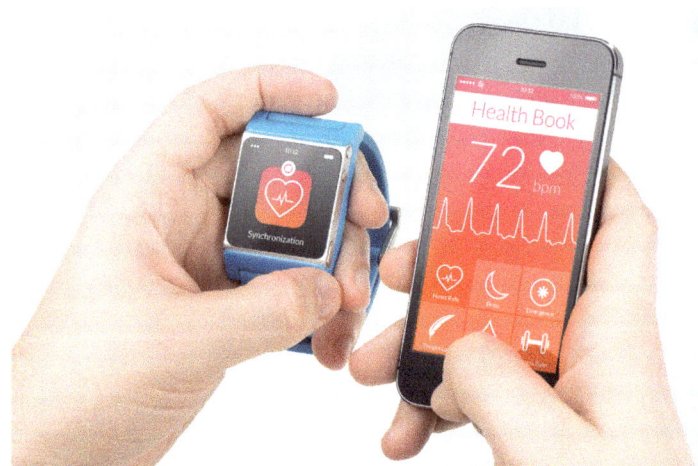

Figure 1.1 An example of how technology can be used to support our health and well-being.

Source: © Image used under license from Shutterstock.com

Why eHealth?

The essence of healthcare is to provide the best care possible that meets the needs of patients and their (social) environments. However, our healthcare system is under pressure. For example, due to declines in birth rates and longer life expectancies, the number and proportion of older people in our society is growing. An ageing population implies an increase in the chances of age-related illnesses like coronary heart disease, diabetes, and/or lung diseases. Many of these diseases are chronic diseases, which means the focus of care is more on managing the disease rather than on curing it. Older people may have more than one of these conditions simultaneously (called 'multi-morbidity'), which makes the demand for high-quality care even more complex. Another factor contributing to the rise of chronic conditions that require long-term care is lifestyle: Many people have unhealthy habits such as smoking, a sedentary lifestyle, or a diet with too much fat and sugar. This is related to problems such as joint pain, lung cancer, or diabetes mellitus type 2. Furthermore, an increase of mental illnesses such as depression and anxiety have been observed in many countries. These factors result in a high demand for good healthcare. Besides that, it is of importance to maintain the feasibility of this level of quality care over time. To this end, efforts are made to limit the demand for care, e.g., by focusing more on prevention of lifestyle-related disease, decreasing relapse in addiction, or to increasing patient satisfaction. This is highly relevant since, at the same time, fewer working-age adults and limited financial resources are available to support the increasing number of people with a need for care. Preserving high standards of patient-centred care with fewer resources is a challenge. This shows that the healthcare system is in great need of innovation.

A particular trend in the world today is that patients and their 'informal caregivers' (such as family members) are more in the lead in taking care of their own health. This is an extension of the traditional model, in which a professional caregiver is in the lead and makes most of the decisions. To allow patients and their informal caregivers to take on a more actively involved role in the management and treatment of their health and well-being, requires a shift in the way the healthcare system is shaped. Researchers and policy makers from all over the world are looking for innovative solutions that support patients and their informal caregivers, and many possible solutions have

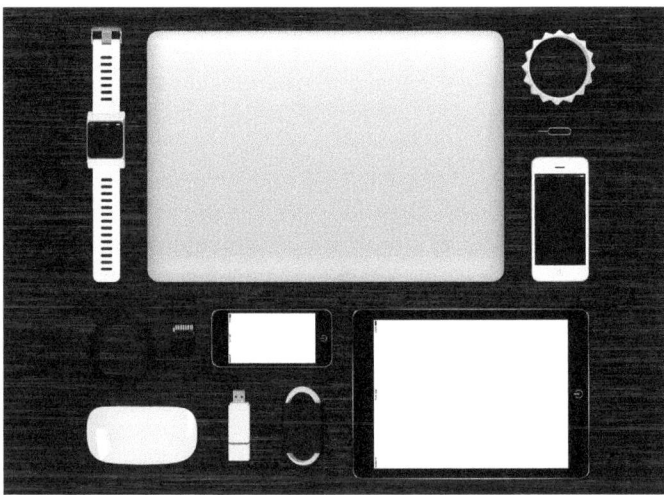

Figure 1.2 Examples of technologies that can be used to improve health and well-being.

Source: © Image used under license from Shutterstock.com

been thought of and tried out in practice. Serious options include de-hospitalization, organizing healthcare into regional networks, adequate homecare, and the concentration of highly specialized, complex care in one location. An integral part of many of these options is the use of technology. A large proportion of the population has access to and uses the Internet in their daily lives, via, for example, a PC, tablet, *wearables*, and/or smartphone (see Figure 1.2). Consequently, the role of technology is emphasized in such solutions, both within and outside healthcare.

Ways of Looking at Using Technology to Support Health

With the introduction of the Internet, eHealth became popular as an instrument for communication between patients and caregivers and for providing health-related information instead of paper-based information and telephone-guided communications. There have been active discussions about views and definitions on eHealth (Oh, Rizo, Enkin, & Jadad, 2005). The definition provided in an influential paper by Eysenbach called 'What is eHealth' in 2001 is still much-used:

> *eHealth is an emerging field in the intersection of medical informatics, public health and business, referring to health services and information delivered or enhanced through the Internet and related technologies. In a broader sense, the term characterizes not only a technical development, but also a state-of-mind, a way of thinking, an attitude, and a commitment for networked, global thinking, to improve healthcare locally, regionally, and worldwide by using information and communication technology.*
>
> (Eysenbach, 2001)

The Eysenbach statement is beyond defining eHealth merely as a tool or a device to change information or to facilitate communication. eHealth disrupts the healthcare infrastructure and delivery, and it implies that people should have the capacities and capabilities to use technology to support self-care and to create novel ways of healthcare delivery; affordable, accessible, and feasible for all. eHealth thus influences and is influenced by the context in which it is used. This context is

Box 1.1 eHealth terminology.

Within this book several terms that are used in the field of eHealth technologies are referred to. Many of them can be applied interchangeably, but they all have their specific meaning, as is explained below:

- *eHealth*: The use of technology to support health, well-being, and healthcare;
- *eHealth technology*: The actual technological system via which health, well-being, and healthcare are supported, often referring to information or communication technology;
- *eHealth intervention*: An eHealth intervention that is delivered through or supported by technology in an existing context by changing behaviour and/or cognitions;
- *Behaviour change interventions*: Behaviour change interventions are interventions designed to intentionally affect the actions that individuals take with regard to their health.

continuously changing due to demographics, changes in roles and role-players in healthcare, and the growing capacities of technology to generate and communicate data, showing the importance of constantly verifying whether eHealth is still optimally aligned with a specific context.

Throughout this book, the term eHealth will be used in multiple forms. Box 1.1 provides a brief overview of the terminology used.

eHealth in Practice

eHealth is increasingly being used in practice. In this section, we will provide several examples to give you an idea of what eHealth can look like. Within the field, there is no one perfect categorization that is always applicable, which has to with the continuously evolving possibilities of technology. In this book, we use a categorization that is based on the way different types of stakeholders are involved: *Self-care and prevention, supportive care,* and *societal health.*

Self-care and Prevention

In this domain, the patient or health consumer is in the lead. eHealth can be used to foster *self-management* in an easy and convenient way (see Figure 1.3 for a visualization). Examples are using a website or app to find health-related information, talking to peers with similar health issues in a discussion forum, or following a self-help course to quit smoking or lose weight. Sometimes a healthcare professional can be involved, for example, when he or she answers a question in an e-consultation or gives feedback within a self-help course, but this is not necessary.

In its simplest form, *self-care and prevention technologies* can be employed to unidirectionally provide information on health and well-being. There are many websites dedicated to offering credible and understandable health information, e.g., on the influence of alcohol on your brain. However, most eHealth technologies not only send information, but also offer an opportunity to interact with the system. Decision aids are one way of allowing the user to interact with information. In their simplest form, it can be question-and-answer systems that help health consumers or patients to decide on what to do with a certain health complaint or disease. Decision aids can help you to decide whether you need to visit a doctor or assist you in choosing the type of therapy that best suits you, for example, whether or not to have surgery for carpal tunnel syndrome. Ideally, these systems are based on medical protocols, and as of recently, they can be supported by artificial

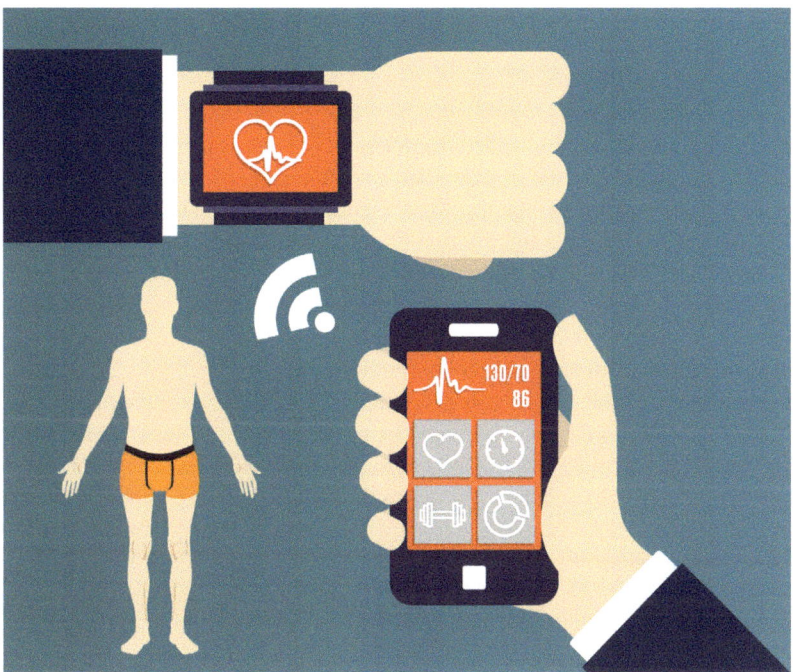

Figure 1.3 An example of how technology, in this case a smartwatch that monitors physical states and an app, can be used to self-manage health.

Source: © Image used under license from Shutterstock.com

intelligence. In addition, technologies such as discussion fora can stimulate interaction with others (e.g., with similar health issues) in multiple ways.

Another form of self-care and prevention can be found in technologies that support (*self*)-*monitoring* via the use of health-related information. Think of wearables like smartwatches that monitor behaviours such as physical activity or sleep. These data can be used to offer individual coaching, e.g., by motivating someone to move more in case of a lower step count, or to go to bed earlier in case of a lack of sleep. Sensors can also be used to collect real-time data about other health-related variables, such as heart rate, blood pressure, or glucose levels. In any case, it is important to interpret these data with care, since they might not always be as valid or reliable as a system might make them out to be. For example, an increased heart rate may be a sign of unhealthy stress, but it might also be an indication of healthy physical exercise.

A last example of self-care and prevention in eHealth technologies are online (self-help) interventions. These exist for many lifestyle areas, such as physical activity, dieting, and smoking, but also for mental health issues, such as (mild) depressive complaints, stress, or anxiety. Ideally, such online interventions are based on evidence-based protocols and are grounded in theories like *Cognitive-Behavioural Therapy*. They often use a fixed structure of lessons. For example, every lesson may start with an explanation of the purpose of the lesson, followed by assignments, exercises, and useful information provided by experts. Many of these interventions can be followed individually, at one's own pace and time, without support from a therapist. There are also online treatments available with therapist- or automated-support, open to anyone, even without a prescription from a healthcare professional. These types of interventions can prevent a further increase of (mental) health complaints by providing low-threshold treatment early on.

Supportive Care

This category of eHealth is characterized by more involvement of healthcare professionals. Ideally, if resources allow it, healthcare professionals and patients work together to manage or improve the health of the patient. In this domain, the care process is often more complex than in self-care and prevention, as caregivers are involved for a longer period of time, or multiple caregivers are involved, as is visualized in Figure 1.4. The care of patients with a chronic disease such as diabetes is an example of this. For instance, eHealth can improve the information exchange across professionals or between professionals and their patients, as well as provide online self-management support, and monitor the performance of disease management programmes.

One of the oldest examples of the role of eHealth in supportive care is *telemedicine*. In 1995, tele-dermatology – a form of telemedicine – became one of the first examples of eHealth among healthcare professionals. In tele-dermatology, telecommunication is used to exchange long-distance medical information, for example, by means of videoconferencing. This can enable a dermatologist to remotely diagnose skin lesions or allow one dermatologist to ask for another colleague's opinion about skin conditions based on actual images. As compared to just a text message or phone call, images can help dermatologists give more reliable advice.

Electronic *personal health records* (PHRs) are another example of eHealth technology for supportive care and chronic disease management. A PHR is an electronic application through which individuals can access, manage, and share their health information and that of others for whom they are authorized, in a private, secure, and confidential environment. Recently, many PHRs have added functionalities in order to support disease management. Besides sharing clinical and personal data (e.g., disease history, test results, treatment plans, and appointments) between patients and healthcare professionals, these systems often include functions to support self-management.

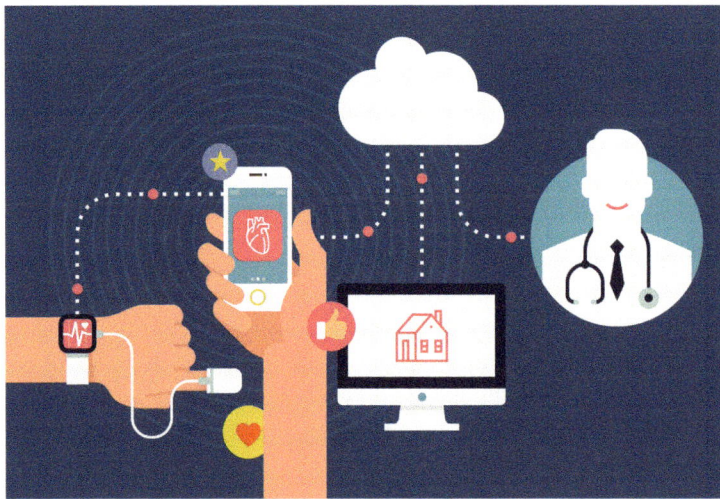

Figure 1.4 An example of the role that technology can play in the healthcare process. Patient data is automatically collected and sent to a general practitioner. It is also stored in a database that saves this information and makes it available to other healthcare professionals.

Source: © Image used under license from Shutterstock.com

Examples are working on health-related goals while being supported by a healthcare professional and/or the system, and facilitating communication between patient and healthcare professional, which allows patients to interact with their healthcare professional or make new appointments.

Societal Health

In this domain, patients and healthcare professionals are both involved, but the lead is at a higher, societal level. *Societal health* focuses on broad health-related issues that might affect individuals, of which the COVID-19 pandemic is an example. However, societal health issues can never be solved by the behaviour of just one individual (like self-care) or by a small group of people (like supportive care). Societal health issues demand that governments and health authorities play a vital role in creating policies and regulations. In turn, healthcare inspectorates must implement and maintain these policies and regulations. Examples of such broad societal health issues are the prevention, spread, and control of diseases and infections, as well as access to healthcare for everyone – which is especially relevant for low-income countries. As you can imagine, due to its large reach, interactivity, and ability to provide easy access to information, eHealth is often seen as a way to improve the health and well-being of individuals on a large scale and thus improve the health of a society as a whole.

First, eHealth can influence the attitude or awareness of individuals about societal health issues. An example of this is the CDC (the U.S. Center for Disease Control and Prevention) 'Solve the Outbreak' game. In this game, you become a disease detective trying to fight an outbreak before it can spread any further. Second, eHealth can be used to support behaviour that is compliant with guidelines that are required to manage broad health-related issues. Technology can help healthcare professionals adhere to policies or guidelines in a care environment, for example, in managing their use of antibiotics in order to decrease the spread of resistant bacteria. This is a societal health issue, where, for example, the government plays an important role in creating the policies on how to deal with this challenge. Technology can assist in translating such policies into action. Third, eHealth can be used to manage the behaviour of individuals during outbreaks of infectious diseases. An example are the mobile contact tracing apps that were introduced during the COVID-19 pandemic in multiple countries. Via Bluetooth, users received a notification when they had been within a specified distance (e.g., 1.5 meters) of an infected person. Finally, technology can support communication between health professionals about societal health issues. An example of this is the risk communication and education of healthcare professionals regarding zoonoses. Zoonoses are infectious diseases that are transmissible between animals and humans, like Lyme disease, MRSA, and COVID-19. Dealing with an outbreak of a zoonotic infection requires acute intensive cooperation between disciplines that do not normally do so. A technology such as a serious game can be used to support this. By simulating an outbreak, awareness of the importance of collaboration is raised among healthcare professionals. If such a game can be deployed in blended form, it can also contribute to low-threshold strengthening of the professional network.

Benefits of eHealth

In the first part of this chapter, we have given a general idea of the potential of eHealth and why it sometimes even seems necessary to use it. In this section, we will discuss in more detail why eHealth can be of added value. eHealth can have different advantages in different contexts and for different people. Therefore, an exhaustive list of all the possible eHealth benefits is impossible to compile. Also, not all benefits will always hold true for every eHealth technology. Again, this is because the technology's added value will vary depending on the context and the people. The benefits below are provided to give an idea of some of eHealth's advantages for healthcare and people in general. They refer to the access to care that eHealth can enhance, the empowerment of patients and healthy people via eHealth, its possibilities for innovating healthcare and the way we look at health and well-being, and its potential for improving quality of care.

Access to Care

Via eHealth, healthcare can become available independent of time and place. People can access it whenever and wherever they need it. An example is someone who has a busy working schedule and has trouble making appointments with his or her diabetes nurse, they can now contact the nurse whenever it suits them through a digital messaging service. Or think of the COVID-19 pandemic: Many people were still able to contact a caregiver via e.g., videoconferencing, despite lockdowns or quarantine. Furthermore, someone living in a remote area might use videoconferencing to contact his or her general practitioner instead of driving for an hour or so.

eHealth can also create a lower threshold to access healthcare, which means that more people have a possibility to access effective healthcare (WHO, 2016). With easier access, healthcare becomes more equally distributed among people, allowing for an improvement in healthcare equity. For example, think about the use of mobile apps for mental healthcare that can freely be used in low-income countries. These types of scalable interventions have the potential to reach thousands or even millions of people in need of care. Other examples are the use of online support groups to enable social networking of isolated individuals, or the use of an anonymous intervention for people with stigmatized illnesses, e.g., sexually transmitted diseases. A patient who may be uncomfortable finding help in person, due to taboos, might be more willing to talk with peers or care professionals online. However, there are preconditions for the actualization of this benefit, such as having access to the Internet and possessing satisfactory digital skills.

Empowerment

Technology may empower people by giving them the opportunity to take more control of their own healthcare. Technology can enable people to choose when and where they want to access care. For example, digital mental health interventions can be used to receive treatment outside of sessions with a psychologist, in a patient's own time. Working independently on (parts of) treatment might allow patients to attribute more positive change to their own effort, as opposed to only their caregivers'. Furthermore, people can be empowered when they are educated about their health and become more aware of their own health data, e.g., data on test outcomes in a personal health record, or data on sleep or steps per day collected by a wearable.

Patient-centredness is a closely related advantage. The patient-specific health data that are collected and analyzed via technology, allows healthcare to more specifically account for the individual patients' health needs and goals. It also facilitates shared decision making, which is a collaborative process through which caregiver and patient together come to a decision about treatment.

Finally, healthcare professionals can be empowered as well. Technology can provide tailored support for medical decision making, for example via *artificial intelligence*. Think of an AI-system that provides doctors with predictions on if and when a patient can best be discharged from a hospital. Furthermore, caregivers can use mobile apps to look at diagnoses or protocols. Quick, valid diagnoses and precise and personalized medicine are made possible by such data-driven systems.

Innovation

New technologies and new applications of technologies open up a whole range of possibilities for improving or even drastically changing healthcare (see Chapter 4). The mere use of technology will not automatically result in long-lasting and positive change, but if it is implemented well, it can provide the groundwork for sustainable change in healthcare. For example, eHealth can support important movements such as towards *patient-centred care* and shared decision making. A straightforward example of this is the opportunity that technology can create for easy communication between different healthcare professionals, e.g., consulting a specialist on a specific disease who lives in another country via videoconferencing. Another example is the use of mobile apps or Internet-based interventions in mental healthcare. These types of innovations can drastically change the role of a therapist, which might shift from being completely in charge regarding the content of treatment, to a more supportive role in which the patient works on large parts of treatment individually.

The possibilities that eHealth offers can be seen as a catalyst for innovation in healthcare. Technology can change the way healthcare is delivered, for example by opening up access to an array of data via the introduction of EMRs, or even by stimulating all involved stakeholders to critically think about how they deliver or receive care. Thus, on the one hand eHealth creates the technological opportunity for innovation, while on the other hand it also provides inspiration to see and discover new possibilities.

Quality of Care

The quality of healthcare can be improved via innovative systems and effective interventions that might result in lower costs and increased safety by reducing human errors. eHealth technologies can incorporate medical guidelines and quality standards for healthcare, for example, via an app that supports nurses in preparing and administering antibiotics to patients at their bedsides. This makes following guidelines or standards independent of individual healthcare professionals' knowledge and an integral part of the regular process. Information systems can even monitor real-time compliance with guidelines, e.g., hand hygiene, to support safety at work.

Effectiveness can also be improved by using the possibilities of technology to improve traditional interventions and treatments. For instance, think of an interactive virtual reality intervention in which patients with aggression-regulation problems can safely practice with remaining calm in different types of settings, together with their therapists. This provides new ways to practice with behaviour, as opposed to only talking about it in a treatment room. Another example is the use of an intervention for stimulating physical activity in patients with obesity, where wearables are used to track a person's activities throughout the day. The collected data can be used to provide tailored coaching – something that current traditional interventions and therapists cannot do.

Efficiency is an important benefit as well, since eHealth can require fewer resources to achieve the same quality of care and effects on health and well-being. For example, tele-dermatology – the use of video communication in the assessment and treatment of skin conditions – can decrease the number of doctor visits, saving costs by delivering high quality of care with fewer personnel. It can even contribute to preventing hospital admissions by catching e.g., skin tumours early on due to a lower threshold for receiving care.

eHealth Barriers

Up until now, we have mostly discussed the advantages of eHealth. However, in practice, eHealth technologies are often not as successful as expected. There are multiple barriers that cause this gap between the current situation and the potential benefits eHealth can bring – if it is used as intended. Furthermore, it is important to not just look at the possibilities of eHealth, but also critically reflect on barriers related to, for example, legislation or ethics. There are many barriers towards eHealth so this is not a comprehensive overview. For overview purposes, we divided them into implementation, ethical, and evidence barriers.

Uptake Barriers

Implementation of eHealth refers not only to the individual uptake in a certain context, but also to the integration in healthcare practices and maintenance for long-term use and upscaling a technology to the market. A successful eHealth intervention should be embedded in practice and used as was intended, but multiple factors can negatively influence its uptake in practice (Greenhalgh et al., 2017; Chapters 13 and 14).

First of all, a lack of incentive to use technology can result in a resistance to use it. For eHealth to be used it should be financially feasible. However, there often are no obvious financial benefits, and it is often not clear enough who pays for what. For example, videoconferencing (e-consultation) was often unsuccessful in reaching sustained use, because the reimbursement for using it in a general practitioners practice was lower than face-to-face visits. Innovative business models are needed to invest in technologies that provide care. For example, the shift from hospital care to homecare and the role of technology in supporting this requires different financing systems.

It is also not always clear if and how people benefit from eHealth: What is the added value? For example, self-management portals to support patients with chronic care, although proven effective, are often not used because patients feel they are not benefitting enough. This may for example be because of a perceived lack of human support. When people's needs are not acknowledged and thought through during the development process, eHealth technology can lack commitment because they do not perceive enough benefits for health or well-being.

Low eHealth literacy can hinder the uptake of eHealth technologies. Merely having digital skills or possessing a smartphone is not a guarantee people have the capacities and skills to manage their own health using technology. For example, people can have difficulty in understanding self-management data visualized via graphs or tables – implying the need for a suitable design that fits people's skills or might simply be a lack motivation to use it. These types of difficulties with using eHealth can further increase the digital divide, since highly educated people often benefit more than people with a lower education level.

Furthermore, there is often a lack of motivation to start or continue using an eHealth technology among users and other stakeholders. eHealth technologies touch the lives and work of many people. When the interests of these people are not acknowledged and thought through, the new eHealth technology can lack support. Think of nurses who have been told to start using an app that they haven't agreed to use in the first place and which may not fit into their individual work routines. Once people have accepted a technology, motivation can still be an issue: Many people stop using a technology prematurely or do not use all of the available opportunities. This issue is called non-adherence and indicates that eHealth interventions are not always motivating enough to use in the long term, which hampers effectiveness (Kelders et al., 2013).

Lack of trust or confidence in eHealth is another barrier. Healthcare providers might fear that they will be substituted by technology, for example, in the case of robots. Also, a well-known problem in practice is the fear that a technology might decrease the quality of treatment: A psychologist might think that the use of an eHealth intervention in treatment could negatively impact the therapeutic relationship with his or her client.

Technologies are developed using different software and hardware elements, with the frequent result of systems not being interoperable. This makes it difficult or even impossible to communicate information from one system to another, since they cannot 'talk' to each other. For example, wearables to monitor behaviour may not be compatible with other apps or personal health records. In particular, the shift from hospital care to homecare requires that standardized labels for treatment are used within systems, which is usually not the case.

Finally, certification of a technology, general data protection regulations (GDPRs), and medical device regulations impact the uptake of eHealth technologies in practice. The certification procedures that are necessary for the medical device regulations that currently often apply to eHealth technologies are time-consuming and associated with high costs. In practice, there is often not enough expertise to comply with certifications and regulations. It is important to account for these types of regulations and responsibilities from the start, since they are often overlooked during development and implementation.

Ethical Barriers

A very important aspect to consider when using (new) eHealth technologies, are ethical points of attention. Of course, ethics is not a new phenomenon with respect to health information, but the introduction and integration of eHealth technology in healthcare raises many new ethical issues that must be accounted for. The process of storing and sharing health data becomes beyond peoples' ability to directly control. This impacts multiple factors that should be addressed to increase the chances of eHealth's success in the long term. Not all ethical barriers have a solution or a clear-cut answer yet. However, it is pivotal to carefully consider the ethical barriers that may arise.

Privacy and security are obstacles people perceive when using technologies to share health or medical information. Patients often do not have enough knowledge about what happens to their data. Who is the owner of the information? And how do we know who has access to the information? Commercial companies might sell personal health data. For example, companies provide technologies to monitor physical activity, sleeping, and eating behaviours with monitoring devices such as smartwatches. These data provide much insight into people's health and, if not protected well, might be misused by, for example, health insurance companies to increase their premiums for people with an unhealthy lifestyle.

A lack of transparency is not a new phenomenon, but the difference is that the 'clinical eye' of a caregiver can be overruled. For example, people receive tailored feedback on their behaviour, but often do not have any idea what decision rules ground the personalized feedback. This highlights the role of 'explainable AI': AI should not be a black box, but it has to be clear on what grounds decisions are made. In line with this: What happens when a 'wrong' decision is provided by an eHealth technology? Who is responsible?

The reliability and accuracy of information provided by an eHealth technology is another important point to consider. To what extent can we trust the information that is provided by the Internet? Think of Wikipedia pages that can provide unreliable and incorrect information about symptoms or treatments, or a system that provides wrong feedback about the amount and intensity of physical activity for a person with obesity and joint problems. This highlights the importance of reliable certification, the importance of involving the perspective of a healthcare professional, and educating the end-user so they are able to critically assess the reliability of provided information or suggestions.

While empowerment via eHealth is an important benefit, it might also have a negative impact on healthcare. People independently use commercial technologies such as wearables or self-testing to improve their health. An issue is how this impacts the autonomy and trustworthiness of healthcare. People adopt self-regulation devices rapidly, and 'infiltration' with medical practices is ongoing. This can create pressure for medical professionals: How should they cope with information from data that is not based on medical standards? How should patients' self-judgements be respected? And how should we use self-test information be used in clinical consultations?

Finally, eHealth always aims a change in cognitions or behaviours, and uses certain persuasive strategies to ensure that users are optimally supported in their desired behaviour change. However, there also is a 'dark side of persuasion'. How far can we go in changing behaviour? When are suggestions provided by an app too intrusive? How can we ensure that the user (or healthcare professional) remains in control, and that the technology does not have an undesired impact on behaviour? It is important to carefully consider how far we can and want to go with the use of each technology.

Evidence Barriers

An important critique on eHealth technologies is the limited large-scale evidence of their *cost-effectiveness*, and the relative scarcity of reliable information on long-term effects on health and healthcare. More such evidence is needed: The more we know about what works, why and for whom, the more we can optimize eHealth.

One of the first barriers is that since eHealth is a relatively new domain, there are not that many studies on its effectiveness compared to other interventions, such as certain types of drugs, treatment for cancer, or cognitive behavioural therapy. The paradox here is that before eHealth is implemented, we need evidence for its effectiveness, but it is difficult to study this effectiveness if eHealth is not implemented well. As the field further progresses and gains some age, more studies are conducted and we learn more about why eHealth does or does not work, but we still need to be careful when drawing conclusions about its effectiveness.

A related barrier can be found in the study designs that are used to evaluate many eHealth interventions, as they do not always address the full picture. In general, the effects of web-based interventions are measured with the gold standards for (clinical) interventions (*Randomized Controlled Trials; RCTs*). While this type of study design is suitable for testing the effectiveness of e.g., drugs or a new type of treatment for cancer or the effectiveness of a face-to-face CBT-intervention for anxiety, the model is not always suitable for determining if an eHealth intervention was successful in improving predetermined outcomes. eHealth interventions differ for everyone through, for example, personalization of the intervention and the fact it is sometimes difficult to control the intervention (like with drugs or a face-to-face encounter with a psychologist). An example would be whether an intervention was successful in reducing depressive complaints or increasing physical activity. Conventional pre-post comparisons do not help us understand what elements of the intervention were and were not used and contributed to outcomes. Factors such as costs, usage of the technology, and other outcome variables should be measured more continuously since they are also really important processes. Furthermore, mere information on effectiveness on specific outcome measures does not suffice for eHealth. Since it is always used within specific contexts and can influence the way healthcare is delivered, information on eHealth's impact on these contexts is required as well. The need for this type of evidence requires other evaluation methods that are more suitable for eHealth (also see Chapter 16).

Another barrier to evidence is related to how eHealth is used. We do not yet have enough knowledge on the process of *adherence*, which refers to the question of whether the technology is used as was intended by the developers. We know that many people are not adherent: They stop using the technology prematurely, or do not use all of its different possibilities, which has a negative influence on an eHealth intervention's impact. More knowledge is required on what impact this non-adherence has on effectiveness and what factors can predict or even influence adherence to eHealth interventions.

Another issue that has to be addressed to ensure that the quality of eHealth evidence increases is related to the way evaluation studies are reported. Many studies have a rather myopic view on technology and evaluation, meaning that they do not provide enough information about matters that need to be reported to ensure replicability of studies and interventions. For example, in most cases it is unclear which software functionalities and development methods have been used to create the technology. Studies do not report why and how a certain technology was used, developed, and implemented: Evaluation is merely outcome-driven and little to no attention is paid to the design and quality of the evaluated technology. As a consequence, it is impossible to identify what specific features of technology could have contributed to the effects of the eHealth interventions, and replication is hardly possible. To overcome this problem, a CONSORT checklist was developed to guide how 'eHealth and mHealth trials should be reported, in particular related to reporting sufficient details of the intervention to allow replication and theory-building' (Boutron, Altman, Moher, Schulz, & Ravaud, 2017).

A final barrier is the need to better combine fundamental and applied research, since we not only need more evidence on effectiveness, but also more insight into the working elements of eHealth interventions. This requires both applied and fundamental research. *Applied research* focuses on matters such as good design, implementation, use in practice, and effectiveness of an intervention, all within specific contexts. *Fundamental research* aims to make generic claims about constructs such as adherence, behaviour change theories, persuasive elements, or *tailoring*. The results of experiments and empirical studies can be used to validate abstract theory-driven behaviour change models or to develop new models to predict reach, usage, and adherence. These models are useful for applied research in which they can be used to, for example, optimize interventions.

eHealth: Technology and People

As can be seen in the previous sections, eHealth cannot exist without people such as patients and healthcare professionals and is also highly dependent on the possibilities of technology (van Gemert-Pijnen et al., 2011). In this final section, we dive into two important concepts for eHealth: Technology and psychology.

eHealth: Technology

eHealth and technology are inseparable, since the first is not possible without the second. Therefore, well-functioning technology is a necessary precondition for any good *eHealth intervention*, and a good design that appeals to *users* is beneficial as well. As a result, it seems logical to pay attention to the role of technology within eHealth, but, unfortunately, this aspect is often overlooked.

Developments in the domain of eHealth are dependent on the development of technologies. The first eHealth technologies were websites with plain text, mainly because technology did not offer many more options. However, eHealth soon became increasingly interactive, making it possible to communicate with its users. Since then, new ways for technology to monitor and coach its users are emerging – think of smartwatches that measure our heartrate variability and send a notification when it exceeds a certain threshold to support us in reducing stress. Technology also offers users the possibility to communicate with each other, for example by enabling patients to contact their physicians or other patients, and the possibilities in this area are still evolving, as became apparent during the COVID-19 pandemic. Technology is increasingly becoming part of us and our daily lives. This humanizing technology is very relevant for eHealth: The 24/7 monitoring of our physical state and behaviour offers many options for supporting improvements in our health and well-being. However, this raises several ethical concerns about how far we can go in this: How reliable should feedback of technology be, and who is the owner of all of the collected data? Another important issue for eHealth is the balance between following the newest trends and innovations in technology – which might have unknown effects – or using well-researched but less state-of-the-art and perhaps less appealing technologies.

An important point regarding any technology is its fit with the user and the context in which it is used. If the users feel like the technology does not match their needs and preferences, or cannot be embedded in their routines, it will not be used. A technology should fit the way people live and work, should be aligned with their skills and socio-economic backgrounds, and has to appeal to way they make decisions about their health and well-being (Beerlage-De Jong, 2016; Wentzel, 2015). To put it bluntly: The better the fit with user and context, the more likely it is that a technology will be used and is effective. To achieve this, a *participatory and interdisciplinary development process* is essential. For instance, system design models for technology are not always suitable for eHealth development, since a focus on matters like user perspective, context, and financing are also needed. To conclude: Technology is essential for eHealth, and developers should always make sure that there is a good fit between the technology, the user, and the context (Van Gemert-Pijnen et al., 2013).

eHealth: Psychology

The goal of eHealth is to improve health and well-being via technologies. Often, a change in people's cognitions and related behaviours is required to achieve this, but changing behaviour has proven to be very difficult. Merely using a well-functioning and nice-looking technology does not suffice: Theories and approaches from psychology should be used to create content for technologies that can enable behaviour change.

Research has shown that eHealth interventions that use theories grounded in behavioural science are more effective in changing attitudes and behaviour than those that do not (Webb, Joseph, Yardley, & Michie, 2010; Carey et al., 2019)). Consequently, approaches such as *behaviour change techniques* (BCTs; Michie et al., 2013) and persuasive features (Oinas-Kukkonen & Harjumaa, 2009) should be integrated in eHealth interventions. BCTs are derived from psychological theories and can be used in interventions (see Chapter 2). For example, the BCT 'reward' can be integrated in an app by providing the user with a compliment after completing a task, e.g., reaching the intended number of steps per day. *Persuasive technology* aims to persuade users in a positive way to make better choices for their health and well-being. It does this by using the characteristics and possibilities of technology, such as cues for communication (text, speech, video, graphics), anonymity, or its possibility to access situations in which human persuaders are not allowed (see Chapter 12). The use of these kinds of approaches in a design increases the chances of effective behaviour change.

Furthermore, eHealth technologies have to be used by people, so they should fit their perspective. Merely using theory doesn't account for this important aspect. When theory-based interventions are created behind a desk, without talking to actual people, chances are that they don't appeal to or fit the user, since the developers can be mirroring themselves and are thus implicitly designing for themselves. Designing for your target group requires knowledge of how people think and behave. Psychological theories and methods can be used to get a grasp of this, since psychology pays a lot of attention to analysing and explaining human behaviour. Also, methods from human-centred design can be used to actively involve the users in the development process via research methods such as interviews, observations, and usability tests (see Chapter 11).

Integrating Psychology and Technology

Psychology and technology are both important ingredients for successful eHealth interventions and should be intertwined. Figure 1.5 visualizes this interrelationship. However, in many cases, the content of an intervention is developed by social scientists, and the technology is created separately, by engineers or technology designers. Understandably, both groups speak different languages, often causing a lack of collaboration or project management. For example, a team of psychologists might have a certain design in mind to deliver the content for an intervention. They communicate this to designers who have to 'translate' the delivered content into a technology that fulfils the need of these content experts. Unfortunately, this often proves to be challenging because of misunderstandings or differences in preferences and perspectives. As a result, content and technology are often developed independently from each other, which can lead to a neglect of perspectives of stakeholders along the way. To prevent this, multi- or interdisciplinary collaboration during development is key. Content and technology developers not only should closely communicate with each other but should also be in frequent touch with users and other stakeholders to

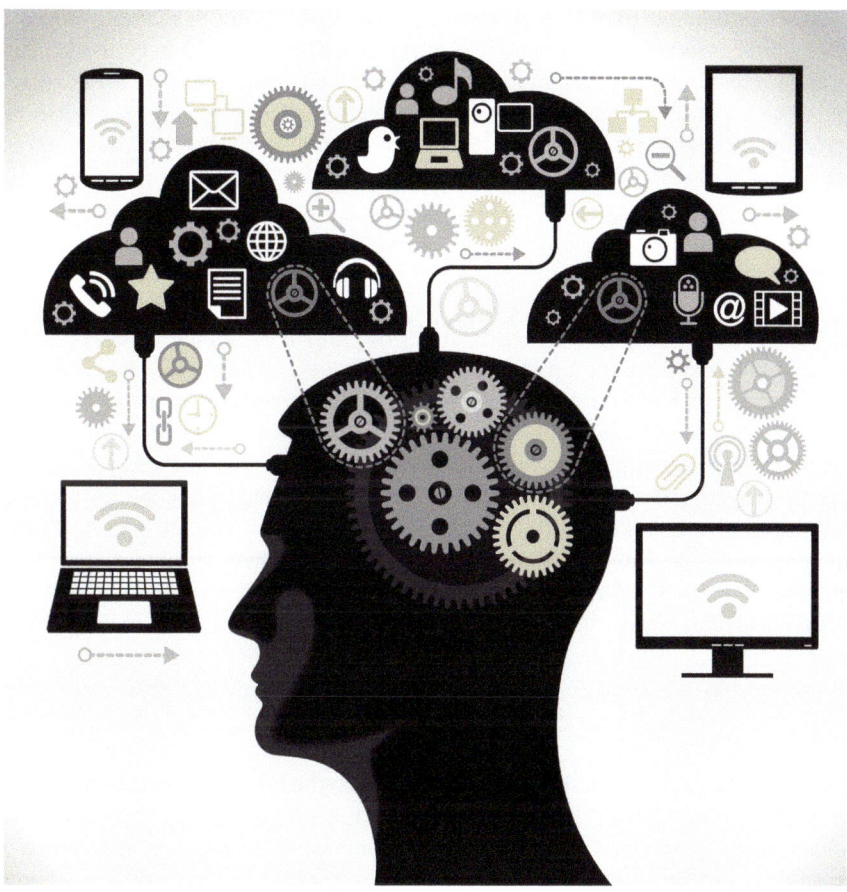

Figure 1.5 Technology can influence our cognitions, and our cognitions influence the way we view and use technology.

Source: © Image used under license from Shutterstock.com

ensure that an eHealth intervention is an integrated whole that fits all stakeholders' needs as closely as possible.

eHealth – A Multidisciplinary Approach

As we have seen, eHealth has many proven and potential benefits, but there are still many barriers that need to be overcome. One way to overcome these barriers is to ensure that enough attention is paid to the development, implementation, and evaluation of eHealth (van Gemert-Pijnen et al., 2011; van Gemert-Pijnen et al., 2013). Participatory development – in which relevant stakeholders are actively involved in creating the technology – is important to ensure that content and design fit their needs. Thorough implementation is essential to ensure that an eHealth technology is used in the long term and that it is financially sustainable. Evaluation is essential to assess the added value of a technology, but also to identify points of improvement. More attention to these processes is paid in Chapter 7. However, what is important to note before diving into this book, is the importance of a multidisciplinary approach. As we have seen, eHealth is not a unidimensional thing or tool: There is a close interrelationship between the design and content of the technology, its end-users, other stakeholders, and the healthcare context in which it will be used. To fully account for all perspectives throughout the development, implementation, and evaluation processes of eHealth, methods, frameworks, and theories from different disciplines need to be used. The most important disciplines that are discussed in this book are psychology, engineering, health sciences, human-centred design, business modelling, and implementation science. It is important to note that in regard to eHealth, these disciplines are not separate entities, but are integrated and interrelated, resulting in a multi- or even interdisciplinary approach in which technology, people, and their context are related.

Roadmap to the Book

The interdisciplinary approach towards eHealth and its development, implementation, and evaluation are central to this book. The first part of the book (Chapters 2 through 6) elaborates on the interdisciplinary background of eHealth by diving into the constructs of human behaviour, the possibilities of technology, and the healthcare system. In this first part, attention is also paid to the current state of affairs regarding the role of eHealth in prevention, and somatic and mental healthcare. The second part of this book (Chapters 7 through 16) pays attention to the development, implementation, and evaluation of eHealth, using frameworks, models, and theories from disciplines such as health psychology, human-centred design, engineering, business modelling, and implementation science. The CeHRes Roadmap (Chapter 7) – a framework for holistic, interdisciplinary eHealth development, implementation, and evaluation, provides the backbone for this part.

Summary

This first chapter introduced the domain of eHealth and described the relationship between technology, psychology, and healthcare. It provided an overview of benefits and barriers related to eHealth and this was illustrated through multiple brief examples. It is important to note that while eHealth has many advantages, many barriers are still experienced in practice. To overcome these barriers and achieve the benefits, an interdisciplinary approach towards development, implementation, and evaluation is advocated. Such an approach will likely result in an eHealth technology that fits people and their environments. The take-home messages for this chapter are:

- eHealth is the use of technology to support health, well-being, and healthcare, and can be categorized into self-care and prevention, supportive care, and societal health;
- Potential benefits of eHealth are related to access to care, patient empowerment, innovation, or quality of care;
- In practice, many barriers to eHealth are experienced with regard to uptake in practice, ethics, and evidence;
- When looking at eHealth, it is essential to consider the perspective and characteristics of the technology, the involved people, and their healthcare context;
- An interdisciplinary development, implementation, and evaluation process can create eHealth technologies that overcome the barriers and achieve the benefits.

Key References for Further Reading

Eysenbach, G. (2001). What is e-health? *Journal of Medical Internet Research*, 3(2).
Greenhalgh, T., Wherton, J., Papoutsi, C., Lynch, J., Hughes, G., Hinder, S., … & Shaw, S. (2017). Beyond adoption: A new framework for theorizing and evaluating nonadoption, abandonment, and challenges to the

scale-up, spread, and sustainability of health and care technologies. *Journal of Medical Internet Research*, 19(11), e367.

Van Gemert-Pijnen, J. E. W. C., Nijland, N., van Limburg, M., Ossebaard, H. C., Kelders, S. M., Eysenbach, G., & Seydel, E. R. (2011). A holistic framework to improve the uptake and impact of eHealth technologies. *Journal of Medical Internet Research*, 13(4).

Van Gemert-Pijnen, J. E. W. C., Peters, O., & Ossebaard, H. C. (Eds.). (2013). *Improving eHealth*. Den Haag, The Netherlands: Eleven International Publishing.

World Health Organization (2016). Global diffusion of eHealth: Making universal health coverage achievable. In *Report of the third global survey on eHealth* (pp. 11–76). Geneva: World Health Organization.

References

Beerlage-De Jong, N. (2016). *eHealth vs. infection: Participatory development of persuasive eHealth to support safe care*. Doctoral dissertation, University of Twente, Enschede.

Boutron, I., Altman, D. G., Moher, D., Schulz, K. F., & Ravaud, P. (2017). CONSORT statement for randomized trials of nonpharmacologic treatments: A 2017 update and a CONSORT extension for nonpharmacologic trial abstracts. *Annals of Internal Medicine*, 167(1), 40–47.

Carey, R. N., Connell, L. E., Johnston, M., Rothman, A. J., de Bruin, M., Kelly, M. P., & Michie, S. (2019). Behavior change techniques and their mechanisms of action: A synthesis of links described in published intervention literature. *Annals of Behavioral Medicine, a Publication of the Society of Behavioral Medicine*, 53(8), 693–707. doi:10.1093/abm/kay078

Eysenbach, G. (2001). What is e-health? *Journal of Medical Internet Research*, 3(2).

Greenhalgh, T., Wherton, J., Papoutsi, C., Lynch, J., Hughes, G., Hinder, S., … & Shaw, S. (2017). Beyond adoption: A new framework for theorizing and evaluating nonadoption, abandonment, and challenges to the scale-up, spread, and sustainability of health and care technologies. *Journal of Medical Internet Research*, 19(11), e367.

Kelders, S. M., Kok, R. N., Ossebaard, H. C., & van Gemert-Pijnen, J. E. W. C. (2012). Persuasive system design does matter: A systematic review of adherence to web-based interventions. *Journal of Medical Internet Research*, 14(6).

Michie, S., Richardson, M., Johnston, M., Abraham, C., Francis, J., Hardeman, W., … & Wood, C. E. (2013). The behavior change technique taxonomy (v1) of 93 hierarchically clustered techniques: Building an international consensus for the reporting of behavior change interventions. *Annals of Behavioral Medicine*, 46(1), 81–95.

Oh, H., Rizo, C., Enkin, M., & Jadad, A. (2005). What is eHealth (3): A systematic review of published definitions. *Journal of Medical Internet Research*, 7(1).

Oinas-Kukkonen, H., & Harjumaa, M. (2009). Persuasive systems design: Key issues, process model, and system features. *Communications of the Association for Information Systems*, 24(1), 28.

Van Gemert-Pijnen, J. E. W. C., Nijland, N., van Limburg, M., Ossebaard, H. C., Kelders, S. M., Eysenbach, G., & Seydel, E. R. (2011). A holistic framework to improve the uptake and impact of eHealth technologies. *Journal of Medical Internet Research*, 13(4).

Van Gemert-Pijnen, J. E. W. C., Peters, O., & Ossebaard, H. C. (Eds.). (2013). *Improving eHealth*. Den Haag, The Netherlands: Eleven International Publishing.

Webb, T., Joseph, J., Yardley, L., & Michie, S. (2010). Using the internet to promote health behavior change: A systematic review and meta-analysis of the impact of theoretical basis, use of behavior change techniques, and mode of delivery on efficacy. *Journal of Medical Internet Research*, 12(1), e4.

Wentzel, M. J. (2015). *Keeping an eye on the context: Participatory development of eHealth to support clinical practice*. Doctoral dissertation, University of Twente, Enschede.

World Health Organization (2016). Global diffusion of eHealth: Making universal health coverage achievable. In *Report of the third global survey on eHealth* (pp. 11–76). Geneva: World Health Organization.

2 Psychological Principles and Health Behaviour Change

Jane Walsh, Eimear Morrissey, Rory Coyne, & Leona Ryan

Introduction

The first chapter introduced eHealth and pointed out its added value for our health, well-being, and the healthcare system. To understand and develop persuasive eHealth interventions, which aim to change behaviour or attitudes, it is essential to get a grasp of the relationship between technology and psychology. Consequently, the main goal of this second chapter is to provide an understanding of the role of psychology in health and illness. In the domain of eHealth, technology and behavioural sciences cannot be viewed separate from each other. In order to grasp this interrelationship, the basics of psychology, health, behaviour, and their relationship should be made clear. There also are links between eHealth technology specific paradigms within psychology such as health and positive psychology. There are many theories that were initially developed for psychology that are important for eHealth interventions as well, such as behaviour change theories. Furthermore, technology offers new and innovative opportunities to enable behaviour change.

This second chapter provides an understanding of the role of psychology in health and illness and in how the behavioural sciences can be integrated with eHealth technologies to enhance health and well-being. To achieve this, the chapter is divided into three sections. The first section introduces the basics of psychology, health, behaviour, and their relationship. Positive psychology and health psychology are briefly explained because of their importance for eHealth interventions. In the second section, the importance of theories to explain and influence behaviour is highlighted. This theoretical approach is connected to interventions that aim to improve health behaviour. The third section of this chapter centres around technology and behaviour change. Opportunities of technology to enable behaviour change are discussed and technology is connected to previously described topics such as positive psychology, behaviour change techniques, and health. After completing this chapter, you will be able to:

- Provide definitions of psychology in general and its subdomains – health psychology and positive psychology – and explain how they relate to health, well-being, and technology;
- Explain how self-management and health behaviours impact health and how and why technology can support these behaviours;
- Provide an overview of the science of health behaviour change with an emphasis on the Behaviour Change Technique Taxonomy and explain its relation to eHealth;

DOI: 10.4324/9781003302049-3

- Discuss developments in eHealth technologies for health behaviour change – both the development and evaluation of health behaviour change models and their application to real-world settings;
- Discuss the challenges associated with the use of eHealth technology to change behaviour.

Health and Psychology

What is Health? Changing Patterns in Health and Illness

In order to understand the relationship between psychology and health, it is important to be clear on the meaning of health. Health is a word that means different things to different people. The most widely recognized definition of health was formulated by the World Health Organization (WHO) in 1948 and defines health as a 'state of complete physical mental and social well-being... not merely the absence of disease or infirmity'. In more recent years, however, Huber et al. (2011) argued that this definition has several limitations, for example, the use of the word 'complete' unintentionally contributes to the over-medicalization of society, as it requires an unrealistic standard. They point out that because of the changing demography of populations, and of disease prevalence, with a shift from acute diseases to *chronic disease* coupled with an ageing population, a move towards effective *self-management* is required. Self-management refers to the individual's ability to manage the symptoms, treatment, physical, and psychosocial consequences, as well as the lifestyle changes inherent in living with a chronic disease. Huber et al. posit that we should move to a view of health characterized as 'the ability to adapt and self-manage'.

This new approach to defining health becomes increasingly applicable when one considers that during the 20th century the leading causes of death have changed from infectious diseases to those that relate to unhealthy behaviour and lifestyle. The leading causes of death in Europe (circulatory diseases, cancer, and respiratory diseases) are strongly related to behaviour (OECD/European Union, 2022). For example, in 2016, the American Heart Association stated that approximately 80% of cardiovascular diseases (CVDs) can be prevented through not smoking, eating a healthy diet, engaging in physical activity, maintaining a healthy weight, and controlling blood pressure, diabetes mellitus, and elevated lipid levels (Mozaffarian et al., 2016). At the same time, healthcare costs have been rapidly increasing, in part because the diseases that are currently most prevalent are chronic in nature and thus require continual treatment and monitoring (also see Chapter 4). This behavioural approach to health is consistent with Huber's definition, in which the ability to adapt and self-manage is central.

Behaviour and Health: Focus on Self-management

It has become increasingly clear from the changing patterns of disease mortality that our health remarkably depends on a capacity to self-manage. *Self-management* involves an individual managing their illness in a way that maximizes control over symptoms and quality of life. Health services often provide self-management support to patients with chronic conditions. These tend to be focused on the provision of education and supportive interventions to increase the patients' knowledge, skills, and confidence in managing their condition. In these cases, the traditional doctor-patient relationship changes into a partnership where the patient is also actively involved in their own care. For example, an individual with arthritis might self-manage through exercise, managing pain, eating healthily, taking arthritis medication, and working with the doctor and healthcare team. This conceptualization of active self-management as a central feature of health and well-being is further emphasized in theoretical and research developments in psychology, particularly in the areas of positive psychology and health psychology, which are outlined in the next section.

What is Psychology?

Psychology can be defined as the scientific study of mental and behavioural functioning. More specifically, psychology aims to describe, explain, predict, and, where possible, intervene to modify behavioural and cognitive processes. The field of applied psychology investigates how empirical psychology can be used in a real-world setting to solve practical problems.

The Role of Psychology in Health

In recent years, the application of psychology to health and well-being has been increasingly recognized. Among other things, psychology can provide insight into issues with our health. Psychological factors (e.g., factors related to life events, stress, emotions, behaviours, and other events in the environment that have an impact on the individual's state of mind) can affect health both directly and indirectly. Direct effects include the negative impact of prolonged elevated levels of stress on immune function (Dhabhar, 2014). Indirect effects include the impact of behaviour on health, such as the harmful effects of smoking and excessive alcohol consumption or the beneficial effects of exercise or a low-fat diet. A biopsychosocial approach is often used in the understanding of health and well-being. For example, health is understood as the product not only of biological processes (e.g., a virus) but also of psychological (e.g., thoughts and emotions), behavioural (e.g., habits), and social processes (e.g., socio-economic status). The field of psychology has made important contributions to our understanding of health; in particular, developments in both positive psychology and the specialized domain of health psychology have provided valuable insights into factors influencing best practices in therapy and in building resilience.

The Emergence of Positive Psychology

Positive psychology was pioneered by Martin Seligman in 1998 and is defined as 'the scientific study of positive human functioning and flourishing on multiple levels that include the biological, personal, relational, institutional, cultural, and global dimensions of life' (Seligman & Csikszentmihalyi, 2000). This field postulates that focusing only on a psychological disorder may result in a limited understanding of a person's health and well-being. In its application to health, positive psychology suggests that positive emotional states have a favourable effect on mortality and survival in both healthy and diseased populations. Studies suggest that happier people seem to live longer, even when health behaviours are controlled for. Intervention studies conducted also indicate that positive affect is associated with greater resistance to common viruses such as colds and flu (Cohen et al., 2006).

There is increasing evidence of a link between positive health behaviour and psychological well-being. Research in positive psychology has found that there is evidence of an association between fruit and vegetable intake and happiness (Boehm et al., 2013; White, Horwath, & Conner, 2013). This finding may not be fully explained by demographic or other variables, including socio-economic status, body mass index, smoking, and exercise, suggesting a possible causal link (Conner et al., 2015). This may be as a result of the protective benefits from both chronic diseases as well as a greater intake of nutrients important for psychological health. These findings further emphasize the importance of developing interventions that target behaviours that promote both physical and psychological well-being. This approach shifts the predominant focus from interventions that mostly address negative health issues or problematic behaviour to interventions that also pay attention to positive aspects of health and well-being, like positive emotions or realizing one's own goals and values.

Health Psychology

Another approach that is important for interventions is health psychology, which examines how psychological factors such as people's behaviour, personality, and emotions influence their health. Matarazzo (1982) defined health psychology as an aggregate field in psychology, involving educational, scientific, and professional contributions, and accomplishing a variety of ends: the promotion and maintenance of health; the prevention and treatment of illness; the identification of etiologic and diagnostic correlates of health, illness, and related dysfunction; and to the analysis and improvement of the healthcare system and health policy formation. A more recent analysis streamlines the definition as 'an interdisciplinary field concerned with the application of psychological knowledge and techniques to health, illness and healthcare' (Marks et al., 2005). The aims of health psychology can be divided into (1) understanding, explaining, developing, and testing theory, and (2) putting theory into practice (Ogden, 2012). One of the key ways that health psychology has developed in applying theory into practice is in attempting to understand and to change health behaviour, with a particular focus on the individual, and not just population-based approaches to health behaviour change. Health psychologists have been developing, implementing, and evaluating many in-person or paper-based interventions over the years. Recently, the field has been acknowledging the added value of technology in interventions to improve health.

Behaviour Change and Interventions

In view of the striking evidence of the link between behaviour and health, it is clear that the implementation of evidence-based practice and public health is highly dependent on behaviour change. Thus, behaviour change interventions are fundamental to the effective practice of public health and clinical medicine. Behaviour change interventions can be defined as coordinated sets of activities designed to change specified behaviour patterns (Michie, van Stralen, & West, 2011). Interventions can be used to increase both uptake and optimal use of effective clinical services (e.g., vaccination, screening) and to promote healthy lifestyles (e.g., increase physical activity, quit smoking).

Many different types of interventions that support health behaviour have been developed in the last decades. Because of this multitude of studies, much knowledge about effective intervention elements and development approaches has been generated. One important conclusion that can be drawn from the body of intervention research is that the use of theory to explain and influence behaviour is of much added value. Theories have been proven to be pivotal in the development of in-person interventions, and an increasing amount of research also shows its importance for eHealth interventions (Moller et al., 2017). There are several reasons for this:

1. Theories can inform the development and design of eHealth interventions so that they are based on our understanding of what drives behaviour change;
2. The use of theory also gives the opportunity to operationalize and measure constructs that can be used as potential moderators and mediators of the intervention's effect on the chosen health outcome;
3. Using common theories across interventions provides a mutual vocabulary which allows comparison and synthesis across studies (Simoni, Ronen, & Aunon, 2018).

In this section, attention will be paid to theories that can be used to explain and influence health behaviour. Knowledge about these theories is important for all intervention developers, regardless of the mode of delivery of the intervention: in-person, via paper or, of course, technology.

Theories of Health Behaviour

A theory can be defined as 'a set of concepts and/or statements which specify how phenomena relate to each other'. In psychology, theory provides an organizing description of a system that accounts for what is known, and explains and predicts phenomena (Davis, Campbell, Hildon, Hobbs, & Michie, 2015). In the case of health behaviour change, theories provide a mechanism to encapsulate existing knowledge about how variations in interventions produce a desired behaviour change. In addition, theories provide explanations and predictions that support the generalization of findings from past work into future areas of inquiry and use (Noar & Zimmerman, 2005). These theories can be used to explain and predict both healthy and unhealthy behaviours that will be targeted by the intervention. A thorough understanding of behaviour and its predictors is required to find out what the intervention should focus on and how this should be done (also see Chapter 7). Theories can guide developers in getting a grasp of the behaviour that their intervention will target.

There are many theories that can be used for this. We shall not discuss all of them, but briefly point out several of the most influential ones. See Table 2.1 for a brief overview of key behaviour change theories. In the last 40 years, considerable progress has been made in understanding and predicting the pursuit of planned, goal-directed behaviour and especially individuals' decision to behave in a healthy way. Also, models of behaviour change and maintenance have been proposed and empirically tested for a variety of health behaviours (Prochaska, 1994). The Theory of Planned Behaviour (TPB) has been the dominant theoretical approach to guide research on health-related behaviour for over 30 years. The TPB proposes that volitional human behaviour is a function of the intention to perform the behaviour and of perceived behavioural control (PBC). Intention is hypothesized to be a function of attitudes towards the behaviour, subjective norms, and perceived behavioural control.

The vast majority of TPB studies have been correlational in nature to examine the associations between TPB cognitions and behaviour (Noar & Zimmerman, 2005). The limitations with using this approach have been outlined by Sniehotta, Presseau, and Araújo-Soares (2014), in particular the limited predictive validity of the TPB. Reviews show clearly that the majority of variability in observed behaviour is not accounted for by measures of the TPB. A single theory often does not

Table 2.1 Summary of key behaviour change theories.

Behaviour Change Theory	Summary
Theory of Planned Behaviour (Ajzen, 1985)	The TPB is a theory that links beliefs and behaviour. The theory states that attitude towards behaviour, subjective norms, and perceived behavioural control together shape an individual's behavioural intentions and behaviours.
Self-efficacy Theory (Bandura, 1986)	Self-efficacy is one's belief in one's ability to succeed in specific situations or accomplish a task. One's sense of self-efficacy can play a major role in how one engages in health behaviours.
Health Belief Model (Janz & Becker, 1984)	The Health Belief Model (HBM) is a psychological model that attempts to explain and predict health behaviours by focusing on the attitudes and beliefs of individuals.
Elaboration Likelihood Model (Petty, 1986)	The Elaboration Likelihood Model is a general theory of attitude change. It provides a framework for organizing, categorizing, and understanding the basic processes underlying the effectiveness of persuasive communications.
Protection Motivation Theory (Rogers, 1983)	The Protection Motivation Theory proposes that people protect themselves based on four factors: the perceived severity of a threatening event, the perceived probability of the occurrence, or vulnerability, the efficacy of the recommended preventive behaviour, and the perceived self-efficacy.

seem to cover the complexity of behaviour: a more theory-overarching approach was required. In recent years, the field has moved from adopting a single theoretical approach focused on a small number of determinants, to an array of theories and models developed in the field of social psychology (Hagger & Chatzisarantis, 2014).

It has become clear that in order to successfully understand and change health behaviour via technology, we must first accurately describe and analyze behaviour and its antecedents, for which the previously described theories can be used. Theories of health behaviour change coupled with evidence from existing intervention studies provide a base for considering key components for a health behaviour change intervention by identifying the core components ('active ingredients') of interventions. As many different theories and models have emerged, recent developments in health psychology have led to systematic guidance and lists of behavioural change techniques. First, these techniques provide a mechanism to develop theory-based behaviour change interventions. Furthermore, they detail the mechanisms through which change is expected to occur, and finally they are also useful to describe intervention content using a shared terminology. The Behaviour Change Wheel (BCW) (see Figure 2.1) of Michie et al. (2011) was developed from 19 frameworks of behaviour change, synthesizing the common features of the framework and linking them to a model of behaviour that was sufficiently broad that it could be applied to any behaviour in any setting (Michie, Atkins, & West, 2014). The main goal of this BCW is to support intervention developers in adding theory-based behaviour change elements to their interventions in order to increase the chances of the intervention successfully changing behaviour. Multiple studies showed that the BCW provides an excellent framework to guide in the development of health behaviour change interventions.

Health Behaviour Change

Michie and colleagues continued to advance our understanding of health behaviour change by developing a taxonomy of behaviour change techniques (BCTs; Michie et al., 2013) that is connected to the BCW. A *BCT* is defined as 'the smallest active component of an intervention

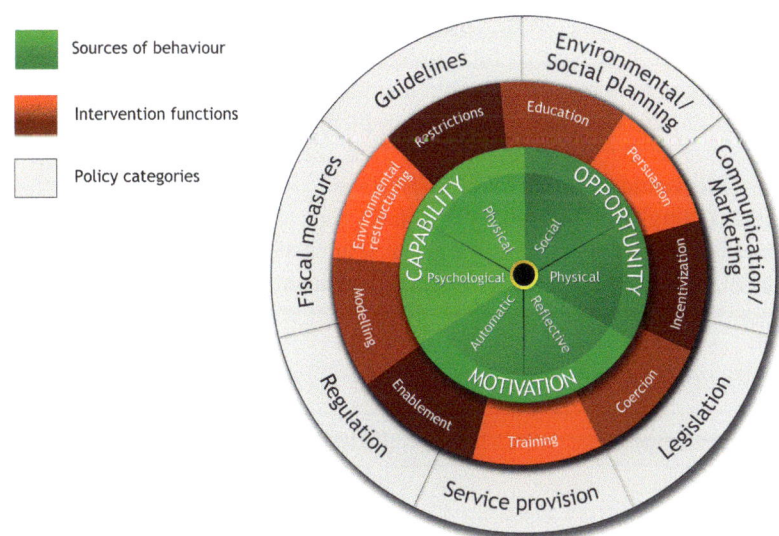

Figure 2.1 Behaviour Change Wheel (Michie et al., 2011).

designed to change behaviour'. They are both observable and replicable components of behaviour change interventions. The Behaviour Change Technique Taxonomy Version 1 (BCTTv1) contains 93 BCTs, the categories of which are provided below:

- **Goals and planning**. Examples are goal setting, action planning, and commitment;
- **Feedback and monitoring**. Examples are self-monitoring, biofeedback, and monitoring of behaviour by others;
- **Social support**. Examples are practical social support and emotional social support;
- **Shaping knowledge**. Examples are introduction, information, and re-attribution;
- **Natural consequences**. Examples are information about health consequences, salience of consequences, and anticipated regret;
- **Comparison of behaviour**. Examples are demonstration of the behaviour, social comparison, or information about other's approval;
- **Associations**. Examples are prompts/cues, associative learning, and exposure;
- **Repetition and substitution**. Examples are behavioural practice, habit formation, and graded tasks;
- **Comparison of outcomes**. Examples are credible sources, pros and cons, and comparative imagining of future outcomes;
- **Reward and threat**. Examples are material rewards, future punishment, or social incentive;
- **Regulation**. Examples are reducing negative emotions, conserving mental resources, or paradoxical instructions;
- **Antecedents**. Examples are restructuring the physical environment, reducing exposures to cues for the behaviour, and distraction;
- **Identity**. Examples are framing/reframing, incompatible beliefs, and valued self-identity;
- **Scheduled consequences**. Examples are reward removal, behaviour cost, or reward alternative behaviour;
- **Self-belief**. Examples are mental rehearsal of successful performance, focus on past success, and self-talk;
- **Covert learning**. Examples are imaginary punishment, imaginary rewards, and vicarious consequences.

In Table 2.2 an example of a worked out BCT is provided.
Several research methods have been successfully used to identify effective BCTs within complex interventions. One example is meta-regression, a statistical technique to analyze evidence across studies (Michie et al., 2014). Relevant BCTs can then be selected based on a review of previous research and serve as the 'active ingredients' of a successful behaviour change (both traditional and digital) intervention, in other words: BCTs are related to intervention effectiveness. For example, 'goal setting' and 'self-monitoring' have been shown to be effective strategies in increasing physical activity in a digital intervention using apps with university students (Walsh, Corbett, Hogan, Duggan, & McNamara, 2016). The BCT taxonomy will be updated and refined as time goes on.

Table 2.2 Example of the BCT Taxonomy (Michie, Atkins, & West, 2014).

Number and Label	Definition	Example
1. Goals and planning 1.1 Goal-setting (behaviour)	Set or agree on a goal defined in terms of the behaviour to be achieved.	Agree on a daily walking goal (e.g., 3 kilometres) with the person and reach agreement about the goal.

Unfortunately, as seen in many articles on health behaviour change interventions, the development of effective interventions is hampered by the absence of a detailed specification and reporting on their content, including the used BCTs. This limits the possibility of replicating effective interventions, synthesizing evidence, and understanding the causal mechanisms underlying behaviour change. When designing the content of an intervention, it is important to base each of the components of the intervention on theory. Guidance on developing interventions requires them to be developed in a systematic and rigorous way (Michie et al., 2011). That requirement involves using the BCW to select one or more 'intervention functions' (e.g., education, persuasion, incentivization, environmental restructuring, modelling) and then choose BCTs that can deliver these functions (Michie, Atkins, & West, 2014). Of course, these abstract BCTs have to be translated into understandable intervention elements (also see Chapter 7).

Originally, these complex interventions were often delivered in person, or through written materials. The reach of such interventions is limited in scope. However, in the appropriate setting, eHealth technologies significantly increase reach and access to the target population by using an easy and relatively low-cost platform to deliver these BCTs (see Chapter 1). For example, smartphone apps to enhance medication adherence often contain BCTs such as 'prompts/cues' in the form of an alarm and 'feedback on behaviour' in the form of an adherence log (Morrissey, Corbett, Walsh, & Molloy, 2016). In the next section, we will elaborate on the relationship between behaviour change and technology.

Behaviour Change and Technology

Technology and Health

There has been rapid growth in the number of 'electronic health' (eHealth) and mobile health (mHealth) interventions in the last few years. Mobile applications (apps), text messages, wearables and sensors, interactive websites, and social media, can improve health by supporting behaviour change involved in disease prevention and self-management, and delivery of evidence-based healthcare.

Technology and Behaviour Change Theory

Recent rapid advances in technology, such as the collection of psychological, social, and contextual variables that are passively recorded or tracked (e.g., GPS location, social media activity), have provided us with a golden opportunity for empirically testing behavioural theories in 'real-world' contexts. Behaviour change theories are the key to effectively personalizing eHealth interventions. eHealth interventions facilitate health promotion by providing support in the 'real world' to change specific behaviours in specific contexts and are used by individuals. The shift from traditional to digital platforms presents researchers with an opportunity to both develop and test BCTs within interventions (Hekler et al., 2016b). For example, goal setting and self-monitoring can be easily achieved by using an app to track step count, enabling users to achieve their goals more readily (Glynn et al., 2014; Walsh et al., 2016). Setting a step count target of 10,000, which can be displayed and monitored visually on an app, can be easier to achieve than a more arbitrary target of 30 minutes of 'moderate exercise' which can be more open to subjective interpretation. See the case study in Box 2.1 for an illustration of this type of BCT-based intervention. There is little doubt that there is an opportunity for eHealth technology to allow for greater specification of behavioural theories and models (e.g., defining how constructs relate to one another and the predicted magnitude and direction of those relations) (Hekler et al., 2016b). However, whilst this is a novel and exciting area of research, many of the early studies have been heavily criticized for lacking a strong evidence base in terms of both design and implementation.

Box 2.1 Case Study: BCT's practical application and evaluation.

Behaviour change techniques can be integrated into a technology in different ways. In this box we provide you with some examples of how they can be integrated in an intervention. Following that, we discuss how to evaluate which BCTs are effective and which ones may not add much value.

Imagine an intervention that aims to improve regular exercising for older persons. This intervention could use a smartwatch and an accompanying app. When looking at Michie's BCT taxonomy, several BCTs could be integrated in this kind of intervention.

1. Monitoring of outcome(s) of behaviour without feedback (BCT 2.5). The smartwatch can track exercising behaviour of the user via combining data on, for instance, taken steps and location;
2. Goal setting (BCT 1.1). The user can set a personal goal about his or her intended exercising behaviour in the app, for example, to undertake at least 60 minutes of moderate physical activity a day;
3. Material reward (BCT 10.2). If the user has been active for at least 60 minutes each day during an entire month, he or she will receive a reward, such as a popular book on healthy cooking;
4. Prompts/cues (BCT 7.1). During the day, at fixed moments, several prompts can be sent to the user via the smartwatch, to remind him or her to engage in physical activity;
5. Anticipated regret (BCT 5.5). The app could potentially contain several short videos in which a virtual avatar asks the person which degree of regret they will feel if they are still unfit in a year.

To determine which BCTs are effective for this target group, three adapted versions of this intervention can be made. In one version, the material reward BCT will be removed, in another one the prompts will be lacking and in the third version there will be no videos to elicit anticipated regret. In a so-called fractional factorial design (see Chapter 16), five groups can be compared to each other: one control group, one group that uses the entire intervention with all BCTs, and the remaining three groups will use one of the three adapted versions. If, for example, the intervention without prompts is less effective than the other versions of the intervention, it might very well be that the prompts contribute to the effectiveness. Through these types of studies, we can gather knowledge on which BCTs are effective for specific groups, and which ones do not contribute much.

Interventions to change behaviours related to health are usually 'complex' in that they comprise several or many components that may interact with each other. These components include BCTs and modes of delivery (e.g., smartphone apps or face-to-face delivery). The interactions among these components create challenges in terms of identifying which techniques are contributing to any effects observed and the mechanisms of action of techniques contributing to the effect. To date, few digital health intervention developers specify how characteristics of their interventions map onto underlying evidence-based theories and techniques (Morrissey et al., 2016). Morrison (2015) suggests that to achieve long-term sustainability of digital interventions more research is required on effective components rather than of effective digital interventions as a whole. She argues that the reach and use of these interventions needs more scientific input to increase the public health impact of Internet-delivered interventions. The application of behavioural science theory provides a useful starting point to develop and evaluate such technological interventions in a similar manner to methods used in the development of standard behaviour change interventions. The case study in Box 2.1 provides a simplified example of what such research on effective elements of an eHealth intervention can look like. By conducting an analysis of previous research, we can begin to understand the factors that predict the target behaviour, and this provides a platform upon which to consider the key elements to target for a behaviour change intervention. Using a theory-based approach to developing digital interventions will enable us to develop and evaluate high-quality effective interventions to change behaviour. Improving this would be expected to increase the effectiveness of interventions and advance our understanding of the underlying theory. For example, a theory that stipulates that a construct such as 'social support' is an important predictor of behaviour can be useful in designing an intervention that seeks to change behaviour (e.g., to reduce alcohol use). Hence, an intervention that is designed to provide targeted appropriate social support should be more effective in reducing binge drinking. By adopting theories and models that are as precise, quantitative, and testable as possible for describing the complexity of behaviour change, we can achieve greater precision in specifying model structures, defining directionality and complex interactions influencing behaviour.

Development

When developing behaviour change interventions, BCTs have to be integrated into the intervention during the development process, not afterwards. There are multiple frameworks that support the systematic integration of these BCTs into behaviour change interventions. Examples of such models are the CeHRes Roadmap (see Chapter 7), Intervention Mapping, and Behavioural Design Thinking Approach (see Box 2.2). A strong theory-based framework can serve as guidance to

Box 2.2 Behavioural Design Thinking Approach.

When merging behaviour change processes with digital solutions, the most successful outputs are those that are designed with the specific needs of the intended user in mind. As mentioned before, there are many approaches to guide this process, but an especially suitable one that can be integrated with BCTs is the Behavioural Design Thinking Approach (see Figure 2.2) This approach uses an innovative framework that synthesises and leverages behavioural science and design thinking processes to optimise digital health interventions by maximising user engagement.

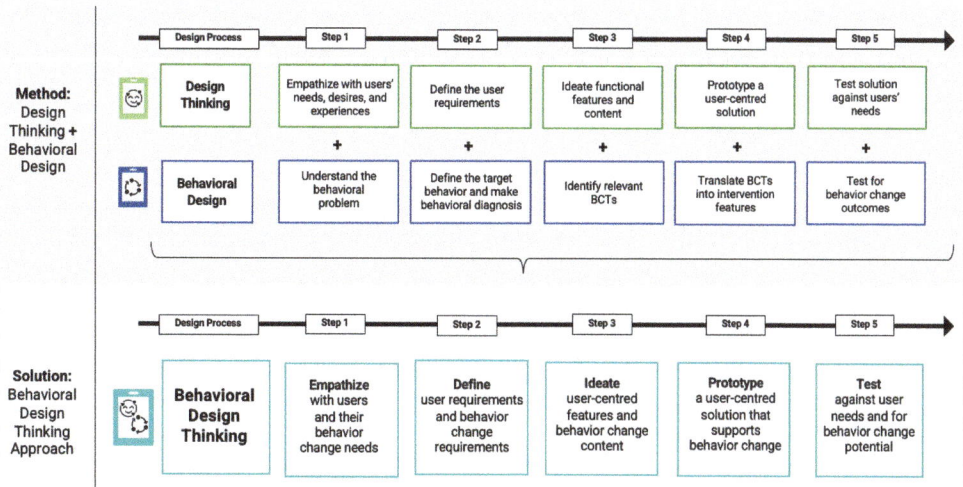

Figure 2.2 Behavioural Design Thinking (Voorheis et al. 2022).

develop an intervention, but it is also important to focus on elements critical to success such as the context the intervention will be delivered in and modes of intervention delivery. If an eHealth intervention does not consider these elements, chances are higher that it will not be used at all, or not in the intended way.

However, in recent years great strides have been made to develop sound scientific methodologies to help developers create effective solutions. In particular, increased recognition and emphasis have been placed on the importance of involving stakeholders in intervention design and implementation from the outset to ensure that an intervention matches their needs and wishes (also see Chapter 7 on the CeHRes Roadmap). One method of approaching this is to take the person-based approach (Yardley, Morrison, Bradbury, & Muller, 2015), which involves in-depth qualitative research conducted with the users before the digital intervention is developed. This data is used to develop 'guiding principles' that state the key intervention design objectives and describe the key features of the intervention required to achieve each objective. Yardley et al. posit that both qualitative and quantitative research is crucial at all stages of intervention development and evaluation, including planning and design, early development, acceptability and feasibility testing, and evaluation in clinical trials and real-life settings. The person-based approach is rooted within the discipline of health psychology and focuses primarily on the BCTs the intervention is intended to deliver, and their implementation by the people using the intervention. However, the person-based approach is highly compatible with the more in-depth approaches that have evolved within the disciplines of information systems and human-computer interaction, such as human-centred design (see Chapter 11). These types of approaches seek to understand the user's knowledge, skills, behaviour, motivations, cultural background, and organizational context, and they involve users iteratively throughout development.

The development of the Behaviour Change Taxonomy, coupled with evidence-based user-centred methodologies (e.g., person-based approach), have helped to create a universal approach to facilitate intervention development. In addition, eHealth interventions should be developed with a clear understanding of which BCTs are to be incorporated and how they link to the theoretically driven mechanisms of change.

Technology and Behaviour Change – Future Directions

Case 1: Machine learning and the Human Behaviour Change Project

In recent years, machine learning models have been given greater attention by behaviour scientists. Machine learning is a branch of artificial intelligence (AI) in which algorithms are trained to make either predictions or classifications through identification of patterns in a dataset. There are two main types of machine learning models. In supervised learning, the researcher directly trains the model to make a correct classification or prediction by 'labelling' the correct result in a training dataset. Unsupervised learning does not rely on labelled data, and instead the model works independently to make classifications or predictions.

One exciting application of machine learning to behaviour science can be seen in the Human Behaviour Change Project (HBCP; Michie et al., 2017). As the scientific literature on health behaviour change is vast and constantly expanding, efforts to quickly synthesise the knowledge that is generated are needed. The HBCP aims to take advantage of machine learning and another branch of AI, natural language processing (the use of AI to comprehend, generate and manipulate language) to extract key information from reports of behaviour change interventions. Once extracted, the goal is for this information to be used to answer important questions about the evidence from interventions, and to make inferences about behaviour change (Michie et al., 2017). This project, currently in progress, is also an example of behaviour scientists collaborating with multidisciplinary stakeholders such as computer scientists and systems architects.

Case 2: Immersive technology

The adaptation of immersive technologies (ImTs) to support BCTs is at the forefront of state-of-the-art research in psychology and human-computer interaction (HCI) studies. ImTs give the user the experience of being immersed in simulated objects and environments (such as virtual and augmented realities). This provides an interesting new context for the delivery of interventions and their associated BCTs. Egenfeldt-Nielsen et al. (2019) outline how a virtual reality-based game could support a rehabilitation regime, where the BCT 'feedback on behaviour' is delivered through congratulatory messages in the game, or vibrational feedback sent to a wearable device such a smartwatch. These types of immersive technologies offer unique affordances by directly supporting engagement and active learning while preserving the fidelity of the effective theoretical principles underlying the intervention (Otkhmezuri et al., 2019). The potential of ImTs for effective behaviour change lies in the interactive and immersive properties of virtual environments (Dirksen et al. 2019). However, while ImTs offer a sophisticated medium to facilitate behaviour change processes, the catalyst for behaviour change is largely dependent on the user's intention and motivation to engage with the content (Lee et al., 2020).

The Importance of Interdisciplinary Collaboration

It is clear that innovations in digital health are emerging on multiple fronts. In order to capitalize on these enormous opportunities for health behaviour change, interventions should be based on state-of-the-art science in medicine, technology, and the social and behavioural sciences. Innovations in digital health must involve close collaboration with disciplines such as health and positive psychology, engineering, human-computer interaction, computer science and technologies. To do this successfully, this requires the application of a multidisciplinary approach. Computer science models can define and test not just interactions between intervention components, methods of presentation and behaviours but also variations across individuals, populations, environments, and time. Data modelling such as this provides enormous opportunity to advance our theoretical understanding of behaviour change so that we can answer with confidence the questions put by health practitioners and policy makers: 'What works, how well, for whom, in what settings, for what behaviours, and why?' (Michie et al., 2017).

Summary

Rapid changes in technology coupled with recent developments in behavioural science provide an excellent opportunity to deliver personalized, evidence-driven behaviour change interventions. In developing effective health interventions, researchers should involve stakeholders at all stages of the development process and should explicitly identify and systematically apply evidence-based BCTs in the intervention. Health psychologists should work closely in multidisciplinary teams to capitalize on the quantity and quality of data generated by new health technology efficiently and effectively. The take-home messages for this chapter are:

- The evidence for the role of eHealth interventions to influence behavioural factors in the development of chronic diseases is becoming increasingly clear;
- Health psychology plays a major role in developing effective technological interventions to promote health behaviour change;
- State-of-the-art scientific methodologies used in health psychology (such as the Behaviour Change Technique Taxonomy and the person-based approach) can provide a valuable contribution to the development of new and emerging technologies;

- Evidence-based eHealth interventions have enormous potential to provide effective personalized solutions to enhance health and well-being;
- The inherent complexity of behaviour change requires input from a multidisciplinary research team and from relevant stakeholders such as end users.

Key References for Further Reading

Blandford, A., Gibbs, J., Newhouse, N., Perski, O., Singh, A., & Murray, E. (2018). Seven lessons for inter-disciplinary research on interactive digital health interventions. *Digital Health*, 4, 2055207618770325.

Hekler, E. B., Michie, S. F., Rivera, D. E., Collins, L. M., et al. (2016). Advancing models and theories for digital behavior change interventions. *American Journal of Preventive Medicine*, 51, 825–832.

Michie, S., Yardley, L., West, R., Patrick, K., & Greaves, F. (2017). Developing and evaluating digital interventions to promote behavior change in health and health care: Recommendations resulting from an international workshop. *Journal of Medical Internet Research*, 19(6), e232.

Michie, S., Thomas, J., Mac Aonghusa, P., West, R., Johnston, M., Kelly, M. P., Shawe

Taylor, J., Hastings, J., Bonin, F., & O'Mara-Eves, A. (2020). The Human Behaviour-Change Project: An artificial intelligence system to answer questions about changing behaviour. *Wellcome Open Research*, 5, 122.

Yardley, L., Morrison, L., Bradbury, K., & Muller, I. (2015). The person-based approach to intervention development: Application to digital health-related behavior change interventions. *Journal of Medical Internet Research*, 17(1), e30.

References

Ajzen, I. (1985). From intentions to actions: A theory of planned behavior. In J. Kuhl & J. Beckmann (Eds.), *Action Control. SSSP Springer Series in Social Psychology.* (pp. 11–39). Berlin, Heidelberg: Springer Berlin Heidelberg.

Bandura, A. (1986). *Social foundations of thought and action: A social cognitive theory*. Englewood Cliffs, NJ: Prentice-Hall.

Boehm, J. K., Williams, D. R., & Rimm, E. B., (2013). Association between optimism and serum antioxidants in the midlife in the United States study. *Psychosomatic Medicine*, 75(1), 2–10.

Cohen, S., Alper, C. M., & Doyle, W. J. (2006). Positive emotional style predicts resistance to illness after experimental exposure to rhinovirus or influenza A virus. *Psychosomatic Medicine*, 68(6), 809–815.

Conner, T. S., Brookie, K. L., Richardson, A. C., & Polak, M. A. (2015). On carrots and curiosity: Eating fruit and vegetables is associated with greater flourishing in daily life. *British Journal of Health Psychology*, 20(2), 413–427.

Davis, R., Campbell, R., Hildon, Z., Hobbs, L., & Michie, S. (2015). Theories of behavior and behavior change across the social and behavioral sciences: A scoping review. *Health Psychology Review*, 9, 323–344.

Dhabhar, F. S. (2014). Effects of stress on immune function: The good, the bad, and the beautiful. *Immunological Research*, 58, 193.

Dirksen, J., Ditommaso, D., & Plunkett, C. (2019). Augmented and virtual reality for behavior change. *The eLearning Guild*. doi:10.13140/RG.2.2.23504.35842

Egenfeldt-Nielsen, S., Smith, J. H., & Tosca, S. P. (2019). *Understanding video games: The essential introduction* (3rd edition). New York, NY: Routledge.

Glynn, L. G., Hayes, P. S., Casey, M., Glynn, F., Alvarez-Iglesias, A., & Newell, J. (2014). Effectiveness of a smartphone application to promote physical activity in primary care: The SMART MOVE randomised controlled trial. *British Journal of General Practice*, 64(624), e384–e391.

Hagger, M. S., & Chatzisarantis, N. L. D. (2014). An integrated behavior-change model for physical activity. *Exercise and Sport Sciences Reviews*, 42(2), 62–69.

Hekler, E. B., Michie, S. F., Rivera, D. E., Collins, L. M., … Spruijt-Metz, D. (2016b). Advancing models and theories for digital behavior change interventions. *American Journal of Preventive Medicine*, 51, 825–832.

Huber, M., Knottnerus, J. A., Green, L., Horst, H., Jadad, A. R., Kromhout, D., Leonard, B., Lorig, K., Loureiro, M. I., Van der Meer, J. W., & Schnabel, P. (2011). How should we define health? *British Medical Journal*, 343, d4163.

Janz, N. K., & Becker, M. H. (1984). The health belief model: A decade later. *Health Education Quarterly*, 11(1), 1–47.

Lee, J., Kim, H., Kim, K. H., Jung, D., Jowsey, T., & Webster, C. S. (2020). Effective virtual patient simulators for medical communication training: A systematic review. *Medical Education*, 54(9), 786–795. doi:10.1111/medu.14152

Marks, D. F., Murray, M., Evans, B., Willig, C., Woodall, C., & Sykes, C. M. (2005). *Health psychology: Theory, research, and practice* (2nd edition). London, UK: Sage Publications.

Matarazzo, J. D. (1982). Behavioral health's challenge to academic, scientific and professional psychology. *American Psychologist*, 37, 1–14.

Michie, S., Atkins, L., & West, R. (2014). The Behavior Change Wheel: A guide to designing interventions. Surrey, UK: Silverback Publishing.

Michie, S., Richardson, M., Johnston, M., Abraham, C., Francis, J., & Hardeman, W. (2013). The Behavior Change Technique Taxonomy (v1) of 93 hierarchically clustered techniques: Building an international consensus for the reporting of behavior change interventions. *Annals of Behavioral Medicine*, 46(1), 81–95.

Michie, S., van Stralen, M. M., & West, R. (2011). The Behavior Change Wheel: A new method for characterising and designing behavior change interventions. *Implementation Science*, 6(1), 42.

Michie, S., Thomas, J., Johnston, M., Aonghusa, P. M., Shawe-Taylor, J., Kelly, M. P., ... & West, R. (2017). The Human Behavior-Change Project: Harnessing the power of artificial intelligence and machine learning for evidence synthesis and interpretation. *Implementation Science*, 12(1), 1–12.

Michie, S., Thomas, J., Mac Aonghusa, P., West, R., Johnston, M., Kelly, M. P., ... & O'Mara-Eves, A. (2020). The Human Behavior-Change Project: An artificial intelligence system to answer questions about changing behavior. *Wellcome Open Research*, 5, 122.

Moller, A. C., Merchant, G., Conroy, D. E., West, R., Hekler, E., Kugler, K. C., & Michie, S. (2017). Applying and advancing behavior change theories and techniques in the context of a digital health revolution: Proposal for more effectively realizing untapped potential. *Journal of Behavioral Medicine*, 40, 85–98.

Morrison, L. G. (2015). Theory-based strategies for enhancing the impact and usage of digital health behavior change interventions: A review. *Digital Health*, 1–10.

Morrissey, E. C., Corbett, T. K., Walsh, J. C., & Molloy, G. J. (2016). Behavior change techniques in apps for medication adherence: A content analysis. *American Journal of Preventive Medicine*, 50(5).

Mozaffarian, D., Benjamin, E. J., Go, A. S., Arnett, D. K., & Blaha, M. J., (2016). American Heart Association Statistics Committee and Stroke Statistics Subcommittee. Heart disease and stroke statistics – 2016 update: A report from the American Heart Association. *Circulation*, 133.

Noar, S. M., & Zimmerman, R. S. (2005). Health behavior theory and cumulative knowledge regarding health behaviors: Are we moving in the right direction? *Health Education Research*, 20, 275–290.

OECD/European Union (2022). *Health at a Glance: Europe 2022: State of Health in the EU Cycle.* Paris: OECD Publishing.

Ogden, J. (2012). *Health psychology: A textbook.* Maidenhead: McGraw-Hill Education.

Otkhmezuri, B., Boffo, M., Siriaraya, P., Matsangidou, M., Wiers, R. W., Mackintosh, B., ... Salemink, E. (2019). Believing is seeing: A proof-of-concept semi-experimental study on using mobile virtual reality to boost the effects of interpretation bias modification for anxiety. *JMIR Mental Health*, 6(2), e11517. doi:10.2196/11517

Petty, R. E. (1986). *Communication and persuasion: Central and peripheral routes to attitude change.* New York: Springer-Verlag.

Prochaska, J. O. (1994). Strong and weak principles for progressing from precontemplation to action on the basis of twelve problem behaviors. *Health Psychology*, 13, 47–51.

Rogers, R. W. (1983). Cognitive and physiological processes in fear appeals and attitude change: A revised Theory of Protection Motivation. In: J. Cacioppo & R. Petty (Eds.), *Social psychophysiology*. (pp. 153–177). New York: Guilford Press.

Seligman, M. E. P., & Csikszentmihalyi, M. (2000). Positive psychology: An introduction. *American Psychologist*, 55(1), 5–14.

Simoni, J. M., Ronen, K., & Aunon, F. M. (2018). Health behavior theory to enhance eHealth intervention in HIV: Rationale and review. *Current HIV/AIDS Reports*, 15, 423–430.

Sniehotta, F. F., Presseau, J., & Araújo-Soares, V. (2014). Time to retire the theory of planned behavior. *Health Psychology Review*, 8(1), 1–7.

Voorheis, P., Zhao, A., Kuluski, K., Pham, Q., Scott, T., Sztur, P., Khanna, N., Ibrahim, M., & Petch, J. (2022). Integrating behavioral science and design thinking to develop mobile health interventions: Systematic scoping review. *JMIR MHealth and UHealth*, 10(3), e35799.

Walsh, J. C., Corbett, T., Hogan, M., Duggan, J., & McNamara, A. (2016). An mHealth intervention using a smartphone app to increase walking behavior in young adults: A pilot study. *JMIR mHealth uHealth*, 4(3), e109.

White, B. A., Horwath, C. C., & Conner, T. S. (2013). Many apples a day keep the blues away – Daily experiences of negative and positive affect and food consumption in young adults. *British Journal of Health Psychology*, 18(4), 782–798.

Yardley, L., Morrison, L., Bradbury, K., & Muller, I. (2015). The person-based approach to intervention development: Application to digital health-related behavior change interventions. *Journal of Medical Internet Research*, 17(1), e30.

3 Opportunities of Technology to Promote Health and Well-being

Saskia M. Kelders

Introduction

> Technology offers many opportunities to improve health and well-being. In this chapter, you will learn that the pace of innovation in technology is very fast, which can make it difficult for eHealth researchers and developers to keep up-to-date with the latest technological developments. However, it is important to have some knowledge of what technology can do. This chapter provides examples of technologies that can be used to promote health and well-being and gives an introduction to the some of the aspects that give technologies these opportunities. Combined with basic knowledge of software development processes, these insights can help you in finding the added value of technology for your specific goal. This knowledge is also helpful – if not essential – in working with the software developers who might be able to develop the technology with you.

In this chapter, we show why and how technology, in particular Information and Communication Technology (ICT), is a very suitable way to promote health and well-being. This is explained by briefly going into the evolution of technologies within the domain of eHealth. Next, the chapter gives an overview of how different types of technology can play a role in supporting health. We also go into some of the advantages and limitations that technologies have compared to humans, and some of the accompanying ethical issues. After that, we explain some technology-related concepts that are important to understand when working in multidisciplinary eHealth teams. Last, we describe different software development models to give insight into the process that leads to these kinds of technologies. After completing this chapter, you will be able to:

- Discuss the evolution of technology, in particular technologies relating to supporting health, healthcare, and well-being;
- Provide different examples of technologies for health and discuss their advantages and limitations;
- Discuss important ethical issues concerning the use of technology, and in particular artificial intelligence (AI), in health;
- Explain the basics of common concepts in technology for health, and AI in particular;
- Name and explain different software design models and explain why they are important for eHealth.

DOI: 10.4324/9781003302049-4

The Evolution of eHealth Technologies

The use of technology for health purposes has risen dramatically in the last decades. One of the reasons for this was the rise of the Internet, but this was not the only cause for the increasing interest in using technology for health. In this section, we give a short overview of important technological developments that have had an influence on healthcare.

In Figure 3.1, a timeline with some important technologies related to health is presented. It is important to note that this timeline is by no means exhaustive: there are many more technologies and events that have had an impact on health and healthcare – it is merely meant to give an idea of the kind of technologies and the pace of innovation. Second, it is important to differentiate between medical technology, used by medical professionals, such as the X-ray and the MRI, and eHealth technologies used for behaviour change, such as the Fitbit, web-based interventions, and apps on a smartphone. Figure 3.1 shows both types of technology – medical and eHealth – to illustrate the breadth of technology used in healthcare. However, the focus of this chapter is on eHealth technologies, which are mainly Information and Communication Technologies (ICTs) with a clear connection to behaviour change.

What becomes clear from this timeline is that the pace of innovation, especially in the Internet era, is very fast. This is often called the 'digital revolution': the very rapid and impactful changes brought about by digital computing and communication technology. Mosaic, one of the early web browsers which made the World Wide Web popular, was only introduced in 1993. And the iPhone, the smartphone that popularized smartphones, was only introduced in 2007. Nowadays, it seems like the Internet, and easy ways to access it, have always been there. The way that the Internet and related technologies are used also changes rapidly. In the early days, the Internet was more of a read-only platform, with only a relatively few people creating content and many people acting merely as consumers of that content. Nowadays, everybody can, and does, create content with social media, such as Facebook, X, and LinkedIn. This so-called Web 2.0 has only been around from about 2004. A more recent step, made more accessible to the public through ChatGPT in 2022, is generative artificial intelligence (AI), in which the system itself generates text, images, or code, based on the users' input. This may have huge implications for how we see and use technology, including eHealth. However, at this point in time, the actual impact remains to be seen and investigated.

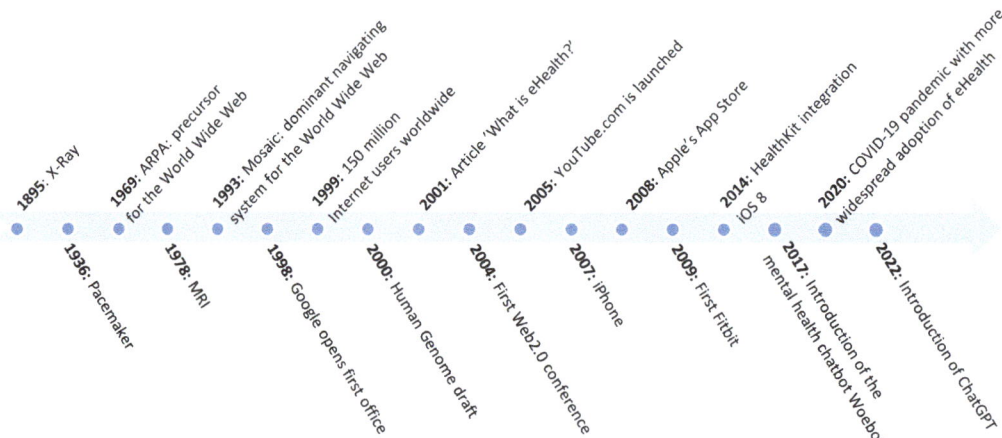

Figure 3.1 Timeline with examples of medical and eHealth-related technologies and events.

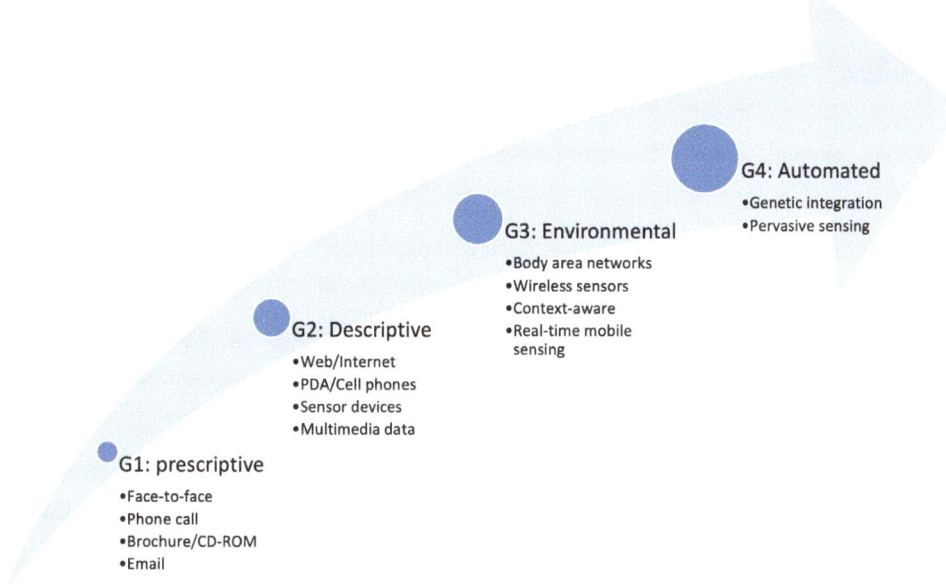

Figure 3.2 Roadmap of evolution of persuasive technologies.

Source: Adapted from Chatterjee and Price (2009).

Figure 3.2 presents a more in-depth overview of the evolution of persuasive technologies (technologies that are designed to change the behaviour or attitudes of people, see Chapter 12) in the context of health (Chatterjee & Price, 2009). This figure shows that eHealth technologies have evolved from prescriptive systems, via descriptive systems, to environmental and automated systems. The early prescriptive systems involved fundamentally human, static one-on-one persuasion where healthcare providers used such technology as telephones and CD-ROMs that could be given to patients for extra information. There was no real interaction with the system or technology itself. Second-generation technologies – descriptive systems – were mainly web-based, where text and, later, multimedia information were shared with and among users. The use of sensors began in the second generation, but evolved in the third generation, in which the data from sensors and other context-aware technologies are used to learn about the current state of the user of the technology (monitoring) so that 'just-in-time' persuasive messages can be given to influence behaviour (coaching). The latest generation of persuasive systems is characterized by more pervasive sensing and the use of smart algorithms using AI, to automatically personalize feedback and support, making human intervention minimal or not needed anymore.

Examples of Technologies for Health and Healthcare

To give an idea of how technology can be used for health and well-being, a non-exhaustive list of technologies that have potential, or are often used for health, well-being, and healthcare is provided below. These examples illustrate the wide spectrum of technological possibilities, aiming to foster a broad perspective on how technology can be used in this area. This broad perspective is useful for each member of an eHealth development team: having at least some basic knowledge of the technology that can be used, helps to understand, and optimally make use of the possibilities of the technology (also see Chapter 7).

Videoconferencing

Videoconferencing is one of the oldest eHealth-technologies and refers to the use of videoconferencing services to connect patients with health care providers, or health providers with each other. This can be valuable for remote consultations, follow-ups, managing chronic conditions, and improving healthcare accessibility. Videoconferencing has been used in healthcare for quite a while already, but it became more commonplace during the COVID-19 pandemic. Overall, research indicates that videoconferencing can be effective in providing remote medical consultations, psychotherapy, and healthcare education. Studies show patient satisfaction and clinical outcomes comparable to in-person visits, especially in mental health care (Hubley, Lynch, Schneck, Thomas, & Shore, 2016; Mallow et al., 2016). However, challenges include privacy concerns, technical issues, and the need for regulatory frameworks (Cowan, McKean, Gentry, & Hilty, 2019). Moreover, research indicated that verbal and non-verbal communication in videoconferencing for health might be different from in-person care (Henry, Block, Ciesla, McGowan, & Vozenilek, 2017). This is an important point of attention, as it influences the quality of care, patient satisfaction, and the effectiveness of remote healthcare interactions.

Web-based Interventions

Web-based interventions are digital platforms that deliver health-related content, tools, and support via the Internet. They provide information, self-help resources and exercises, and interactive features like symptom tracking or virtual coaching to address various health concerns, often by means of multiple (interactive) lessons. They are often based on existing treatment protocols, such as cognitive behavioural therapy (CBT) or mindfulness. Web-based interventions are some of the earliest and most-used eHealth technologies and have been shown to be effective for many health concerns, including mental health, chronic diseases, and lifestyle changes (Beatty & Lambert, 2013; Joseph, Durant, Benitez, & Pekmezi, 2014; Karyotaki et al., 2021). They offer accessibility, convenience, and the potential for personalized support, empowering individuals to manage their health, make informed decisions, and connect with a broader healthcare community.

Mobile Apps

Mobile apps for health, often referred to as mHealth, are software applications, designed for mobile devices such as smartphones and tablets, that focus on promoting health and well-being. These apps encompass a wide range of functionalities and purposes, including health tracking, medication management, and self-help interventions. Essentially, they can do everything web-based interventions can (although on a smaller screen) but are on a device that people always carry with them, providing opportunities to intervene 'just-in-time'. Furthermore, an important characteristic of mobile apps is that they often have one main focal point, as opposed to many different lessons, which is often the case in web-based interventions. Moreover, they can make use of sensors embedded in a smartphone, giving even more opportunities, e.g., tracking of physical activity and providing just-in-time tailored feedback. However, challenges such as data privacy, design quality, and regulatory oversight must be addressed. Additionally, disparities in app access and usage among different populations require attention (Marzano et al., 2015; Mohammadzadeh & Safdari, 2014).

Virtual Reality (VR)

Virtual reality (VR) creates immersive, computer-generated environments, allowing for a 'sense of presence' in its user, which means the user feels as if they are actually in the virtual environment. This phenomenon is also referred to as VR being 'immersive'. In healthcare, VR can be used, e.g., for pain management during procedures, exposure therapy for phobias, rehabilitation exercises, or practicing social skills. It can also be used in training of health care professionals. Some advantages of VR are that users can practice in a safe environment, and that this environment can be controlled by the user or a health care provider. An example of how VR is used in practice is described in Box 3.1.

Box 3.1 Example of the use of VR in practice.

One concrete example of a VR application for health is 'VR for Pain Management' used in paediatric healthcare settings (Chan et al., 2019). This eHealth technology is employed to help children manage pain and anxiety during medical procedures, such as vaccinations or the placement of an intravenous (IV) line.

How it works:

- Before the procedure, a child puts on a VR headset, immersing themselves in a virtual environment, i.e., an underwater environment (see Figure 3.3);
- The VR experience serves as a distraction, engaging the child's attention away from the medical procedure;
- The child interacts with the virtual world, focusing on exploring and enjoying the experience rather than on the pain or discomfort of the procedure.

This intervention has been shown to reduce pain perception and anxiety levels in paediatric patients during medical procedures. Moreover, almost all children wanted VR for future needle procedures, indicating their positive evaluation of the VR intervention.

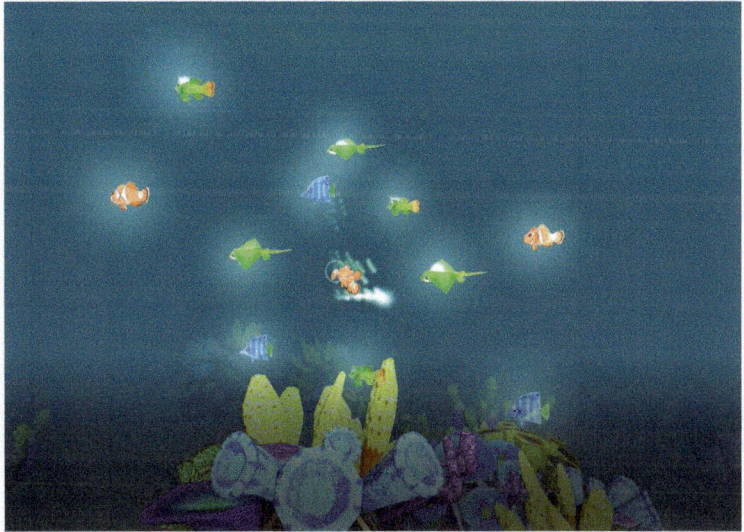

Figure 3.3 The underwater VR environment.

Source: Chan et al., 2019.

Augmented Reality (AR)

Augmented reality (AR) overlays digital information onto the real world. For example, surgeons can use AR headsets to visualize patient data during surgery, potentially raising situational awareness, and save time (Yoon et al., 2018). Another example of AR is smart glasses that can help children with Autism Spectrum Disorder to correctly identify emotions in other people, or help focus their visual attention on another person's face (Liu, Salisbury, Vahabzadeh, & Sahin, 2017). AR can also be used in exposure therapy, e.g., by projecting a spider on a patient's hand (Baus & Bouchard, 2014) in the treatment of arachnophobia (a fear of spiders).

Wearables

Wearables are portable electronic devices that individuals can wear on their bodies to monitor various health-related parameters. These devices include smartwatches, smart rings, and even smart clothes such as socks or vests with sensors. They can collect data on physical activity, heart rate, sleep patterns, and more. Because they are often worn on the body of the user, they can collect more information than smartphones. Wearables provide real-time insights into indicators for an individual's health and wellness, helping users track fitness goals, detect anomalies, and make informed lifestyle choices by providing users with feedback. The goal of such so-called 'biofeedback' is to help individuals understand and regulate these physiological processes, which can lead to improved health and well-being. Wearables can also facilitate remote monitoring by healthcare providers and enable early detection of health issues, enhancing preventive care. Although research highlights the effectiveness of wearables in tracking physical activity, heart rate and sleep, there are challenges, related to validity and reliability of data, privacy concerns, and implementation of these devices in (regular) healthcare (Smuck, Odonkor, Wilt, Schmidt, & Swiernik, 2021). Often, wearables are coupled with mobile apps, making the distinction between these two categories less clear, or even obsolete.

Social Media and Online Communities

Online communities and social platforms enable patients to connect, share experiences, and seek support from peers with similar experiences. Healthcare professionals can also use these platforms for health campaigns and patient education. Anonymity and a wider reach can make it easier for patients to find peer support, especially for issues that are rare or carry stigma. Overall, these platforms can empower patients and bring them into contact with peers that would otherwise have been hard to reach, but challenges include the spread of misinformation and privacy concerns (Johansson, Islind, Lindroth, Angenete, & Gellerstedt, 2021; Moorhead et al., 2013). Ongoing research explores strategies for enhancing the credibility of health information and maximizing the benefits of these online communities for patient empowerment and well-being.

Serious Games

Serious games for health, also referred to as 'health games' or 'medical games', are interactive digital applications, designed with the primary purpose of promoting health, education, and behaviour change in a gamified way. These games leverage the engaging and immersive nature of gaming to deliver health-related messages, teach new skills, or address specific medical conditions. Serious games can cover a wide spectrum of topics, from physical fitness and nutrition to mental health and chronic disease management. They encourage players to make

Box 3.2 Example of a serious game for health.

One concrete example of a serious game for health is SPARX developed by the University of Auckland, New Zealand. SPARX is designed to address mental health issues, particularly depression in adolescents.

How It Works:

Objective: SPARX is an adventure game where players take on the role of a character who explores a virtual world to combat their 'gloomy thoughts'.

Gameplay: Players complete challenges and activities, such as solving puzzles and engaging with characters, to overcome negative emotions.

Cognitive Behavioral Therapy (CBT): The game incorporates principles of CBT, a well-established therapeutic approach for depression, into its gameplay and story.

Emotional Regulation: Players learn skills to manage their emotions and confront depressive thoughts in a safe and supportive virtual environment.

Research has shown that SPARX can be as effective as traditional therapy in reducing symptoms of depression in young people (Merry et al., 2012). Moreover, adolescents enjoyed SPARX and adherence to the program was high.

informed choices about their health by presenting challenges, providing feedback, and rewarding progress. For example, a game might simulate a fitness routine, monitor a player's exercise, and offer advice on improving performance. Their goal is to make learning and behaviour change enjoyable, motivating individuals to adopt healthier habits. Research has shown their potential effectiveness in improving health outcomes, increasing health knowledge, and enhancing patient engagement – making them especially suitable for hard-to-involve patient populations (or healthcare professionals) with less intrinsic motivation (Lau, Smit, Fleming, & Riper, 2016; Papastergiou, 2009; Primack et al., 2012). An example of one such serious game for patients is provided in Box 3.2.

Robotics

Robotics can be used in healthcare to improve patient outcomes by supporting behaviour change or enhancing medical procedures. In rehabilitation, robotic exoskeletons may aid patients in regaining mobility and strength after injuries or surgeries (Shi, Zhang, Zhang, & Ding, 2019). In elderly care, social robots can be used. These are robotic devices designed to provide companionship, emotional support, and social interaction to the user. These robots are equipped with sensors, artificial intelligence, and human-like features to engage with seniors in a way that promotes mental and emotional well-being (Broekens, Heerink, & Rosendal, 2009). One example is the 'Paro' robot, a therapeutic robot designed to resemble a baby seal. Paro responds to touch and sound, allowing it to bond with seniors by reacting to their interactions. It can mimic the behaviour of a live animal, providing comfort and companionship to those who may be isolated or suffering from conditions like dementia or depression. Paro has been used in nursing homes and healthcare facilities worldwide, and has the potential to reduce stress, anxiety, and loneliness among elderly individuals (Jung, van der Leij, & Kelders, 2017).

Chatbots and Conversational Agents

A chatbot or conversational agent is a system that can converse and interact with users using spoken, written, and visual language. Sometimes these systems are based on a decision tree, where the user selects the most appropriate question or answer from a list, and the chatbot responds to that; and sometimes these responses are AI-based, where users can communicate with the chatbot in natural language. These chatbots can be used for multiple purposes, e.g., to deliver accurate and up-to-date medical information; to help users better understand their health conditions, treatment options, and medications; to conduct symptom assessments to provide initial guidance on potential health issues; to recommend self-care measures, or advise users to seek professional medical attention when necessary; to facilitate the booking of medical appointments, reducing administrative burdens for healthcare providers and improving patient access to care; and to offer mental health support, by giving psychoeducation and exercises in a conversation with a user (see also Chapter 5). The possible benefits of healthcare chatbots include accessibility, 24/7 availability, cost-efficiency, and the potential to reduce the burden on healthcare providers. However, ensuring the accuracy of messages, maintaining data privacy and security, and addressing ethical considerations are critical challenges (Abd-Alrazaq, Rababeh, Alajlani, Bewick, & Househ, 2020; Wilson & Marasoiu, 2022).

Advantages of Technology for Health

Now that we know more about the types of technology applied and know *how* technology can be used, it is time to look at *why* technology can be suitable to improve health, healthcare, and well-being. We start with looking at how computers work, to provide more insight into the underlying system that ensures a technology functions.

What Computers Do

To understand how computers work, we'll look at three related concepts: binary code, programming languages, and software. These are integral components of computer technology, working together to enable computers to process information and execute tasks.

- **Binary Code**. Computers communicate internally using binary code, a system of representing data with two symbols: 0 and 1. Each 0 or 1 is a 'bit', and groups of 8 bits form a 'byte'. Binary code encodes all data, instructions, and memory in a computer. For instance, the number 7 is represented as '0111' in binary. Computers use electronic circuits to interpret and manipulate these binary patterns, with electrical voltages representing 0s and 1s;
- **Programming Languages**. Programming languages are intermediary tools that allow humans to communicate with computers. They consist of human-readable syntax and semantics that represent the underlying complex binary code. Programmers write code using programming languages to instruct computers. For example, in Python, 'print("Hello, World!")' instructs the computer to display a greeting. The computer then uses a different tool (called compiler or interpreter) to translate this human-readable code into binary code the computer can execute;
- **Software**. Software is the practical application of programming languages. It is a collection of coded instructions created by programmers. Software serves various functions, from simple utilities like calculators to complex systems like operating systems, applications, and video games. When software is run, the computer's central processing unit (CPU) reads the binary instructions generated from the programming language, processes data, and performs the intended tasks;

- **Application Programming Interface (API)**. An API is a set of rules and protocols that allows different software applications to communicate and interact with each other. It enables developers to access certain features or data from a service or platform, making it essential for building software applications that can integrate with external services or systems;
- **Graphical User Interface (GUI)**. A GUI is a visual interface that allows users to interact with software or devices through graphical elements like windows, buttons, and icons, rather than text-based commands. GUIs make software more user-friendly and accessible, allowing users to perform tasks with a point-and-click approach, common in modern operating systems and applications.

So, to summarize binary code is the computer's native language, programming languages bridge the gap between humans and computers, and software is the tangible product of this interaction, enabling computers to perform the tasks we require them to do. APIs can be used to let different software applications communicate and a GUI is the interface of the software that you see on your screen.

With this basic knowledge of how computer technology works, we can better understand what kind of tasks computers can execute quite easily, compared to humans. Their strengths lie in:

- **Data processing**: computers can swiftly analyse vast datasets, allowing them to work with lots of data from, e.g., electronic patient records, sensors, or usage of health technologies;
- **Complex calculations**: computers perform intricate mathematical calculations with very high accuracy, which can be used, for example, for creating personalized treatment plans;
- **Automation**: computers excel at repetitive tasks, for example, sending reminders to the right people at the right time;
- **Storage and retrieval**: computers efficiently store and retrieve vast amounts of information, facilitating data management for, for example, electronic patient records, wearables, and domotics;
- **Pattern recognition**: machine learning and artificial intelligence algorithms enable computers to recognize patterns in data, making them proficient in image and speech recognition (e.g., in diagnostics), recommendation systems (e.g., personalized medicine), and much more;
- **Connectivity**: computers seamlessly communicate over networks, enabling global connectivity, online collaboration, and real-time information exchange;
- **Information access**: computers grant rapid access to vast online resources, serving as tools for (psycho)education, online interventions, and other information dissemination.

Together, these skills can give computers capabilities that mimic (parts of) human intelligence, so called artificial intelligence (AI). AI is a multidisciplinary field of computer science that focuses on creating machines or systems capable of emulating human-like intelligence and decision-making processes. These systems are designed to process and interpret vast amounts of data, enabling them to perform tasks that traditionally require human cognition. AI is used more and more in the health domain, for example in medical imaging, personalized medicine, but also in mental health. AI encompasses various subdomains, including:

Machine Learning: this subset of AI focuses on developing algorithms and models capable of learning from data and making predictions or decisions without being explicitly programmed. Basically, they learn patterns and relationships from large datasets. They identify these patterns through statistical analysis and adjust their internal parameters to improve their performance. Machine learning is behind many AI applications, such as recommendation systems, fraud detection, and speech recognition.

Natural Language Processing (NLP): NLP enables machines to understand, interpret, and generate human language in a way that is both meaningful and contextually relevant. NLP techniques involve tasks like text and speech recognition, language translation, sentiment analysis, and chatbot development. NLP algorithms use linguistic rules, statistical models, and machine learning to process and analyze vast amounts of natural language data. It is used in chatbots, language translation apps, and sentiment analysis tools.

Computer vision: computer vision empowers computers to interpret and understand visual information from the world, much like humans do with their eyes and brains. It involves developing algorithms and models that enable computers to analyze images and videos, extract meaningful data, and make decisions based on visual input. Computer vision applications range from object recognition and tracking to facial recognition, medical image analysis, autonomous vehicles, and even industrial quality control. It relies on techniques like image processing, machine learning, and pattern recognition to transform pixels into actionable insights, enabling machines to 'see' and comprehend the visual world.

Why Computers can be Persuasive

With these basic and more advanced skills, computers can also play a role in helping people change their behaviour or cognitions. As we have seen in Chapter 2, this is a key concept within health and well-being. According to Fogg – one of the founders of the field of Persuasive Technology – there are six reasons why technology can sometimes be better than human persuaders at influencing attitudes and behaviour (Fogg, 2002). These are presented below, and as you can see, many of them are directly related to the tasks that computers excel at.

Technology is more persistent than human beings

After a while, humans will get tired of trying to persuade someone. Technology, of course, does not have this fatigue, as it can continue to persuade its users indefinitely. Of course, this also raises an ethical issue: if the technology doesn't automatically stop trying to persuade after a while, how do we prevent that persuasion becomes too invasive?

Technology offers greater anonymity

When talking to a human persuader in person, it is difficult, if not impossible, to stay anonymous. With technology, this is easier. For example, many behaviour change apps offer the possibility to sign up anonymously, which can be a huge advantage for sensitive subjects like psychological problems or substance abuse.

Technology can manage huge volumes of data

Humans can process a lot of data, but when it comes to managing huge volumes of data (Big Data), technology has a clear advantage. This can give technology more persuasive power, because technology can back up a certain message with the data that supports it and it can quickly identify patterns within these large datasets, allowing for personalized, just-in-time feedback.

Technology uses many modalities to influence

Technology can present information in many different ways, including text, audio, and video. Because of this, technology can match the persuasive methods it uses to each person's individual preferences and skills.

Technology is scalable

This may be the largest and most practical advantage. People can only reach a limited number of other people. By using technology, many more people can be reached without a large increase in cost. Especially in public health, this is a major advantage, and this is the argument that is most often used for delivering a behaviour change programme by means of technology, also to, for example, lower income countries.

Technology can go where humans cannot go or may not be welcome

Technology can be, and is, everywhere, even in places that you would not allow a human persuader to be, such as in one's bathroom. We know that for many behaviour change techniques to be effective, timing is important. For example, consider changing your tooth-brushing behaviour. Having the dentist telling you how to brush your teeth may be persuasive when you are in the dental chair, but chances are you will have forgotten about it when you are at home and ready to brush your teeth. But technology, like a smart toothbrush, can persuade you to continue brushing your teeth for a while longer that night in your own bathroom. Imagine the dentist doing that!

These reasons why computers can be persuasive shows some of the specific opportunities of technology that we may be able to harness to improve health and healthcare. It is good to note that this list is not exhaustive. Persuasiveness in this way, is mainly focused on getting the attention of users and helping them make a (healthier) decision. However, sometimes, the power of technology is that you don't even notice that it's there. This is called unobtrusive technology, i.e., technology that is integrated seamlessly into our environment and daily lives without being obtrusive or disruptive. An example of a (near) unobtrusive technology is a wearable fitness tracker. A glance on your wearable might be sufficient to know whether you are on track to reach your fitness goals, which can be very persuasive, without the need to ask for a lot of your attention.

Limitations of Technology

While there are many things that technology can do really well, it is also important to understand that there are some things that technology is less good at. These aspects often require the input of humans, and arguably this will remain so, at least for the foreseeable future. Some of these important aspects are:

- **Contextual understanding**. Computers can struggle to grasp the nuances of human language, making it difficult to understand sarcasm, humour, metaphors, and idiomatic expressions, which most humans can interpret effortlessly through cultural and contextual knowledge;
- **Common sense reasoning**. While humans possess common sense and intuitive reasoning abilities, computers lack this innate understanding, making them prone to misinterpretation and errors, especially in situations where context matters;
- **Creativity and innovation**. Computers can generate content based on patterns and data, but at this point in time, they often struggle to exhibit *true* creativity, innovation, or emotional intelligence;
- **Adaptation to ambiguity**. Humans are able to adapt to ambiguous or unfamiliar situations, drawing from their diverse experiences and emotions. Computers require clear instructions and structured data, struggling when faced with unanticipated scenarios;
- **Learning from limited data**. Humans can learn from small amounts of data or a single experience, adapting quickly to new situations by drawing on, e.g., previous experiences. In contrast, computers often require extensive training data for machine learning algorithms to generalize effectively.

A last limitation, or at least point of attention, in using technology in health, are ethics. As we have seen, there are many ways of using technology to support health, healthcare, and well-being. Each of these ways of using technology will bring their own unique ethical issues. However, some issues play a role in almost any form of eHealth. In an integrative review on ethical issues related to eHealth from the users' perspective, the following four ethical themes were found to be most prominent (Jokinen, Stolt, & Suhonen, 2021):

- **Privacy**. Users expressed concerns about the privacy of their health information in eHealth technologies. They emphasized the importance of controlling with whom their information is shared and the need for informed consent to share their data;
- **Beneficence and non-maleficence**. Users generally viewed eHealth technologies as beneficial, empowering them to take a more active role in their healthcare. However, concerns included potential harm resulting from the misuse of personal health information, such as discrimination or stigma;
- **Justice**. Challenges related to equality and equity in accessing eHealth services were highlighted. Issues such as poor Internet access, limited digital skills, and the cost of devices and Internet access hindered equitable use of eHealth services;
- **Trust**. Users expressed concerns about the competence of healthcare professionals in managing eHealth data, including accuracy, legitimacy, and data security. Moreover, they emphasized the importance of maintaining human contact in healthcare.

As indicated, apart from these more general ethical concerns, most technologies also bring their own ethical challenges. It is beyond the scope of this chapter to go into all of these, but because of the rise in artificial intelligence (AI), we will go into some more specific challenges that are related to this, based on a recent systematic review in this area (Karimian, Petelos, & Evers, 2022).

Preservation of human autonomy. When using AI, it is important to ensure that patients retain control over their medical decisions. This challenge highlights the importance of shared decision making between patients and healthcare providers, perhaps supported but not dominated by AI. Patients (or healthcare professionals) should not feel that their autonomy is compromised by AI recommendations, but rather that AI enhances their ability to make informed choices about their care. Consequently, the challenge lies in striking a balance between the efficiency of AI systems and respecting patients' values, preferences, and unique needs.

Explainable AI. Explainable AI is all about making AI systems transparent and interpretable. It addresses the 'black-box' problem, where complex AI algorithms are hard to understand for users and it is not clear on what a specific recommendation is based. In healthcare, it's vital for healthcare providers and patients to grasp why AI makes certain recommendations. This transparency builds trust and allows for effective communication. Moreover, it ensures accountability, making it clear who is responsible when AI-driven decisions result in harm for patients.

Fairness. Fairness in AI means that AI systems treat individuals or groups equitably and without bias. Biases in AI algorithms can arise from biased training data (which is a common problem) and can perpetuate discrimination in healthcare. The goal is to prevent such biases and ensure that AI doesn't unfairly advantage or disadvantage specific demographics such as neighbourhood, gender, or race. Fair AI promotes equal access to healthcare resources and treatment outcomes, regardless of demographic and socioeconomic factors. Achieving fairness involves addressing bias in AI algorithms, using diverse and representative data, and actively monitoring for disparities in AI-driven decisions.

Working in Multidisciplinary Teams

As can be seen, there are many barriers that are related to technology. One way to address this, is by joining forces via multidisciplinary collaborations. As you will read throughout the book, it is necessary to work in multidisciplinary teams when developing, implementing, and evaluating eHealth. Working in such teams works best when everyone at least has a basic understanding of each other's areas of expertise. Therefore, the remainder of the chapter is focused on the software development process.

Software Development

In this section, we will cover a few well-known and much-used software development models, i.e., Waterfall and Spiral models, Agile, and the Scrum framework.

Waterfall and Spiral design models

The *Waterfall Model of System Development* (Figure 3.4) is one of the earliest software development models. It is essentially a sequential model: once a phase is finished, you move on to the next phase. The process starts with requirements specification, moves on to designing, implementing (coding), verification (testing), and finally maintenance. Although this model is often used for large projects, it has received a lot of criticism, mainly because of the rigid nature of a sequential model: no changes are possible later because the requirements are finalized in the first stage and because testing is done at a late stage, it is harder to fix possible issues (Petersen, Wohlin, & Baca, 2009). Because of this, adaptations to the Waterfall Model have been proposed (e.g., adding feedback loops between the phases), leading, for example, to the *Spiral design model* (Boehm, 1988). The Spiral Model is also a sequential model, but it involves iterative cycles of the sequential phases. This way, the model can cope with more complex projects where not all the requirements are known in advance, or where the requirements may change due to feedback on prototypes or new insights. The Waterfall and Spiral models are more traditional methods of software development and are used less and less in current practice.

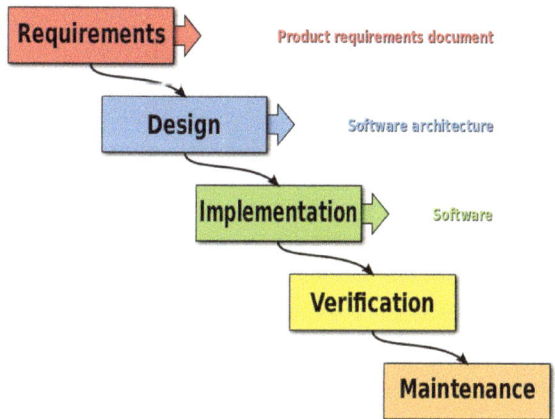

Figure 3.4 The Waterfall Model of system development.

Source: © Peter Kemp/Adapted from Paul Smith's work at Wikipedia.

Agile software development and Scrum

In 2001, different software development practitioners shared their view on what software development should be like in the 'Manifesto for Agile software development' (Beck et al., 2001). Since then, numerous methods and practices have surfaced that share the values and principles stated in this manifesto. Agile development focuses on fast development of small pieces of software that eventually make up one software application. By taking smaller steps, the approach is more adaptive and able to deal with change. Core values are collaborative development, a 'lean' mentality where unnecessary work is minimized, more stakeholder involvement, and the acceptance of uncertainty by developers, which encourages a rapid and flexible response to change (Dingsøyr, Nerur, Balijepally, & Moe, 2012).

According to the *Agile Manifesto*, there are four core values:

1. **Individuals and interactions over processes and tools**. An Agile approach prioritizes human communication and collaboration among team members over relying solely on formal processes or tools, e.g., for documentation and bug-tracking. It recognizes that effective teamwork is essential for successful software development;
2. **Working software over comprehensive documentation**. While documentation is important, Agile development emphasizes that the primary measure of progress should be functional software. Excessive documentation can slow down development and may become outdated quickly;
3. **Customer collaboration over contract negotiation**. Agile development encourages continuous customer involvement throughout the entire project. Rather than rigid contracts, it favours ongoing collaboration to ensure that the software meets the customer's evolving needs;
4. **Responding to change over following a plan**. Agile development acknowledges that change is inevitable in software development. It values the ability to adapt to changing requirements and priorities over rigidly sticking to a predefined plan.

According to a review on Agile software development (Al-Saqqa, Sawalha, & Abdel-Nabi, 2020), an Agile approach aims to build trust between customers and development teams by delivering working software early and often, allowing customers to provide feedback early on and to prioritize requirements. It promotes adaptability to changing requirements, encourages collaboration, and focuses on delivering value to the customer. Agile teams are self-organizing and emphasize technical excellence. The advantages of an Agile approach may include improved communication, quicker releases, flexible design, and a more reasonable development process. It excels in handling changes efficiently, reducing the cost and time impact of late-stage alterations compared to traditional development processes. Agile is not a rigid methodology but a set of practices, values, and principles that promote agility and responsiveness in software development. However, an Agile development approach also has some pitfalls. First, if teams are new to this approach, inadequate understanding of the approach, methods, and tools, but also unrealistic expectations, may hamper the effectiveness of the approach. Second, Agile development promotes adaptive planning, but being overly optimistic about what can be achieved in each iteration can lead to missed deadlines and frustration. Moreover, the adaptive planning can make it difficult to paint a clear timeline and total costs of a project. Last, the Agile approach relies heavily on collaboration among team members. Poor communication, conflicts, or lack of trust within the team can hinder progress.

Scrum

One way to ensure a systematic approach to Agile development, is via development frameworks. One of the most widely used Agile development frameworks is *Scrum*. In Scrum, developers work in teams of around three to nine people and break up their work into short cycles, called sprints.

SCRUM FRAMEWORK

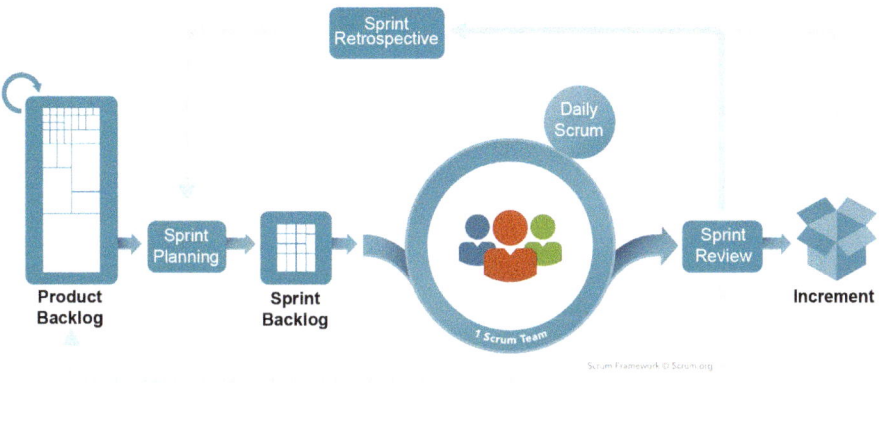

Figure 3.5 Scrum framework.

The work that needs to be done is collected in the product 'backlog': a list of everything that might be needed in the product. A few notable activities (e.g., 'events') are (Figure 3.5):

- **Sprint**: a short period of often two weeks in which a usable and potentially releasable product (increment) is developed. During a sprint, no changes are made that endanger the sprint goal, and the quality goals may not be decreased. However, the scope may be clarified or renegotiated when new insights are learned;
- **Sprint planning**: a longer meeting (maximum eight hours) of the Scrum team to set the sprint goal and to determine how the needed work can be achieved;
- **Daily scrum**: a short meeting (15 minutes), or stand-up, of the development team at the beginning of the day to check whether they are still on their way to achieve the sprint goals and to synchronize the activities of the day.

Agile approaches to technology development like Scrum are increasingly considered to be appropriate for the development of eHealth technology. The reasons for this are the often-complex context that the technology needs to fit in, the large number of different stakeholders, and the difficulty of specifying each requirement for the technology in advance (also see Chapter 7). Moreover, there has been a call not only to apply these principles in the development of eHealth technology, but also to use them in the way research into eHealth technology is conducted and disseminated (Hekler et al., 2016).

Summary

In this chapter, you have seen that technology offers many opportunities to improve health and well-being. Characteristics of technology such as persistence and being able to deal with large amounts of data can make technology an effective persuader. We have seen that the pace of innovation in technology is very rapid. This makes it difficult, if not impossible, for researchers and practitioners in related fields to keep up-to-date with all of the latest technological developments. However, it is important for everyone in the field of eHealth to have some basic knowledge of what technology can do. One of the things technology can do is be 'smart', using artificial intelligence, and this chapter has given an introduction to some of the building blocks of AI, including an overview of some important ethical issues. Combined with the basic knowledge of Agile software development processes, these insights can help you in finding the added value of technology for your specific goal and in working with the software developers who might be able to develop the technology with you. The take-home messages for this chapter are:

- Technology offers specific opportunities to be an influential persuader with its persistence, anonymity, ability to deal with large amounts of data, use of many modalities, its scalability, and its being able to be everywhere;
- Concepts that are good to know when working in multidisciplinary eHealth teams are AI, machine learning, image recognition, NLP, generative AI, API, and GUI;
- There are many types of (rapidly developing) technologies that are useful for eHealth, including VR, AR, web-based interventions, mobile apps, serious games, biofeedback, and chatbots;
- There are numerous ethical challenges when working with technology in health, healthcare, and well-being, including those related to privacy, beneficence and non-maleficence, justice, and trust; and specifically for AI, preservation of human autonomy, explainability, and fairness;
- As opposed to more sequential software development models such as Waterfall and Spiral models, Agile software development, such as Scrum, is much more flexible and able to deal with change, making it more suitable for the development of eHealth technologies.

Acknowledgement

We would like to acknowledge the use of ChatGPT (GPT-3.5, OpenAI) to generate a first draft of some paragraphs of this chapter, and for improving the writing style. SK reviewed, edited, and revised the ChatGPT-generated texts to their own liking and take ultimate responsibility for the content of this chapter.

Key References for Further Reading

Abd-Alrazaq, A. A., Rababeh, A., Alajlani, M., Bewick, B. M., & Househ, M. (2020). Effectiveness and safety of using chatbots to improve mental health: Systematic review and meta-analysis. *Journal of Medical Internet Research*, 22(7), e16021. https://doi.org/10.2196/16021

Al-Saqqa, S., Sawalha, S., & Abdel-Nabi, H. (2020). Agile software development: Methodologies and trends. *International Journal of Interactive Mobile Technologies*, 14(11).

Karimian, G., Petelos, E., & Evers, S. M. A. A. (2022). The ethical issues of the application of artificial intelligence in healthcare: A systematic scoping review. *AI and Ethics*, 2(4), 539–551.

Marzano, L., Bardill, A., Fields, B., Herd, K., Veale, D., Grey, N., & Moran, P. (2015). The application of mHealth to mental health: Opportunities and challenges. *The Lancet Psychiatry*, 2(10), 942–948.

Smuck, M., Odonkor, C. A., Wilt, J., Schmidt, N., & Swiernik, M. A. (2021). The emerging clinical role of wearables: Factors for successful implementation in healthcare. *NPJ Digital Medicine*, 4.

References

Abd-Alrazaq, A. A., Rababeh, A., Alajlani, M., Bewick, B. M., & Househ, M. (2020). Effectiveness and safety of using chatbots to improve mental health: Systematic review and meta-analysis. *J Med Internet Res*, 22(7), e16021. doi:10.2196/16021

Al-Saqqa, S., Sawalha, S., & Abdel-Nabi, H. (2020). Agile software development: Methodologies and trends. *International Journal of Interactive Mobile Technologies (iJIM)*, 14, 246. doi:10.3991/ijim.v14i11.13269

Baus, O., & Bouchard, S. (2014). Moving from virtual reality exposure-based therapy to augmented reality exposure-based therapy: A review. *Front Hum Neurosci*, 8, 112. doi:10.3389/fnhum.2014.00112

Beatty, L., & Lambert, S. (2013). A systematic review of internet-based self-help therapeutic interventions to improve distress and disease-control among adults with chronic health conditions. *Clin Psychol Rev*, 33(4), 609–622. doi:10.1016/j.cpr.2013.03.004

Beck, K., Beedle, M., Van Bennekum, A., Cockburn, A., Cunningham, W., Fowler, M., … & Jeffries, R. (2001). Manifesto for Agile software development. *The Agile Manifesto*.

Boehm, B. W. (1988). A Spiral Model of software development and enhancement. *Computer*, 21(5), 61–72.

Broekens, J., Heerink, M., & Rosendal, H. (2009). Assistive social robots in elderly care: A review. *Gerontechnology*, 8, 94–103. doi:10.4017/gt.2009.08.02.002.00

Chan, E., Hovenden, M., Ramage, E., Ling, N., Pham, J. H., Rahim, A., . . . Leong, P. (2019). Virtual reality for pediatric needle procedural pain: Two randomized clinical trials. *J Pediatr*, 209, 160–167.e164. doi:10.1016/j.jpeds.2019.02.034

Chatterjee, S., & Price, A. (2009). Healthy living with persuasive technologies: Framework, issues, and challenges. *Journal of the American Medical Informatics Association*, 16(2), 171–178.

Cowan, K. E., McKean, A. J., Gentry, M. T., & Hilty, D. M. (2019). Barriers to use of telepsychiatry: Clinicians as gatekeepers. *Mayo Clin Proc*, 94(12), 2510–2523. doi:10.1016/j.mayocp.2019.04.018

Dingsøyr, T., Nerur, S., Balijepally, V., & Moe, N. B. (2012). A decade of Agile methodologies: Towards explaining agile software development. *Journal of Systems and Software*, 85(6), 1213–1221.

Fogg, B. J. (2002). Persuasive technology: Using computers to change what we think and do. *Ubiquity*, 2002(December), 5.

Hekler, E. B., Klasnja, P., Riley, W. T., Buman, M. P., Huberty, J., Rivera, D. E., & Martin, C. A. (2016). Agile science: Creating useful products for behavior change in the real world. *Translational Behavioral Medicine*, 6(2), 317–328.

Henry, B. W., Block, D. E., Ciesla, J. R., McGowan, B. A., & Vozenilek, J. A. (2017). Clinician behaviors in telehealth care delivery: A systematic review. *Adv Health Sci Educ Theory Pract*, 22(4), 869–888. doi:10.1007/s10459-016-9717-2

Hubley, S., Lynch, S. B., Schneck, C., Thomas, M., & Shore, J. (2016). Review of key telepsychiatry outcomes. *World J Psychiatry*, 6(2), 269–282. doi:10.5498/wjp.v6.i2.269

Johansson, V., Islind, A. S., Lindroth, T., Angenete, E., & Gellerstedt, M. (2021). Online communities as a driver for patient empowerment: Systematic Review. *J Med Internet Res*, 23(2), e19910. doi:10.2196/19910

Jokinen, A., Stolt, M., & Suhonen, R. (2021). Ethical issues related to eHealth: An integrative review. *Nurs Ethics*, 28(2), 253–271. doi:10.1177/0969733020945765

Joseph, R. P., Durant, N. H., Benitez, T. J., & Pekmezi, D. W. (2014). Internet-based physical activity interventions. *Am J Lifestyle Med*, 8(1), 42–68. doi:10.1177/1559827613498059

Jung, M. M., van der Leij, L., & Kelders, S. M. (2017). An exploration of the benefits of an animallike robot companion with more advanced touch interaction capabilities for dementia care. *Frontiers in ICT*, 4. doi:10.3389/fict.2017.00016

Karimian, G., Petelos, E., & Evers, S. M. A. A. (2022). The ethical issues of the application of artificial intelligence in healthcare: A systematic scoping review. *AI and Ethics*, 2(4), 539–551. doi:10.1007/s43681-021-00131-7

Karyotaki, E., Efthimiou, O., Miguel, C., Bermpohl, F. M. G., Furukawa, T. A., Cuijpers, P., . . . Forsell, Y. (2021). Internet-based cognitive behavioral therapy for depression: A systematic review and individual patient data network meta-analysis. *JAMA Psychiatry*, 78(4), 361–371. doi:10.1001/jamapsychiatry.2020.4364

Lau, H. M., Smit, J. H., Fleming, T. M., & Riper, H. (2016). Serious games for mental health: Are they accessible, feasible, and effective? A systematic review and meta-analysis. *Front Psychiatry*, 7, 209. doi:10.3389/fpsyt.2016.00209

Liu, R., Salisbury, J. P., Vahabzadeh, A., & Sahin, N. T. (2017). Feasibility of an autism-focused augmented reality smartglasses system for social communication and behavioral coaching. *Front Pediatr*, 5, 145. doi:10.3389/fped.2017.00145

Mallow, J. A., Petitte, T., Narsavage, G., Barnes, E., Theeke, E., Mallow, B. K., & Theeke, L. A. (2016). The use of video conferencing for persons with chronic conditions: A systematic review. *Ehealth Telecommun Syst Netw*, 5(2), 39–56. doi:10.4236/etsn.2016.52005

Marzano, L., Bardill, A., Fields, B., Herd, K., Veale, D., Grey, N., & Moran, P. (2015). The application of mHealth to mental health: Opportunities and challenges. *Lancet Psychiatry*, 2(10), 942–948. doi:10.1016/s2215-0366(15)00268-0

Merry, S. N., Stasiak, K., Shepherd, M., Frampton, C., Fleming, T., & Lucassen, M. F. G. (2012). The effectiveness of SPARX, a computerised self help intervention for adolescents seeking help for depression: Randomised controlled non-inferiority trial. *British Medical Journal*, 344, e2598. doi:10.1136/bmj.e2598

Mohammadzadeh, N., & Safdari, R. (2014). Patient monitoring in mobile health: Opportunities and challenges. *Med Arch*, 68(1), 57–60. doi:10.5455/medarh.2014.68.57-60

Moorhead, S. A., Hazlett, D. E., Harrison, L., Carroll, J. K., Irwin, A., & Hoving, C. (2013). A new dimension of health care: Systematic review of the uses, benefits, and limitations of social media for health communication. *J Med Internet Res*, 15(4), e85. doi:10.2196/jmir.1933

Papastergiou, M. (2009). Exploring the potential of computer and video games for health and physical education: A literature review. *Computers & Education*, 53(3), 603–622. doi:https://doi.org/10.1016/j.compedu.2009.04.001

Petersen, K., Wohlin, C., & Baca, D. (2009). *The Waterfall Model in large-scale development*. Paper presented at the PROFES.

Primack, B. A., Carroll, M. V., McNamara, M., Klem, M. L., King, B., Rich, M., . . . Nayak, S. (2012). Role of video games in improving health-related outcomes: A systematic review. *Am J Prev Med*, 42(6), 630–638. doi:10.1016/j.amepre.2012.02.023

Shi, D., Zhang, W., Zhang, W., & Ding, X. (2019). A review on lower limb rehabilitation exoskeleton robots. *Chinese Journal of Mechanical Engineering*, 32(1), 74. doi:10.1186/s10033-019-0389-8

Smuck, M., Odonkor, C. A., Wilt, J., Schmidt, N., & Swiernik, M. A. (2021). The emerging clinical role of wearables: Factors for successful implementation in healthcare. *npj Digital Medicine*, 4. doi:10.1038/s41746-021-00418-3

Wilson, L., & Marasoiu, M. (2022). The development and use of chatbots in public health: Scoping review. *JMIR Hum Factors*, 9(4), e35882. doi:10.2196/35882

Yoon, J. W., Chen, R. E., Kim, E. J., Akinduro, O. O., Kerezoudis, P., Han, P. K., . . . Quinones-Hinojosa, A. (2018). Augmented reality for the surgeon: Systematic review. *Int J Med Robot*, 14(4), e1914. doi:10.1002/rcs.1914

4　Healthcare and Digital Transformation

Laura Kooij & Wim H. van Harten

Introduction

Worldwide, the population is ageing, more people have one or multiple chronic condition(s), and healthcare costs are increasing. This in turn causes an increased demand on healthcare services and rising concerns related to the shortage of healthcare personnel. The pressure on the healthcare system is mounting, and transformation is inevitable to meet up to those challenges. The use of eHealth technologies is very promising, for example to deliver more care in the home setting. In this chapter, we provide an update on digital transformation in healthcare, with a specific focus on hospital care.

This chapter starts with background information on different healthcare systems, followed by a reflection on the main challenges healthcare is facing. Subsequently, digital health technologies and relevant concepts for digital transformation are described, and finally relevant theoretical models are explained. After reading this chapter, you will be able to:

- Understand and explain the basics of healthcare systems from different countries;
- Explain the main challenges facing healthcare;
- Explain the relevant developments in healthcare in terms of healthcare transformation and eHealth technology;
- Explain the need for digital transformation and name important factors that affect this digital transformation;
- Explain and describe relevant theoretical models to explain technology acceptance and implementation of eHealth technology in healthcare practice.

Healthcare Systems

Healthcare systems are complex, involving various organizations, healthcare providers, and insurers. Payment structures and coverage policies are very influential in shaping innovation and dissemination, also in terms of eHealth technology. In order to understand how to design and organize digital transformation, it is essential to understand the specific healthcare systems, especially as the delivery of healthcare and funding are organized differently throughout the world. In this section, we will shortly explain different healthcare systems. We provide a more concrete example: the Netherlands, because this is one of the frontrunners in terms of digital transformation.

DOI: 10.4324/9781003302049-5

Healthcare in the United States

In the United States there is not one uniform healthcare system; rather, it consists of multiple payor-systems, in which governmentally financed insurance coexists with private insurance.

Overall, health insurance in the US can be divided in private, e.g., through employment or public insurance such as Medicare and Medicaid. Medicare, a social healthcare insurance for people older than 65 years, and Medicaid, available for people with low-incomes, were the first federal health insurance programmes and appeared in the mid-1960s (Rice et al., 2020). Healthcare insurance is mostly arranged through employment, but this is not obligatory and part of the population is uninsured (Keisler-Starkey & Bunch 2022; Rice et al., 2020). General practice care is scattered and does not cover the whole population. There is free access to specialist care and no gatekeeper system for hospital- or medical specialist care referrals. The private insurance-based domain especially leaves a lot of space for innovation and implementation of innovative technology. This shows that, if a new digital innovation is introduced, the healthcare context that has to be accounted for is entirely different from that of countries such as the Netherlands and has different implications for the development and implementation of technology. Different digital technologies relevant for healthcare will be described later in this chapter.

Healthcare in the European Union

Healthcare systems differ among European Union (EU) countries. The EU does not have the mandate to regulate healthcare. Each country is responsible for financing, purchasing, and providing healthcare services for their citizens. Healthcare costs are universally covered in nearly all EU countries, with mostly a defined package of services including, e.g., consultations with medical professionals, tests, and hospital care. The main system choices are either a national health system approach (combining coverage and provision) or a social insurance approach in which either private or for-profit agencies are executing the health care insurance and providers are organized as separate entities. In most countries, it is possible to purchase additional private health insurance, such as for dental care or physiotherapy, this is done by over half the population in the Netherlands, Belgium, Luxembourg, France, and Slovenia but is done (much) less in other countries (OECD & European Union, 2022). Below, a worked-out example of healthcare in the Netherlands is provided.

Example: Healthcare in the Netherlands

In the Netherlands, by law, everybody has the right to receive healthcare. Therefore, accessible, affordable, and high-quality care is important. Healthcare services are delivered in primary, secondary, and tertiary care. Primary care is accessible without referral and provided by, e.g., general practitioners, physiotherapists, and social workers. Secondary care involves care by physicians for which a mandatory referral from a general practitioner is needed, such as hospital-, mental-, or rehabilitation care. Specialized or academic hospital care is referred to as tertiary care.

Everybody living or working in the Netherlands is legally obligated to have healthcare insurance, as mandated by the Health Insurance Act. This healthcare insurance consists of a standard basic package that is shaped by the government, is equal for everybody, and covers a wide range of services, for example medical care by a medical specialist or general practitioner, or mental healthcare. Additional insurance is optional, for example for dental, alternative, or maternity care. Healthcare insurers are responsible for the quality of the care that is delivered, purchasing of healthcare services, and agreements with healthcare institutions (Ministerie van Volksgezondheid, 2016).

It is important to understand the structure and funding of the healthcare system, to be able to understand how and why the development and dissemination of new healthcare concepts, such as digital health technology, are or are not (yet) realized. To begin with, often no reimbursements

Box 4.1 Example: Patient journey in the Netherlands.

One way to describe healthcare is by means of patient journeys. The patient journey encompasses a sequence of different phases, events, and other elements a patient experiences in a healthcare setting. We will provide a concept example of a patient journey in hospital care. To receive specialist in- or outpatient hospital care, referral from a general practitioner is needed, which can be seen as a first phase in the patient journey in hospital practice. In acute situations, people can also visit or be transported by ambulance to the emergency room or, if the complaints are not life-threatening, they can visit a general practice centre. After a patient is registered in the hospital, the 'patient journey' consists of different phases and elements, including diagnostics (e.g., radiology), diagnosis, treatment, and follow-up. Treatment can be given on a daycare basis or a patient can be admitted to the hospital, for example, for surgery. Care is also increasingly provided in the home setting. A care pathway in which a patient has consultations with different healthcare professionals such as medical specialist, nurse practitioner, nurse, and other professionals is different for each patient. To provide high-quality care, in line with patients' needs and wishes, (digital) tailored information should be accessible and provided throughout the patient journey. Increasingly, digital care is replacing elements in the care pathway, such as follow-up visits, and self-management and self-monitoring activities are becoming part of those pathways.

are available for these new digital health technologies and finances have to be sought to perform proof-of-principle and effectiveness studies. This can have an impact on the pace of the development of digital transformation and dissemination of this type of innovation in healthcare and will be explained in more detail in the section about digital transformation discussed further on in this chapter.

Challenges Facing Healthcare

In the next part of this chapter, we will describe the challenges facing healthcare in order to highlight the need for digital transformation in healthcare. The information is initially described from the viewpoint of the Dutch healthcare system but reflects the situation in many countries.

Shortages in the Labour Market

In almost all countries in the EU, and even worldwide, shortages in the labour market exist, most prominently in nursing. This was especially clear during the COVID-19 pandemic, when a high increase in care had to be delivered by the same or even fewer healthcare professionals. The increasing demand for care in general, especially due to the ageing population and increasing number of people with a chronic disease, causes an increasing pressure on healthcare delivery. To meet these challenges the delivery of healthcare should be organized differently and more efficiently. This can be supported by eHealth technologies.

Healthcare Costs

In the European Union, healthcare expenditures vary among countries, but usually take a higher percentage of the Gross Domestic Product (GDP) among high-income countries (OECD/European Union, 2020). As in most countries, annual healthcare expenditure in the Netherlands is increasing (OECD and World Health Organization, 2021). Benchmarks between Western countries show interesting differences in relative spending: Dutch hospitals were generally cheaper than in most other Westerns countries, whereas the relative part of the total budget that is spent on chronic care is much higher. These differences can partly be explained by looking per country into degrees of efficiency, exact coverage terms, and social factors especially in dealing with the elderly. Healthcare costs are increasing due to factors such as the ageing population and rising number of people with a chronic disease, who require (more) care. Also, because of better detection and treatment, more people receive care with often expensive accompanying medication and technology.

Ageing Population

Worldwide populations are aging. For example, in the Netherlands, 20% of the population was older than 65 years (January 2023) (Centraal Bureau voor de Statistiek, 2023), and is expected to grow. The proportion of the elderly in the total population is increasing and also the population is ageing, for example because of successful prevention and treatment of diseases. This demographic development is an important reason for the increasing number of people with a chronic disease or multimorbidity (Milieu, 2018).

Increase in Number of People with a Chronic Disease

Chronic diseases are long-term conditions that cannot be cured but can be managed. Examples of common chronic disease are diabetes mellitus, coronary heart disease, asthma, and COPD (Rijksinstituut voor Volksgezondheid en Milieu, 2021a). Almost 60% of the Dutch population had one or more chronic condition(s) at the start of 2021, this was 96% among the population over 75 years of age (Rijksinstituut voor Volksgezondheid en Milieu, 2022). Having a chronic condition has a major impact on people's lives, as they need to manage their condition and symptoms, apply lifestyle adjustments, and adhere to a medication regimen (Wagner et al., 2001).

Chronic disease care can be quite complex, amongst other things because it is often provided by multiple healthcare professionals such as general practitioners and medical specialists. The high prevalence of chronic diseases also has a substantial impact on the demand for care and leads to increasing pressure on hospitals and healthcare expenditures. The organization of care for people with a chronic disease is explained in the Chronic Care Model (CCM), developed in the 1990s by Wagner et al. (2001). The CCM consists of six key elements that can contribute to the improvement of outcomes for patients with a chronic disease. The CCM illustrates the health system, with healthcare organizations to deliver care services, and the community, as a caring for patients with a chronic disease also requires community resources. This underlines the importance of the connection and collaboration between care and welfare institutions. Self-management support is needed because patients are responsible for their own health and disease management, including physical activity, good nutrition, and medication intake. Patients, and their families, should receive support and tools for such self-management. The delivery system design involves the organization of care in healthcare practice for chronically ill patients, such as a care team with a focus on health outcomes and for self-management support. To enable care that is supported by evidence-based protocols and guidelines, decision support is needed with a clinical information system, for example, registration and access to patient-related data (Bodenheimer, Wagner, & Grumbach, 2002; Wagner et al., 2001).

Since the development of the Chronic Care Model, eHealth has been increasingly used in healthcare to support chronic disease management. For example, to support self-management interventions, for the provision of tailored information, and for communication purposes. The use of eHealth is missing in the CCM model but is covered in the updated version of the CCM; the eHealth Enhanced Chronic Care model (eCCM) (see Figure 4.1) (Gee, Greenwood, Paterniti, Ward, & Miller, 2015). The eCCM consists of several elements: self-management support, delivery system

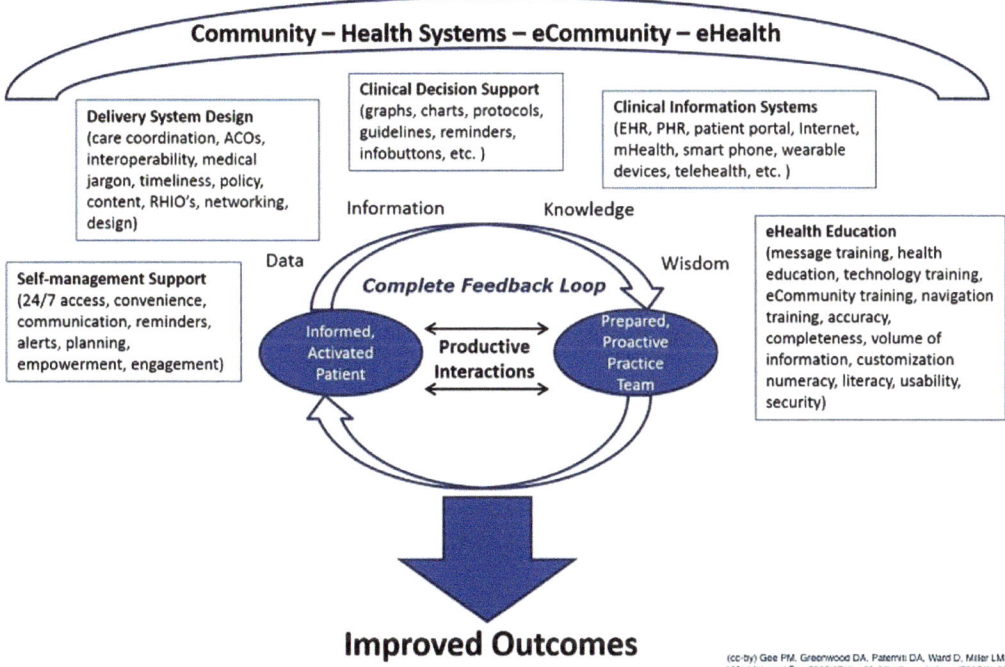

Figure 4.1 eHealth Enhanced Chronic Care model, created by Gee et al. (Gee et al., 2015).

design, clinical decision support, clinical information system, and eHealth education. According to the model, health systems should use eHealth to improve patient self-management and satisfaction. In the eCCM, the community is extended to the online community and social networks for health purposes. In the CCM, the clinical information systems mainly included databases and registries. In the eCCM, this is extended with Electronic Health Records, Patient Portals, and telehealth solutions. Also, education is extended with eHealth (and technology) training for which health literacy is also necessary.

The eCCM also includes the use of data and information, resulting in knowledge and eventually leading to wisdom, including a complete feedback loop. This can eventually lead to improved health outcomes. Thus, the model indicates that the use of eHealth can support interactions between patients and professionals and improve health outcomes (Gee et al., 2015).

Relevant Concepts for Digital Transformation in Healthcare

As becomes clear from the paragraphs above, the current healthcare system is under pressure, and (digital) transformation of care is necessary to maintain high-quality, accessible, and affordable care both now and in the future. Important developments in this regard are provided below.

Care in the Home Setting

Care is increasingly being provided closer to people's homes and there is a permanent trend in reducing the length of hospital stay or the number of hospital visits. This can be supported by eHealth solutions such as digital self-management interventions, remote patient monitoring, and other mHealth solutions. But also, physical consultations in the hospital are replaced by virtual care, such as via video consultations. This may eventually contribute to reducing the pressure on healthcare institutions such as hospitals. A relevant example of this is the Dutch 'right care at the right place' initiative, focused on preventive care and providing care closer to peoples' homes, with the aim to maintain or improve patient care while preventing more expensive care (Ministerie van Volksgezondheid, 2018; The Netherlands Authority for Consumers and Markets, 2019). However, there also are concerns, as digital access might also mean easier access and generate needs that were 'latent, earlier; the aspect of appropriateness in digitalizing care needs further evaluation in the coming years.

Patient-centred Care and Shared Decision Making

Patient-centred care is focused on the individual patient and their needs, including physical, emotional, and others. Patients are involved in their own care and receive care that is accessible and coordinated (Catalyst, 2017; Håkansson Eklund et al., 2019). An important concept within patient-centred care is shared decision making in which patients, their healthcare professionals, and caregivers participate in making decisions about a patient's health and care (Légaré et al., 2018).

Integrated and Shared Care

Multiple healthcare professionals care for patients with a chronic disease. This may lead to fragmentation of care. To deliver efficient and high quality care, shared care between these different healthcare providers such as from secondary (e.g., hospital) and primary care (e.g., general practitioner) should be coordinated (Shaw, Rosen, & Rumbold, 2011). Shared care, which can be defined as 'the joint participation of general practitioners and hospital consultants in the planned delivery of care for patients with a chronic condition, informed by an enhanced information exchange over and above routine discharge and referral letters' (Hickman, Drummond, & Grimshaw, 1994), is a way to improve integration between primary and secondary care.

Self-management

The term self-management has been mentioned before. Several definitions of the concept exist, but one commonly used definition is an 'individual's ability to manage the symptoms, treatment, physical and psychosocial consequences, and lifestyle changes inherent in living with a chronic condition' (Barlow, Wright, Sheasby, Turner, & Hainsworth, 2002). Self-management also includes medical-, role-, and emotional management and requires different skills: problem solving, decision making, resource utilization, patient-provider partnership, and taking action (Lorig & Holman, 2003). Self-management is especially important for people with a chronic disease: they are responsible for their daily disease management, for example related to nutrition and medication intake, and must deal with a multitude of healthcare providers (e.g., general practitioners, hospital specialists) that are involved in their care. Self-management interventions are often supported by eHealth technologies, such as mobile applications. The PRISM taxonomy provides an extensive overview of elements for self-management support for people with long-term conditions and consists of 14 items including information about condition or management, social support, and lifestyle advice. The PRISM taxonomy presents a framework that can be used by researchers, for example to prepare and describe interventions and to integrate evidence (Pearce et al., 2016).

Prevention: Focus on Health Instead of Only Disease

Preventive care with focus on health instead of only disease is important as well. This includes stimulating a healthy lifestyle to keep people healthy and to prevent illness, and also involves considering peoples' social situation and environment. Care should also be provided with and around the patient and in the home setting if possible. In this way hospital care may be prevented (Ministerie van Volksgezondheid, 2018; The Netherlands Authority for Consumers and Markets, 2019). The positive health concept can be used to assess positive health and consists of six dimensions: bodily functions, mental functions and perception, spiritual/existential dimension, quality of life, social and societal participation, and daily functioning. This can be useful for patients and healthcare professionals during consultations, for example, for shared decision making and identifying what support is needed and in what domains (Positieve Gezondheid – Institute for Positive Health (IPH), 2023).

eHealth Technologies in Healthcare

Healthcare transformation is often supported by the use of technology. eHealth encompasses a wide range of digital solutions such as the Electronic Medical Record (EMR), patient portals, video consultation, telehealth, mobile health, and decision-support software (also see Chapters 1 and 3). In this section, different eHealth technologies and solutions are described. Subsequently, factors that affect their use in hospital practice will be outlined to illustrate the importance of their implementation in practice.

Electronic Medical Record

The Electronic Medical Record (EMR) is considered the primary system in hospitals and many primary care practices and is 'an electronic record of an individual's health-related information that can be created, gathered, managed, and consulted by authorized clinicians and staff within one health care organization' (US Department of Health Human Services, 2008). The EMR includes medical data, contact information with patients and even Patient Reported Outcome Measures, to assess health outcomes such as health-related quality of life and symptoms (Churruca et al., 2021). The amount of structured data, such as quantitative questions or selection fields, and unstructured data, such as notes in text boxes covered by an average EMR is huge. This is increasingly described as a 'data lake' with 'real world evidence' that can be explored and has to be managed by the healthcare professionals.

Patient Portal and Personal Health Record

A patient portal is a personal, secured online environment for patients. A patient portal can have multiple features (Goldzweig et al., 2013), including access to information from the medical record such as test and survey results, information, and education material. Patients are also able to view, and sometimes schedule, appointments and to send digital messages to their care provider using e-consultation. Patient portals are directly linked to a hospital's EMR and are managed by the hospital. Personal Health Records (PHRs) also are personal digital environments but are managed by individual patients. In a PHR, a person can collect, manage, and share their own health- and medical data, for example from different healthcare providers, in a private and secure environment (Tang, Ash, Bates, Overhage, & Sands, 2006).

Telehealth

Telehealth is referred to as healthcare provided over a distance using Information and Communication Technology (ICT) to enable interaction between patients and health professionals (Lindberg, Nilsson, Zotterman, Söderberg, & Skär, 2013). It is a broad term encompassing, e.g., telemonitoring (explained below) and video consultation. The latter refers to 'technology used to realize a real-time visual and audio patient assessment with a geographical distance' (Kitamura,

Zurawel–Balaura, & Wong, 2010). Patients can have a videocall with their healthcare provider to replace a visit to the hospital. Until now, evidence on the efficacy on telehealth is limited and predominantly evaluated specifically for COPD and heart failure (Peters, Kooij, Lenferink, Van Harten, & Doggen, 2021). During the COVID-19 pandemic, physical contact and hospital visits had to be limited, and the use of digital solutions such as e-consultation and video-consultation increased substantially (Rijksinstituut voor Volksgezondheid en Milieu, 2021b). However, widespread use and upscaling remains complex due to several factors such as reimbursement issues, costs (James, Papoutsi, Wherton, Greenhalgh, & Shaw, 2021), and technology characteristics. Implementation is complex and requires change on multiple levels (see also Chapter 13) (Greenhalgh, Wherton, Shaw, & Morrison, 2020).

Remote Patient Monitoring

Remote patient monitoring is an example of telehealth in which patients' vital signs, such as heart rate or blood pressure, are monitored using devices such as blood pressure monitors and pulse oximeters. Wireless wearable sensors attached to the body, also referred to as biosensors, can continuously (on average with a data-interval of several minutes) monitor vital signs, for example heart rate and respiratory rate. The devices are connected to an app for patients to transfer their measurements either manually or automatically. The data generated by these devices enables healthcare professionals to monitor patients' health data using a digital platform. The data can be used to detect deterioration, get insight in patients' health status, and to decide if an actual consultation (in the hospital) is necessary. Patients also have access to a mobile application with mostly access to information and education, questionnaires and, sometimes, access to their own monitoring data.

mHealth

Mobile health, mHealth, is referred to as medical and public health practice supported by mobile devices such as mobile phones, patient monitoring devices, and other wireless devices and can be used for communication, information access, and health monitoring (World Health Organization, 2011).

Ubiquitous Healthcare (uHealth)

uHealth technology can be used independently from time and place and can be incorporated into people's lives (Sneha & Varshney, 2006; Weiser, 1999). An example is the use of sensors attached to the body, to gather information on different vital signs such as blood pressure, heart rate, and temperature (Brown & Adams, 2007).

Digital Healthcare Transformation

Although eHealth technologies, such as mobile devices, are already used widely in everyday life, their application in healthcare settings is lagging behind. As mentioned before, the use of eHealth technologies such as video consultation and telemonitoring increased significantly during the COVID-19 pandemic, to limit the number of physical visits to healthcare professionals and organizations. This is further illustrated in the case below.

Case 1 – Digital Transformation during the COVID-19 Pandemic

The COVID-19 pandemic gave the use of digital solutions a boost. Before the pandemic, most use of digital solutions occurred within pilots. During the pandemic, the number of hospital visits needed to be reduced and because of the high pressure on hospital (capacity), patients had to be treated and monitored at home if possible. Remote patient monitoring was used to monitor COVID patients' vital signs, especially saturation and heart rate using pulse oximeters. This was often combined with contact with a healthcare professional in the hospital using video consultation. Besides that, information that was usually gathered via questionnaires was now, as much as possible, gathered digitally using digital platforms such as patient portals. However, a digital transformation such as this case does not only involve the implementation and introduction of a (new) technology. It also has an impact on patients, healthcare professionals, care processes, and the hospital organization itself. For patients, it means that their way of communicating with healthcare professionals changes; they can access their information 24/7 via the patient portal, ask questions using e-consultations in the patient portal, and can have video consultations with their medical professionals or nurses while they are in their own environment. For healthcare professionals, it means a change in their profession; they care for patients remotely and rely on video connection, digital applications and devices, and the use of data. New protocols have to be developed and implemented. Also, new skills are needed to conduct these tasks often resulting in a new team or a new task for an existing department. It also requires a new care process or redesign of existing care processes and different allocation of resources and budget.

The use of eHealth is promising – not only in that it offers the opportunity to exchange physical contact for digital encounters or activities, but also since it provides the opportunity to completely redesign processes to improve efficiency and patient satisfaction. Thus, digital health can become instrumental in the movement of healthcare transformation. In Box 4.1, a Patient Journey example in the Netherlands is described. The entire patient journey (or care process) can be supported with eHealth technology. For example, before a hospital visit it is possible for patients to fill in questionnaires (if needed) online, this will save time for both patients and healthcare professionals. Consultations will be digital as much as possible, and when patients do have a consultation in the hospital, for example for a physical examination, they can announce their presence at a registration pillar. Their (medical) information, questionnaires, education, and appointments are available in their personalized digital patient portal. This also offers them the opportunity to send messages to healthcare professionals, referred to as an e-consult. In case of admission to the hospital, early discharge might be possible with remote patient monitoring of vital signs and regular questionnaires using an app. Remote patient monitoring can be used to prevent hospital re-admissions or unnecessary visits, for example if patient's vital signs are good regular hospital visits might not be needed.

Implementation and widespread use of eHealth technology in healthcare are complex processes, because they are affected by multiple factors and involve a variety of stakeholders (also see Chapters 13 and 14). To illustrate this, think of remote patient monitoring using an app and monitoring devices, such as heart rate monitors, to deliver care at home as much as possible. This way of using technology impacts the delivery of healthcare on multiple levels. For patients it will change the way their care is delivered as contact with healthcare professionals is more time- and place-independent. For healthcare professionals, this can change the way they deliver care because they have to rely on data and virtual communication such as video consultation. For organizations it requires redesign of care pathways and a different allocation of budget and resources. On a governmental level, policy and guidelines are required, for example to enable new types of reimbursements.

To achieve upscaling, constant evaluation and optimization of the use of technology in practice are needed. Due to advancing insights, it may appear that a technology is not the right fit (anymore) for a problem or need. To clarify, the use of video consultation increased rapidly during the COVID-19 pandemic but did not fully progress afterwards. This was due to multiple reasons, such as technical issues, travel time, or an increase in workload. Also, face-to-face or phone consultation may be easier or more useful (Salisbury, 2023).

To accelerate the implementation of innovative eHealth solutions, collaboration with third parties such as software suppliers is often needed. The use of a variation of eHealth technologies, for different purposes, results in a fragmented and sometimes vulnerable landscape of health information systems. In many countries (including the US and the Netherlands) EMRs are provided by a few large software suppliers that often hold a monopoly position. For other features such as remote patient monitoring, additional eHealth technologies are provided by other software suppliers. These innovative technologies are mostly delivered by technology start- or scale-ups. Therefore, careful decision making about technology set-up, priority, and budget allocation is required in a healthcare organization.

Although the trend towards digitalization of care is inevitable and its added value in terms of service improvement and client choice are quite clear, the evidence on its added value in terms of cost reduction is scant. In a review on digital care implementation it was found that reductions in capacity use are possible, but to translate this into actual cost reduction is an issue (Peters et al., 2021). This was also the result of a budget impact study on virtual hospital care using continuous monitoring of vital signs (Peters, Doggen, & Van Harten, 2022). This shows the importance of gathering evidence on the cost-effectiveness of digital innovations.

Factors that affect Digital Transformation in Healthcare

Widespread use of eHealth technologies remains challenging in daily clinical practice. To realize it, requires multiple stakeholders to be involved, such as medical doctors, general practitioners, and IT staff. In addition to that, implementation and use are also affected by multiple factors. This is further illustrated by Case 2 below. After this case, some of these important factors are explained (also see Chapters 13 and 14 on implementation).

Case 2 – R&D in Hospital Practice: Factors affecting eHealth Implementation

The implementation of eHealth in clinical practice faces several barriers and facilitators. We evaluated these aspects for patient portal implementation among different stakeholders including healthcare professionals, managers, and IT personnel. Patient portal implementation is a complex process. Not only technologically speaking but also because it affects the organization and its staff. We found that the main facilitators for implementation included perceived usefulness (e.g., less paperwork) and a positive attitude. The main barriers were a lack of resources (e.g., staff), financial difficulties (e.g., lack of reimbursements), and guaranteeing privacy and security (Kooij, Groen, & van Harten, 2018). In the last few years, the implementation and use of patient portals increased and in 2021 the majority of general practitioners (79%) and medical specialists (75%) reported that patients were provided with a patient portal (Rijksinstituut voor Volksgezondheid en Milieu, 2021b). A more recent development is the use of wireless wearable sensors. Their use on nursing wards was evaluated with nurses. Factors positively or negatively affecting use on nursing wards were found on different levels. Implementation can be positively influenced by perceived advantages such as the ability for early detection of deterioration, patients' needs and resources (e.g., patients feel safe), and personal attributes (e.g., experience with intervention). Negative aspects include complexity of the intervention (e.g., the number of process steps), compatibility with the work process (e.g., change in work for professionals), and facilitating conditions (e.g., bad Wi-Fi connection) (Kooij, Peters, Doggen, van Harten, 2022). Both studies show that the implementation of eHealth solutions is affected by a wide range of factors which should be considered during development and implementation. To eventually realize digital transformation, it is very important to take these factors into account, to involve multiple stakeholders, to integrate new technologies in care processes, and to acknowledge that successful implementation is more than just the implementation of a technology itself.

Human Factors

To support use, eHealth solutions should be adapted to the skills, needs, and knowledge of patients and healthcare professionals. eHealth literacy is an important factor and is defined as the ability to seek, find, understand, and appraise health information from electronic sources and apply this knowledge to address or solve a health problem. This can be influenced by the educational background or health status of an individual, or by the technology used (Norman & Skinner, 2006b). Assessment of patients' digital health literacy is important to be able to match skills and technology. An example of a tool that can be used for such assessments is the eHealth literacy scale (eHEALS). The eHEALS consists of eight items used to assess an individual's perceptions about their knowledge and skills to search for, appraise, and apply digital health related information (Norman & Skinner, 2006a).

Organizational Factors

Research on barriers and facilitators of, e.g., patient portal implementation showed that implementation is not only a technical process, but also has an impact on the organization and its staff. Multiple stakeholders identified several organizational aspects as barriers for implementation such as lack of resources and lack of suitable specialist staff (Kooij et al., 2018). A major challenge lies in the integration of eHealth technologies in work processes and existing information systems. Successful implementation, adoption, and upscaling requires redesign of care processes, instead of adding a new technology to an already existing process (Kooij, 2021). In the design of digital care, the (expected) frequency of contact and interaction between healthcare professionals and patients, and the technical complexity of the required infrastructure are important factors to consider when deciding on how to organize these services.

Technology Factors

Technology in general is developing at a rapid pace and is already used on a wide scale in daily life. However, as stated before this has not been accomplished yet for eHealth technologies. The way eHealth technology is implemented in a healthcare organization can affect its use. A new eHealth technology could be implemented by truly 'integrating' it in a hospital infrastructure, this is a more long-term solution but more expensive and time intensive. An example is connecting an eHealth solution, such as an application for remote patient monitoring, to a healthcare organization's EMR. This new solution can also be implemented 'standalone', this means relatively independent from an existing infrastructure, for example not connected to the EMR. Implementation is less resource- and time intensive. However, in practice this would mean healthcare professionals need to use different systems for different tasks. For example, the EMR for medical information and registration and an eHealth solution for remote patient monitoring information. A standalone solution can be useful if the added value of the new eHealth solution has not yet been demonstrated and if feasibility needs to be established, whereas an integrated solution is beneficial to achieve upscaling.

Financial Factors

To implement a new eHealth solution in healthcare practice, sufficient budget, resources, and time are needed. This requires decision making in an organization about the allocation of (human) resources and budget, especially since reimbursement for new digital health innovations is often not available.

Regional Factors: Collaboration between Care Partners

As said, a single patient may simultaneously be treated by different healthcare professionals from different organizations, such as primary care physicians and hospital medical doctors. Additionally, social welfare services may be required or desired. This is especially the case for patients with a chronic disease. Collaboration among these different care professionals is required to ensure coordinated and patient-centred care, and eventually realize digital healthcare transformation. Oftentimes, these healthcare professionals may be geographically close, yet not efficiently digitally connected. To make matters even more complex, different healthcare providers have their own electronic information system, which are not automatically connected. Additionally, several technologies are used for referral between primary and secondary care, or for communication between healthcare professionals. The fragmentation of eHealth technologies within and between different healthcare organizations complicates their upscaling in practice. Collaboration is challenging because every care institution has their own eHealth technologies, research and development agenda, and organizational and technological priorities.

Evidence Development Factors

There is a gap between research and uptake of eHealth technologies in clinical practice (Baker, Gustafson, & Shah, 2014). First of all, technology is developed at a rapid pace whereas conducting research takes time, especially when conducting large scale studies such as randomized controlled trials (Peterson & Harrington, 2018) (also see Chapter 16). For example, mobile devices are widely used in daily life, but widespread use in clinical practice is lagging behind. More pragmatic research approaches for evaluation of new eHealth technologies and solutions in clinical practice can contribute to evidence-development and application of these findings to clinical practice. In healthcare practice, evidence on new (digital) solutions is important for healthcare professionals' and patients' acceptance and support and to accomplish successful implementation.

Relevant Theoretical Models

Several theoretical models are available to be used as instruments to assist and guide implementation and evaluation, thus increasing the chances of success for digital health technologies. They can also be used to assess technology acceptance and adoption. Some relevant models are described in more detail below.

Technology Acceptance Models

To increase successful use of eHealth technology in healthcare practice it is important that the technology is accepted by its users. Several models have been developed to evaluate the use of technology. Two of them are described in more detail below.

UTAUT model

The Unified Theory of Acceptance and Use of Technology (UTAUT) model has been developed to assess technology acceptance and use. Multiple models exist to evaluate acceptance and use of technology. The UTAUT model is based on eight other models, including the Theory of Reasoned Action (TRA), Technology Acceptance Model (TAM), and Theory of Planned Behavior (TPB), derived from social psychology (Venkatesh, Morris, Davis, & Davis, 2003). For example, according to the Technology Acceptance Model (Davis, Bagozzi, & Warshaw, 1989), *external variables* can affect users' beliefs, attitudes and also intentions.

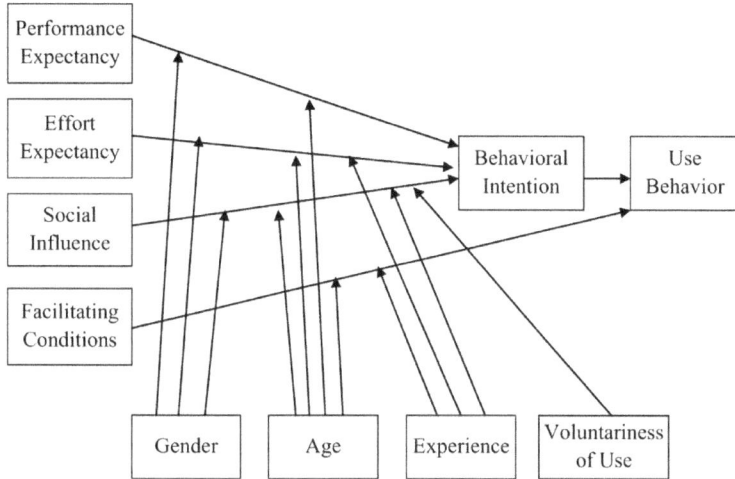

Figure 4.2 The UTAUT model (Tan, 2013).

The UTAUT model (see Figure 4.2) consists of four key elements explaining behavioural intention and use. *Performance expectancy* describes the degree to which an individual believes that using the system will improve job performance. *Effort expectancy* refers to the ease of use of the system. *Social influence* concerns an individual's perception on what others think about them using the system. Finally, *facilitating conditions* include an individual's belief that the system is supported by the organizational and technical infrastructure. These four key elements predict behavioural intention and eventual use. At the same time, the correlation between each of the mentioned predictors and behavioural intention or actual use can be influenced by the determinants gender, age, experience, and voluntariness of use (Venkatesh et al., 2003).

Although, the UTAUT model is used in many studies it also has its limitations. The UTAUT model is, for example, criticized for its large number of variables (Bagozzi, 2007), but also because it may lack completeness of constructs to explain use behaviour. For example, individual characteristics such as attitude of the (future) user of the technology are missing. The moderating elements (gender, age, experience, and voluntariness) may not always be relevant in every context. For example, in some cases the use of a technology may be an obligatory part of the care process, making voluntariness obsolete. Also, previous research did not use all variables of the UTAUT-model (Dwivedi, Rana, Jeyaraj, Clement, & Williams, 2019).

Of course, there are more models and frameworks in healthcare to support eHealth technology implementation and evaluation, some of which are briefly described below.

Models and Frameworks to Support Adoption, Implementation, and Evaluation of eHealth Technology

Several factors should be taken into account in order to stimulate digital healthcare transformation as previously described. Successful uptake of technology is dependent on, among other things, the person, technology, and organizational aspects. Implementation and use of (eHealth) technology in healthcare practice is complex because it is affected by multiple, often interacting, aspects. The interrelatedness of these factors is also shown in several models. For example, the Fit between Individuals, Task and Technology (FITT) framework can be used to assess IT adoption in clinical practice. This framework emphasizes the importance of the interaction between individual users (e.g., motivation), technology aspects (e.g., usability), and clinical tasks and processes (e.g., complexity) (Ammenwerth, Iller, & Mahler, 2006).

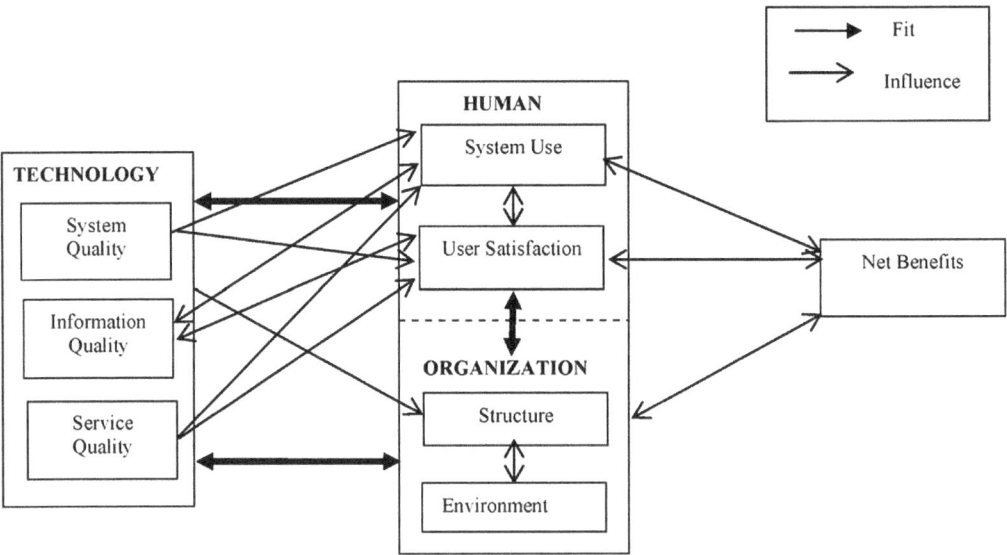

Figure 4.3 The (HOT)-Fit framework (Yusof, Kuljis, Papazafeiropoulou, & Stergioulas, 2008).

With the Human, Organization, and Technology (HOT)-Fit framework (see Figure 4.3), health information systems can be evaluated according to three relevant aspects: human (consisting of system use and user satisfaction), organization (including structure and environment), and technology (Yusof, Kuljis, Papazafeiropoulou, & Stergioulas, 2008; Yusof, Paul, & Stergioulas, 2006). In this model, technology consists of different elements: system quality (referring to system performance), information (referring to the information processed by the system), and service quality (referring to service or technical support). These are still broad terms and each of them encompasses multiple factors.

Finally, the upscaling of eHealth solutions appears to be complex, as many initiatives remain in the pilot phase. This complexity is also pointed out in the Nonadoption, Abandonment, Scale-up, Spread and Sustainability (NASSS) framework (see Chapter 13). This framework can be used to analyze the level of complexity of seven domains: condition, technology, value proposition, adopters, organization(s), wider system, and embedding and adaptation over time. The NASSS framework is useful to analyze technology adoption or abandonment of individuals and also to assess aspect related to upscaling, spreading, and sustainability of technology in clinical practice (Greenhalgh & Abimbola, 2019).

Future Perspective

Although technologies, such as mobile devices, are widely used in daily life, widespread use in healthcare is lagging behind. Therefore, it is important to focus on the upscaling of eHealth in healthcare in general and in hospital practice in particular, taking several factors into account such as personal, organizational, process factors, and technology characteristics. Involvement of relevant stakeholders – such as medical professionals, primary care physicians, and patients – during development and implementation can also contribute to successful uptake of eHealth technologies in practice. With the increasing use of innovative technologies such as sensors for remote patient monitoring, increasing amounts of data are becoming available. The application and use of data analytics and new AI solutions are becoming increasingly relevant and important. This will also have an effect on the delivery of healthcare services and can support patient-centred care, because more personal data will be available to tailor care to a patient's specific needs. Generating evidence on added value and cost reduction possibilities is important in order to convince providers to actually change their practices and support upscaling. However, especially related to digital care, there is still a gap between the development and characteristics of technology and the way research is conducted. Therefore, more pragmatic research approaches conducted in daily healthcare practice are needed to speed up the process and gain more evidence from use in practice (see also Chapter 16).

Summary

This chapter has shown that there are different types of healthcare systems in different countries, but most of them face similar challenges. eHealth technologies such as EMRs, patient portals, video consultations, and remote patient monitoring can be used to address these challenges. In this chapter, several relevant concepts for digital transformation were described, and an overview of factors that affect the large-scale uptake of eHealth in healthcare practice have been explained. It becomes clear that eHealth technologies have a lot of potential to improve healthcare, but there still is much room for improvement.

The take-home messages of this chapter are:

- Globally, there are several challenges with which healthcare systems are faced, including an ageing population, increasing healthcare costs, and labour shortages;
- The use of eHealth technology is promising and can stimulate healthcare transformation to achieve accessible, affordable, and (high) quality care;
- Relevant concepts for digital transformation in healthcare include providing care in the home setting, patient-centred care and shared decision making, integrated and shared care, self-management, and prevention;
- eHealth implementation is affected by several factors that should be accounted for throughout development, implementation, and evaluation of eHealth technologies in healthcare practice: individual characteristics, organizational aspects, financial aspects, and technology aspects;
- Several theoretical models such as the UTAUT can be used for the purpose of implementation, technology acceptance, and evaluation of eHealth technologies in healthcare practice.

Key References for Further Reading

Baker, T. B., Gustafson, D. H., & Shah, D. (2014). How can research keep up with eHealth? Ten strategies for increasing the timeliness and usefulness of eHealth research. *Journal of Medical Internet Research*, 16(2), e36.

Kooij, L. (2021). *Digital transformation in hospital care: Implementation and evaluation of eHealth in clinical practice: The effects on patients, healthcare professionals and hospital organizations.* University of Twente. https://doi.org/10.3990/1.9789036552875

Kooij, L., Vos, P. J., Dijkstra, A., & van Harten, W. H. (2021). Effectiveness of a mobile health and self-management app for high-risk patients with chronic obstructive pulmonary disease in daily clinical practice: Mixed methods evaluation study. *JMIR mHealth and uHealth*, 9(2), e21977.

Peters, G. M., Doggen, C. J., & Van Harten, W. H. (2022). Budget impact analysis of providing hospital inpatient care at home virtually, starting with two specific surgical patient groups. *BMJ Open*, 12(8), e051833.

Peters, G. M., Kooij, L., Lenferink, A., Van Harten, W. H., & Doggen, C. J. (2021). The effect of telehealth on hospital services use: Systematic review and meta-analysis. *Journal of Medical Internet Research*, 23(9), e25195.

References

Ammenwerth, E., Iller, C., & Mahler, C. (2006). IT-adoption and the interaction of task, technology and individuals: A fit framework and a case study. *BMC Medical Informatics and Decision Making*, 6(1), 3. doi:10.1186/1472-6947-6-3

Bagozzi, R. P. (2007). The legacy of the technology acceptance model and a proposal for a paradigm shift. *Journal of the Association for Information Systems*, 8(4), 3.

Baker, T. B., Gustafson, D. H., & Shah, D. (2014). How can research keep up with eHealth? Ten strategies for increasing the timeliness and usefulness of eHealth research. *Journal of Medical Internet Research*, 16(2), e2925.

Barlow, J., Wright, C., Sheasby, J., Turner, A., & Hainsworth, J. (2002). Self-management approaches for people with chronic conditions: A review. *Patient Education and Counseling*, 48(2), 177–187.

Bodenheimer, T., Wagner, E. H., & Grumbach, K. (2002). Improving primary care for patients with chronic illness. *JAMA*, 288(14), 1775–1779.

Brown, I., & Adams, A. A. (2007). The ethical challenges of ubiquitous healthcare. *The International Review of Information Ethics*, 8, 53–60.

Catalyst, N. (2017). What is patient-centered care? *NEJM Catalyst*, 3(1).

Centraal Bureau voor de Statistiek. (2023). Ouderen. Retrieved from https://www.cbs.nl/nl-nl/visualisaties/dashboard-bevolking/leeftijd/ouderen

Churruca, K., Pomare, C., Ellis, L. A., Long, J. C., Henderson, S. B., Murphy, L. E. D., . . . Braithwaite, J. (2021). Patient-reported outcome measures (PROMs): A review of generic and condition-specific measures and a discussion of trends and issues. *Health Expect*, 24(4), 1015–1024. doi:10.1111/hex.13254

Davis, F. D., Bagozzi, R. P., & Warshaw, P. R. (1989). User acceptance of computer technology: A comparison of two theoretical models. *Management Science*, 35(8), 982–1003.

Dwivedi, Y. K., Rana, N. P., Jeyaraj, A., Clement, M., & Williams, M. D. (2019). Re-examining the unified theory of acceptance and use of technology (UTAUT): Towards a revised theoretical model. *Information Systems Frontiers*, 21, 719–734.

Gee, P. M., Greenwood, D. A., Paterniti, D. A., Ward, D., & Miller, L. M. S. (2015). The eHealth enhanced chronic care model: A theory derivation approach. *Journal of Medical Internet Research*, 17(4), e4067.

Goldzweig, C. L., Orshansky, G., Paige, N. M., Towfigh, A. A., Haggstrom, D. A., Miake-Lye, I., . . . Shekelle, P. G. (2013). Electronic patient portals: Evidence on health outcomes, satisfaction, efficiency, and attitudes: A systematic review. *Annals of Internal Medicine*, 159(10), 677–687.

Greenhalgh, T., & Abimbola, S. (2019). The NASSS framework – A synthesis of multiple theories of technology implementation. *Stud Health Technol Inform*, 263, 193–204.

Greenhalgh, T., Wherton, J., Shaw, S., & Morrison, C. (2020). Video consultations for covid-19. In *BMJ*, (Vol. 368): British Medical Journal Publishing Group.

Håkansson Eklund, J., Holmström, I. K., Kumlin, T., Kaminsky, E., Skoglund, K., Höglander, J., . . . Summer Meranius, M. (2019). "Same same or different?" A review of reviews of person-centered and patient-centered care. *Patient Educ Couns*, 102(1), 3–11. doi:10.1016/j.pec.2018.08.029

Hickman, M., Drummond, N., & Grimshaw, J. (1994). A taxonomy of shared care for chronic disease. *J Public Health Med*, 16(4), 447–454. doi:10.1093/oxfordjournals.pubmed.a043026

James, H. M., Papoutsi, C., Wherton, J., Greenhalgh, T., & Shaw, S. E. (2021). Spread, scale-up, and sustainability of video consulting in health care: Systematic review and synthesis guided by the NASSS framework. *Journal of Medical Internet Research*, 23(1), e23775.

Keisler-Starkey, K., & Bunch, L. N. (2022). Health insurance coverage in the United States 2021: Current population reports. Retrieved from https://www.census.gov/content/dam/Census/library/publications/2022/demo/p60-278.pdf

Kitamura, C., Zurawel–Balaura, L., & Wong, R. (2010). How effective is video consultation in clinical oncology? A systematic review. *Current Oncology*, 17(3), 17–27.

Kooij, L. (2021). *Digital transformation in hospital care: Implementation and evaluation of eHealth in clinical practice: The effects on patients, healthcare professionals and hospital organizations*. (Dissertation). University of Twente. Retrieved from https://research.utwente.nl/en/publications/digital-transformation-in-hospital-care-implementation-and-evalua

Kooij, L., Groen, W. G., & van Harten, W. H. (2018). Barriers and facilitators affecting patient portal implementation from an organizational perspective: Qualitative study. *J Med Internet Res*, 20(5), e183. doi:10.2196/jmir.8989

Kooij, L., Peters, G. M., Doggen, C. J. M., & van Harten, W. H. (2022). Remote continuous monitoring with wireless wearable sensors in clinical practice, nurses perspectives on factors affecting implementation: A qualitative study. *BMC Nursing*, 21(1), 1–13.

Légaré, F., Adekpedjou, R., Stacey, D., Turcotte, S., Kryworuchko, J., Graham, I. D., . . . Elwyn, G. (2018). Interventions for increasing the use of shared decision making by healthcare professionals. *Cochrane Database of Systematic Reviews* (7).

Lindberg, B., Nilsson, C., Zotterman, D., Söderberg, S., & Skär, L. (2013). Using information and communication technology in home care for communication between patients, family members, and healthcare professionals: A systematic review. *International Journal of Telemedicine and Applications*, 2013.

Lorig, K. R., & Holman, H. R. (2003). Self-management education: History, definition, outcomes, and mechanisms. *Annals of Behavioral Medicine*, 26(1), 1–7.

Milieu, R. v. V. e. (2018). Synthese. De impact van vergrijzing. Retrieved from https://www.vtv2018.nl/impact-van-de-vergrijzing

Ministerie van Volksgezondheid, W. e. S. (2016). Het Nederlandse zorgstelsel. Retrieved from https://open.overheid.nl/documenten/ronl-5f6ea9d9-c8b5-4f2a-903b-1732d9579578/pdf

Ministerie van Volksgezondheid, W. e. S. (2018). De juiste zorg op de juiste plek. Retrieved from https://www.dejuistezorgopdejusteplek.nl/

Norman, C. D., & Skinner, H. A. (2006a). eHEALS: The eHealth literacy scale. *Journal of Medical Internet Research*, 8(4), e507.

Norman, C. D., & Skinner, H. A. (2006b). eHealth literacy: Essential skills for consumer health in a networked world. *J Med Internet Res*, 8(2), e9. doi:10.2196/jmir.8.2.e9

OECD & European Union. (2022). *Health at a Glance: Europe 2022*.

OECD and World Health Organization. (2021). State of health in the EU. Nederland. Landenprofiel Gezondheid 2021. Retrieved from https://health.ec.europa.eu/system/files/2022-01/2021_chp_nl_dutch_0.pdf

OECD/European Union. (2020). Health at a glance: Europe 2020: State of health in the EU cycle. Retrieved from https://health.ec.europa.eu/system/files/2020-12/2020_healthatglance_rep_en_0.pdf

Pearce, G., Parke, H. L., Pinnock, H., Epiphaniou, E., Bourne, C. L., Sheikh, A., & Taylor, S. J. (2016). The PRISMS taxonomy of self-management support: Derivation of a novel taxonomy and initial testing of its utility. *Journal of Health Services Research & Policy*, 21(2), 73–82.

Peters, G. M., Doggen, C. J., & Van Harten, W. H. (2022). Budget impact analysis of providing hospital inpatient care at home virtually, starting with two specific surgical patient groups. *BMJ Open*, 12(8), e051833.

Peters, G. M., Kooij, L., Lenferink, A., Van Harten, W. H., & Doggen, C. J. (2021). The effect of telehealth on hospital services use: Systematic review and meta-analysis. *Journal of Medical Internet Research*, 23(9), e25195.

Peterson, E. D., & Harrington, R. A. (2018). Evaluating health technology through pragmatic trials: Novel approaches to generate high-quality evidence. *JAMA*, 320(2), 137–138.

Positieve Gezondheid – Institute for Positive Health (IPH). (2023). Retrieved from https://www.iph.nl/

Rice, T., Rosenau, P., Unruh, L. Y., & Barnes, A. J. (2020). United States: Health system review. *Health Systems in Transition*, 22(4), 1–441.

Rijksinstituut voor Volksgezondheid en Milieu. (2021a). Welke aandoeningen komen het meeste voor? Retrieved from https://www.vzinfo.nl/ranglijsten/voorkomen

Rijksinstituut voor Volksgezondheid en Milieu. (2021b). E-healthmonitor 2021 Stand van zaken digitale zorg. Retrieved from https://www.rivm.nl/documenten/e-healthmonitor-2021-stand-van-zaken-digitale-zorg

Rijksinstituut voor Volksgezondheid en Milieu. (2022). Chronische aandoeningen en multimorbiditeit | Leeftijd en geslacht. Retrieved from https://www.vzinfo.nl/chronische-aandoeningen-en-multimorbiditeit/leeftijd-en-geslacht#:~:text=Ruim%2010%20miljoen%20mensen%20met,uitzicht%20is%20op%20volledig%20herstel.

Salisbury, H. (2023). Helen Salisbury: What happened to the video revolution? *BMJ*, 382, p. 1706. doi:10.1136/bmj.p1706

Shaw, S., Rosen, R., & Rumbold, B. (2011). What is integrated care? London: Nuffield Trust, 7, 1–23.

Sneha, S., & Varshney, U. (2006). Ubiquitous healthcare: A new frontier in e-health. *AMCIS* 2006 proceedings, 319.

Tan, P. J. B. (2013). Applying the UTAUT to understand factors affecting the use of English e-learning websites in Taiwan. *SAGE Open*, 3(4), 2158244013503837. doi:10.1177/2158244013503837

Tang, P. C., Ash, J. S., Bates, D. W., Overhage, J. M., & Sands, D. Z. (2006). Personal health records: Definitions, benefits, and strategies for overcoming barriers to adoption. *J Am Med Inform Assoc*, 13(2), 121–126. doi:10.1197/jamia.M2025

The Netherlands Authority for Consumers and Markets. (2019). The right care in the right place. Retrieved from https://www.dejuistezorgopdejuisteplek.nl/.uc/fcef77d2b01028d5c0000bd7ca7026baaac90942d76c900/The%20right%20care%20in%20the%20right%20place_report%20taskforce.pdf

US Department of Health Human Services. (2008). The National Alliance for Health Information Technology Report to the Office of the National Coordinator for Health Information Technology. Retrieved from https://www.nachc.org/wp-content/uploads/2016/03/Key-HIT-Terms-Definitions-Final_April_2008.pdf

Venkatesh, V., Morris, M. G., Davis, G. B., & Davis, F. D. (2003). User acceptance of information technology: Toward a unified view. *MIS Quarterly*, 425–478.

Wagner, E. H., Austin, B. T., Davis, C., Hindmarsh, M., Schaefer, J., & Bonomi, A. (2001). Improving chronic illness care: Translating evidence into action. *Health Affairs*, 20(6), 64–78.

Weiser, M. (1999). The computer for the 21st century. *ACM SIGMOBILE Mobile Computing and Communications Review*, 3(3), 3–11.

World Health Organization. (2011). mHealth: New horizons for health through mobile technologies: Second global survey on eHealth. Retrieved from https://apps.who.int/iris/handle/10665/44607

Yusof, M. M., Kuljis, J., Papazafeiropoulou, A., & Stergioulas, L. K. (2008). An evaluation framework for health information systems: Human, organization and technology-fit factors (HOT-fit). *International Journal of Medical Informatics*, 77(6), 386–398.

Yusof, M. M., Paul, R. J., & Stergioulas, L. K. (2006). Towards a framework for health information systems evaluation. Paper presented at the Proceedings of the 39th annual *Hawaii International Conference on System ciences* (HICSS'06).

5 Mental Health and eHealth Technology

Jacob Pitkow & Stephen M. Schueller

Introduction

Previous chapters pointed out that eHealth technologies have the potential to address many health-related issues including public, somatic, and mental health. This chapter focuses on the use of eHealth technology to support or improve mental health, or eMental health, which includes both psychological well-being and mental health disorders. Originating as computer and web-based interventions mostly for depression and anxiety, their scope has expanded rapidly in recent years to include more target conditions, diverse populations, and more advanced technology including wearables and virtual and augmented reality (VR/AR). Evidence supports that eMental health interventions can effectively address a range of mental disorders and a growing body of literature suggests that they can be successfully implemented and integrated into real-world clinical settings. Increased implementation will nevertheless require diligent adherence to implementation frameworks (see Chapter 13) to ensure alignment of interventions, invested parties, and contextual attributes.

eMental health refers to the use of eHealth in mental healthcare. In this chapter, we provide an overview of eMental health as well as a discussion of its practical applications, supporting evidence, limitations, and ethical considerations. This chapter offers an introduction to eMental health in the hope of educating the reader about what kinds of interventions exist, the therapies and theoretical principles underlying these interventions, where these interventions have been provided, their effectiveness and limitations, and what kind of support is needed for users to benefit from eMental health. The chapter provides explanations and examples of interventions within eMental health organized by style of care: Self-guided interventions with no human support, guided interventions incorporating human support, and virtual care platforms. The chapter ends with potential implications of recent trends, predictions for the future of eMental health, and practical and ethical concerns. Consequently, after completing this chapter, you will be able to:

- Describe the predominant models of care incorporating eMental health interventions;
- Reflect on the efficacy, limits, and ethical implications of eMental health interventions;
- Explain the differences between unsupported, supported, and virtual care models of eMental health interventions;
- Explain the potential for eMental health interventions to overcome barriers to traditional treatments;
- Discuss deficits in eMental health intervention research and practice.

DOI: 10.4324/9781003302049-6

Mental Health and eHealth Technology

As work in eHealth expands, eMental health is growing in interest. eMental health refers to the use of digital tools for increasing psychological well-being and treating and preventing mental health disorders. What began over two decades ago, as mostly a translation of self-help tools like pamphlets and books into digital formats like websites, has rapidly expanded to a domain that includes novel technologies including mobile apps, wearable devices, digital games, social media, chatbots, virtual reality (VR), and augmented reality (AR). Tens of thousands of eMental health resources exist, although their quality varies considerably. eMental health tools have demonstrated effectiveness for a variety of conditions (Andersson, 2018; Linardon et al., 2019), with most evidence in the areas of depression, anxiety, and posttraumatic stress disorder (Mohr et al., 2021). These results in research trials have led to implementations in various settings such as the MindSpot Clinic in Australia (Titov et al., 2020) and the Improving Access to Psychological Therapies (IAPT) programme in the UK (Nguyen et al., 2022). The primary value in eMental health is not displacing traditional treatments, but offering patients a form of support when they might otherwise receive none. However, evaluations have also demonstrated that when it comes to eMental health something may not necessarily be better than nothing and not all interventions are effective (Simon et al., 2022). Thus, an important task is separating effective eMental health interventions from ineffective ones.

eMental health programmes are designed for a broad range of contexts and settings. Some are intended to function as replacements for face-to-face therapy – either moving treatment from clinical offices to people's homes and daily lives, or to provide mental health services in settings where they would otherwise not exist (like primary care clinics). Others, however, are intended to be used in addition to face-to-face services; to increase the efficacy or the efficiency of treatment, making it more impactful or less costly. The use of face-to-face services in combination with eMental health technologies is often referred to as blended care (Wentzel, van der Vaart, Bohlmeijer, & van Gemert-Pijnen, 2016). In general, blended care aims to increase the impact of interventions by shifting the responsibilities for some of the aspects of care to the eMental health platform. In an evaluation of patients' and therapists' opinions of blended care programmes, it was found that they preferred practical elements of therapy (e.g., psycho-education and homework assignments) to be accomplished through the technological intervention (van der Vaart et al., 2014). In an evaluation comparing standard therapy with computer-assisted therapy, it was found that patients receiving the computer-assisted programme reported greater knowledge of therapy skills and larger decreases in symptoms (Wright et al., 2005). These findings suggest that the computer-assisted treatment may provide better learning of basic techniques, not only because it enables a clinician to spend more therapy time focusing on more advanced topics, but also because technological tools often emphasize self-management of the patient and allow for repeated practice.

The field of eMental health has reached a crucial point. While these tools have demonstrated the ability to provide effective, low-cost, and scalable treatment and prevention to people all over the world, they yet remain encumbered by policy (e.g., unfavourable regulation and reimbursement), economic (e.g., tools requiring significant fees for use, unequal access to technology), and substantive (e.g., poorly incorporated evidence-based practices, lack of clinical evaluation) issues. These issues readily map onto the ethical principles enumerated in the Belmont Report (Adashi, Walters, & Menikoff, 2018) – respect for persons, beneficence, and justice – providing a framework for future research and implementation planning which will be discussed in more detail later in this chapter.

Models of Care in eMental Health Interventions

Nearly any condition treatable through psychosocial intervention like cognitive-behavioural therapy (described in more detail below) has been demonstrated to be treated through eMental health interventions. For example, Andersson (2018) identified that research evidence supports the effectiveness of eMental health for anxiety, depression, eating disorders, encopresis, erectile dysfunction, obsessive-compulsive disorder, panic disorder, insomnia, irritable bowel syndrome, perfectionism, posttraumatic stress disorder, procrastination, social phobia, smoking cessation, specific phobia, and tinnitus. This list was not intended to be an exhaustive review of the field, but to demonstrate the breadth of potential use cases.

Practitioners of eMental health use various technologies to make mental health resources more accessible, engaging and/or impactful. The following sections focus on the current dominant models of care incorporating eMental health interventions. Self-guided eMental health interventions allow for the direct provision of behavioural interventions with no support from a clinician. Guided eMental health interventions include some human support to improve user engagement or tool effectiveness, usually from a coach, paraprofessional, or mental health professional. Virtual care services allow mental health professionals to provide direct services through technology such as video visits or text-messaging based care.

For depression and anxiety, self-guided interventions are associated with small-to-medium effect sizes (Linardon et al., 2019), while effect sizes for guided interventions can be much larger and equivalent to those found in face-to-face treatments (Andersson, Cuijpers, Carlbring, Riper, & Hedman, 2014). However, including support tends to reduce the scalability of such interventions in ways that are inconsistent with the promise of eMental health interventions to expand access and provide resources to people who may be unable to receive other psychological services. It has been suggested that eMental health interventions offer a 'non-consumable' alternative to traditional 'consumable' face-to-face interventions for mental health (Muñoz, 2010). Consumable interventions are those that once used will never be able to benefit another person, such as an hour of a therapist's time providing face-to-face treatment or a dose of a medication. Non-consumable interventions are those that can be used repeatedly without losing their therapeutic power to help additional people, such as a self-guided eMental health intervention. As such, even eMental health interventions which can reliably produce small effect sizes might have an important public health impact when provided to a large population. Put another way, when the goal is to reach and improve the lives of as many people as possible, self-guided interventions may be superior to guided interventions due to their scalability.

Self-Guided Interventions

Many eMental health interventions are self-guided. In self-guided interventions, a user will interact solely with digital tools, typically working through a combination of automated assessments, educational sections, and interactive elements to support their learning. Most self-guided interventions are educational, teaching skills so that users might better help themselves. The primary value in self-guided eMental health interventions is their low cost, scalability, potential fidelity to evidence-based practices, trialability, and brevity. This section will provide an overview of the most typical self-guided interventions, and several more nascent technologies.

Self-Guided Web and App-Based Interventions

Typical self-guided eMental health interventions are web- or app-based tools, tailored to address a specific condition, set of conditions, or health behaviour. The distinctions between web- and app-based tools have become largely meaningless, as developers are increasingly creating tools for both platforms or mobile-responsive websites that function as either. As such, although we discuss these technologies separately, the benefits and pitfalls of web and app interventions are largely the same.

Mobile applications

Mobile applications (also known as 'apps') are software programmes that run on smartphone devices and are used for a variety of functions, including communicating, accessing information, shopping, and banking. As the number of people who own and use smartphones increases, an increasing amount of time is also being spent on these apps. Indeed, in many places, especially developing countries and low-income populations, desktop computing has been entirely passed over, and smartphone devices are people's only method of accessing the Internet. An estimated 60% of people around the world use the Internet, and by 2025 3.7 billion people are projected to get online exclusively via a mobile device ('Nearly three quarters of the world will use just their smartphones to access the internet by 2025', 2019). As such, an increasing proportion of work in eMental health involves the development of apps, with the intention of efficiently reaching the largest possible group of people. Also, compared to desktop computers or laptops, people are more likely to be able to access apps throughout the day, which allows for new styles of interactions that may be better integrated into the context of daily life. These new styles of interaction are critical for interventions that try to change what a person thinks, feels, and does in a variety of different settings and situations, beyond therapy rooms and clinical settings.

Mobile app interactions tend to be quite different from those with desktop computers. People use desktop computers for various tasks at the same time (e.g., checking email, surfing the web, listening to music) and interactions tend to be longer, whereas people on mobile devices tend to cycle through different apps for specific tasks. As such, use of mobile apps tends to be shorter but more frequent, with some people reporting checking some apps over 50 times per day (Vaish, Wyngarden, Chen, Cheung, & Bernstein, 2014).

A definitive estimate of the number of smartphone apps for mental health is hard to provide, especially because app marketplaces undergo frequent changes (Larsen, Nicholas, & Christensen, 2016). Nevertheless, recent estimates put the number of health apps available for download in the United States at over 350,000, and approximately 20,000 of those are estimated to be specifically built for mental health ('Consumer Health Apps and Digital Health Tools Proliferate, Improving Quality and Health Outcomes for Patients, Says New Report from IQVIA Institute', 2021). Although apps can offer self-guided, guided, or virtual care opportunities, the majority of apps are self-guided such that they can be downloaded and used directly by a consumer. Despite the large number of available apps, few are used. Nearly 90% of all downloads of eMental health apps are of Headspace or Calm, which are mindfulness and meditation apps (Wasil et al., 2019). Cognitive behavioural therapy (CBT)-based apps are also quite popular, with at least five apps offering self-guided tools and training focused on CBT having over 1 million downloads on the Google Play Store alone (Wasil et al., 2019). CBT is based on the notion that one's thoughts, behaviours, and feelings are connected and that changing one's thoughts and behaviours is necessary for subsequent improvement. Core skills within CBT include self-monitoring, goal setting, cognitive restructuring, and problem solving, which for eMental health interventions are translated into digital formats, including lessons and interactive tools.

The content within these CBT apps would be familiar to any provider who has delivered face-to-face CBT, including skills such as cognitive restructuring, behavioural activation, relaxation, and sleep management (e.g., see Andersson, Estling, Jakobsson, Cuijpers, & Carlbring, 2011). Figure 5.1 displays a screenshot from Sanvello, a modular web-based cognitive-behavioural app. Sanvello consists of interactive tools around mood tracking, thoughts, feelings and emotions, and didactic lessons related to mental health challenges. The screenshot below demonstrates how it includes different activities to try to improve one's mood including addressing one's thoughts.

One area of growth in self-guided eMental health interventions has been in the increased use of artificial intelligence (AI) and automated conversational interfaces known as 'chatbots'. Chatbots are software programs which allow users to engage in conversations with virtual agents that can

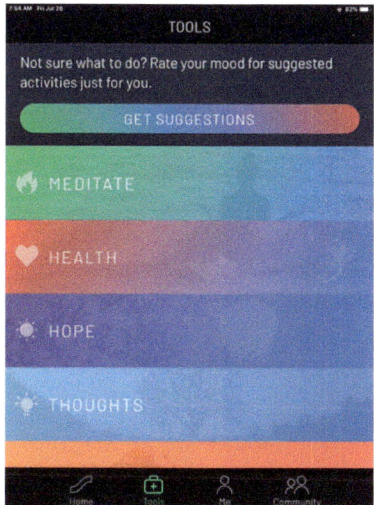

Figure 5.1 Screenshot from Sanvello app.

provide human-like responses through text. AI has allowed these chatbots to create more human-like interactions by adapting the responses to what a user inputs. In the area of eMental health interventions, two popular mental health chatbots are Woebot and Wysa. Both Woebot and Wysa have demonstrated potential to reduce mental health symptoms (Fitzpatrick et al., 2017; Inkster et al., 2018). Both Woebot and Wysa have similarities in their interactions in that users can access them at any time to discuss their thoughts and feelings, learn strategies and coping skills, and be directed towards resources and live providers if necessary. However, despite promising efficacy data, these tools have some challenges that limit their usefulness as clinical services. For example, in tests run by the British Broadcasting Corporation (BBC), Woebot and Wysa failed to identify signs of child sexual abuse (White, 2018). Although both products adjusted their technology and policies in light of this research, anticipating all clinical edge cases is a major challenge that technologies will always have a hard time addressing. This mirrors previous work on conversational agents like Siri's responses to various health concerns (Miner et al., 2016). As such, although chatbots might mirror human interactions in some ways, they face similar limitations as other self-guided interventions and are not yet intended to supplant traditional human care.

Thus, although self-guided interventions are effective for various mental health concerns, they are merely an additional option, not a solution, for the challenges facing mental health services. Neither websites nor mobile apps are necessarily the best treatment overall, nor for any given person. As such, the use of technology should be considered in the context of available resources, target populations, and overall treatment goals. For example, self-guided interventions might serve as a safety-net where no other resources exist (Muñoz, 2010), or could serve as the initial entry point into mental health services such as in stepped care models (March et al., 2019), or as an option for people who are on waiting lists for subsequent care (Peipert, Krendl, & Lorenzo-Luaces, 2022). The use cases for self-guided eMental health interventions (i.e., how it is envisioned they will integrate into care) can help guide decisions around types of technologies and features. Future research should explore if certain features are more effective for specific groups of people and develop best practices for these various use cases to maximize their public health impact.

Although numerous factors will impact the effectiveness of a particular tool, one significant issue facing self-guided eMental health interventions is adherence. Like face-to-face treatments, where many individuals drop-out early, many users of eMental health interventions fail to return after an initial download or use, or do not use the product enough to accrue therapeutic benefits. Insufficient usage is a frequently demonstrated phenomenon yet varies as a function of feature-set and product design characteristics (Baumel et al., 2019b; Baumel & Kane, 2018). Furthermore, multiple studies have emerged demonstrating the disparity in user engagement and adherence to self-guided eMental health interventions when in the context of a trial (Baumel et al., 2019a; Fleming et al., 2018). A systematic review of usage and adherence of self-guided eMental health interventions for depression, anxiety, and/or low mood by Fleming et al. (2018) concluded that while completion rates for self-help tools in research can vary between 44% and 99%, that figure can drop to between 1% and 28% in real-world use. Low levels of engagement and adherence have led to research into how to improve these issues (see e.g., Chapter 15). Responsiveness to user behaviour by customizing their content or experience for them (Balaskas et al., 2022), and further personalizing their experience with the added attention provided by social functionality and clinical support, have recently been proposed as effective mechanisms to remedy these concerns (Balaskas et al., 2021).

Ethical Considerations of Self-Guided Interventions

The most valuable attributes of self-guided interventions also create unique ethical problems, and researchers and practitioners will need to address them. We frame our discussion of ethical considerations using the principles enumerated in the Belmont Report of autonomy, beneficence, and justice (Adashi et al. 2018). Autonomy, or the right to make an informed choice free from undue influence, is often threatened by the unconstrained practices of the businesses who make and disseminate these tools. Many of the promotional materials for apps overstate their efficacy and their empirical basis (Larsen et al., 2019). As well as violating the principle of autonomy, these kinds of business practices violate the principle of beneficence, or the right of persons to be protected from harm and to have their well-being supported, as they allow likely inert and potentially harmful interventions being made available. Although these concerns weigh on the use of all types of interventions which are disseminated by organizations with a profit motive, self-guided interventions do not have a feedback loop between consumers and professionals that would allow for treatment plans to be reconsidered and adapted.

Concerns around access and privacy pervade eMental health interventions regardless of their level of support but are of particular concern for self-guided interventions given their intended use as a first-line, free-to-access tool for consumers who do not have access to resource-intensive alternatives. Despite recent efforts on the part of the Apple App Store and Google Play Store to create greater transparency around privacy, developers are still building interventions which collect far more data than is strictly necessary, creating risks which users are often not aware of (Torous et al., 2018), are informed of in ways that are beyond the patient's reading levels (Powell et al., 2019), or informed of only after data collection (O'Loughlin et al., 2019). Sometimes users are engaging with a program entirely without their consent, as has been the case with Facebook's suicide screening efforts which were deployed on Facebook without user consent and scanned their content for potentially concerning words (Barnett & Torous, 2019). These concerns violate the principle of autonomy, but also that of justice, or the right to fair and equitable access and treatment as some people are provided treatment, but others not. The principle of justice can be violated when tools are made inaccessible. This might be by making the content or supporting materials, like privacy policies, unintelligible at a patient's reading level or in limited languages, or by requiring the use of expensive devices beyond the means of many users.

Guided Interventions

Many interventions include some form of human support (e.g., for provision of feedback, additional skills training or clinical intervention, and technical support) based on findings that guided interventions tend to produce greater benefits and obtain higher rates of adherence (e.g., more logins, time on intervention, completion of intervention content) than self-guided interventions (Baumeister, Reichler, Munzinger, & Lin, 2014). The reliability and efficacy of guided interventions has become so well-established, a statement by a global group of experts of eMental health recently concluded that 'Guided [Digital Mental Health Interventions] should be offered as a treatment option to *all* patients experiencing depression, anxiety disorders, and posttraumatic stress disorder' (Mohr et al., 2021). Similarly, the National Institute for Health and Care Excellence in the UK gave partial support to the adoption of a digital CBT platform into clinical care, with the caveat that it was suitable for use, provided with monitoring, and as flexibility in terms of the amount of human support (NICE, 2020). Guidance is not solely included to increase intervention effectiveness, but also because many payment models require human involvement to be reimbursable (Powell et al., 2019). The role of human supporters in eMental health interventions varies and more details about the specifics of these interactions will be provided later in the chapter. Even when human support is included, however, the intervention itself is conceptualized to be the major agent of therapeutic benefit and change. Users are expected to engage in a great deal of independent practice and self-management to benefit.

The most influential model of support is the 'Swedish Model', which has been used in several randomized controlled trials for a variety of mental health concerns (Andersson et al., 2008). In this model, a user is expected to read lessons and complete activities each week and then provide a summary of their experiences and questions to a therapist. The therapist reads this summary and composes brief feedback usually devoting about 5–15 minutes per patient. This feedback is intended to validate and normalize the experiences of the user, to correct any issues that arose, and to prepare users for upcoming material in the programme. A similar model is the Macquarie University Model (MUM). MUM also tries to encourage engagement with the programme. It aims to practice and integrate skills into one's daily life (Titov et al., 2015). The major difference between the MUM and the Swedish Model is that the MUM uses messages and phone calls from the clinician, while the Swedish Model relies on an asynchronous mode of communication leveraging the summaries provided by the users. The Efficiency Model of Support (Schueller, Tomasino, & Mohr, 2017) builds on both models, but attempts to operationalize why support is provided to better guide the actions of supporters. In the Efficiency Model of Support, human support is doled out on an 'as needed' basis in response to failure points emerging from usability, engagement, fit, knowledge, or implementation. Support in this model is influenced by monitoring the actions and progress of the end user and only intervening among those people who are experiencing failures in the programme. This model draws on findings (e.g., Baumeister et al., 2014; Gellatly et al., 2007) that the number of sessions, type of personnel, content of guidance or mode of contact have no significant influence on the outcome. The Efficiency Model of Support attempts to better quantify the type, quantity, timing, and quality of support that will lead to the best outcomes for each individual while balancing that support, which is essentially a limited resource.

Meta-analyses demonstrate that support is generally beneficial (Baumeister et al., 2014), and that guided eMental health interventions are associated with larger effect sizes than self-guided DMHIs (Linardon et al., 2019). However, neither the supporter's level of expertise nor the amount of time users are supported are predictive of outcomes (Baumeister et al., 2014; Gellatly et al., 2007; Newman, Szkodny, Llera, & Przeworski, 2011). In some cases, increasing support may even reduce the benefits accrued from these interventions (e.g., Newman et al., 2011). It is possible that too much support might impact a patient's motivation, reduce autonomy and opportunities for learning, or introduce additional barriers that eMental health interventions should conceivably overcome (e.g., having to communicate with a provider at a specified time). Many of the activities supporters do can be accomplished by automated features such as chatbots and other conversational interfaces, although the quality of these features vary, especially compared to human support. Indeed, one study found that designing automated features from the framework of persuasive technology resulted in similar rates of adherence and effectiveness across supported and unsupported interventions (Kelders, Bohlmeijer, Pots, & van Gemert-Pijnen, 2015). As technology further develops, it might be possible to adopt more persuasive features as automated technological features and thus increase the adherence to and effectiveness of unsupported interventions (see Chapter 12).

Support may also improve adherence. One intervention built with adherence in mind is IntelliCare (Mohr et al., 2017; Lattie et al., 2016), which includes 13 'mini' apps, each focused on a singular behaviour change technique such as cognitive restructuring, goal setting, or relaxation. IntelliCare apps have very little didactic content and instead are focused on providing features to facilitate practice of skills. For example, instead of explaining why progressive muscle relaxation might be worthwhile, how it relates to causes and symptoms of anxiety, and how to perform progressive muscle relaxation, users are simply provided with an audio track that guides them through a progressive muscle relaxation exercise. Figure 5.2 displays screenshots from the Daily Feats app, one app from the IntelliCare suite that encourages users to incorporate worthwhile and productive activities into their day.

An initial trial of IntelliCare found that users who received the apps along with human support experienced significant and large reductions in depression and anxiety and that use of the apps was

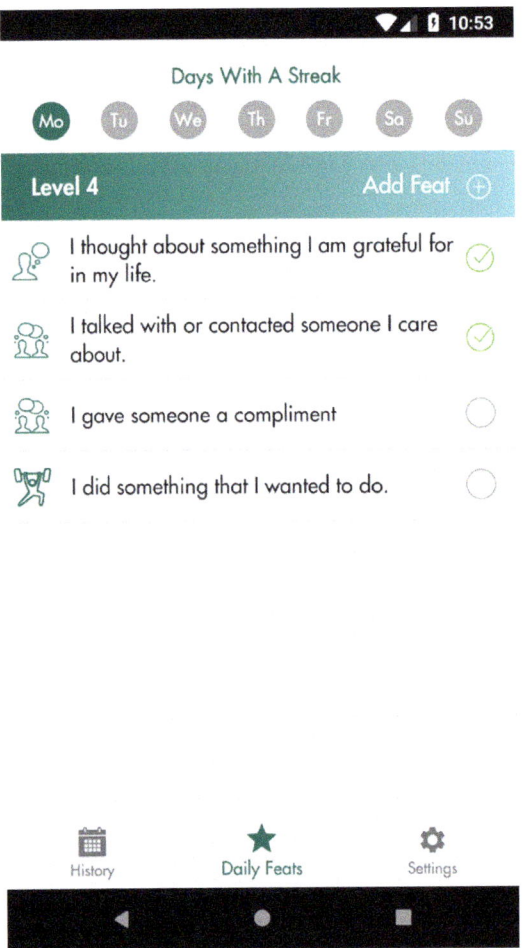

Figure 5.2 Screenshots from Daily Feats, one of the 13 apps in the IntelliCare suite.

high. Participants opened the apps on average 191.4 times over an eight-week period, but what was perhaps most surprising was that apps were used more often in week eight than week one, peaking in week six (Mohr et al., 2017). This is especially surprising when compared to usage rates and patterns of other eMental health interventions that often have considerable rates of non-adherence over time (Eysenbach, 2005). As an example, despite a large number of initial downloads, PTSD Coach, a mobile app targeted towards individuals with PTSD, maintains only 52.1% of users beyond the first week of download (Owen et al., 2015). A systematic review of real-world mental health app usage indicated that the median retention rate was 3.9% after 15 days and 3.3% after 30 days (Baumel et al., 2019b). It is worth noting, however, that the study design and the inclusion of human support in the IntelliCare study meant it was not possible to determine if the interaction style or human support was responsible for the sustained use of the system.

Ethical Considerations of Guided Interventions

Many of the ethical implications of the use of guided eMental health interventions are much the same as those previously discussed around self-guided eMental health interventions. Overstated claims of efficacy, a lack of research on the real-world effectiveness of specific interventions, design and content constructed without consideration for accessibility and acceptability across cultures and socioeconomic contexts, inscrutable and troubling data collection and retention practices, and business decisions prioritizing recurring subscription and ad revenue potentially at the expense of users, are all issues which are not dictated by degree of support.

However, unique to the consideration of guided eMental health interventions is who is providing the guidance, how much guidance they provide, and how to ensure that clinical diligence is assured in digital spaces. As noted earlier, research does not suggest that eMental health interventions are more effective when guidance is provided by a professional. As such, guidance is often provided by paraprofessionals such as coaches or peers. These professional roles may not be well understood by consumers using these interventions, and they may expect that the person delivering care is a licensed professional. Furthermore, while research studies must ensure coaches or other supporters have undergone training and supervision to ensure fidelity with research protocols, the training and supervision of these individuals in real-world settings is poorly defined and unregulated. Although the use of professionals may be costly and professionals may not necessarily be trained to deliver the types of interventions and support that are parts of guided programmes, professionals do have regulatory and ethical guidelines they follow as part of their profession. Furthermore, professionals are trained in crisis management and other complex situations that might arise while providing support. A significant ethical consideration is determining where the regulatory burden falls for guided eMental health interventions when support does not come from a professional. Likely this decision will differ across countries, but making this determination is an important step to supporting consumer confidence and safety.

Virtual Care

In March 2020, the COVID-19 pandemic forced nearly all consumers engaging with ongoing therapy to abandon in-person sessions. Some practitioners simply modified their practice and began seeing their patients using videoconferencing software like Zoom, WebEx, and Doxy for teletherapy. But for consumers seeking treatment, or practitioners seeking new clients, virtual care platforms have become a new pathway for bringing these groups together. Unlike self-guided and guided interventions, eMental health virtual care platforms provide a digital therapeutic experience which is engineered to approximate in-person care. However, the transition to a digital medium does have numerous ramifications for therapeutic practice.

Many virtual care platforms exist, with some of the most well-known operated by large private companies (e.g., BetterHelp, TalkSpace, Blue Cross Blue Shield). Smaller platforms targeting specific demographics also exist (e.g., Pride Counseling, ReGain, Faithful Counseling that focus on LGBTQ+, couples, or Black populations). The offerings of these platforms are similar, matching consumers with practitioners who provide services via video, text messages, phone, or chat tools. Despite the large and growing utilization of virtual care platforms, reimbursement from insurers vary, with some health systems developing or purchasing virtual care platforms themselves, and other platforms seeking opportunities for reimbursement through different insurers (Burgoyne & Cohn, 2020).

A clear benefit of virtual care platforms is in their ability to increase access across geographic space. Enabling consumers to visit with practitioners without the need to commute enables people and communities which are under-served and/or isolated to find care. Visiting a practitioner is no longer contingent on where you live, an invaluable benefit as practitioner availability often does not match the geographic dispersion of people. For example, in the United States over 80% of counties are designated as mental health practitioner shortage areas (Ku et al., 2021). Additionally, virtual care platforms enable consumers to seek practitioners with particular areas of expertise – such as training in specific evidence-based practices or specific cultural knowledge or background – which serves to improve quality and equity of access to care.

A considerable body of literature has emerged supporting the clinical effectiveness of virtual care and demonstrating that patients find virtual care acceptable. Individual studies (Carlbring et al., 2018; Alavi et al., 2016) and meta-analyses (Hilty et al., 2013) demonstrate that virtual care platforms for eMental health are equivalent to offline, in-person care options in terms of their effectiveness across disorders, degrees of severity, settings, and populations.

Despite the broad basis of acceptability and effectiveness of virtual care platforms, they are not without their limits. Nonverbal cues from both consumers and practitioners are limited by the medium, making the subtle task of demonstrating engagement and empathy difficult (Burgoyne & Cohn, 2020). Engaging in therapy via a computer or smartphone opens the patient up to a host of distractions (e.g., push notifications, social media) that are less prominent otherwise. Consumers may also have difficulty in finding and maintaining privacy outside the confines of the therapist's office and may be distracted or withholding for fear of being heard. For some consumers, even having a space for a private session without a therapist's office might prove challenging. Furthermore, newer ways of interacting through virtual care platforms, like text messaging or other text-based chat options, may differ more significantly from traditional therapy. Although the 'talking cure' has a long tradition in psychotherapy, the 'texting cure' does not, and it remains unclear to what extent practitioners maintain their effectiveness in this medium, or the additional training and competencies required to do so.

Ethical Considerations of Virtual Care

Virtual care platforms also present significant ethical implications. Many patients using virtual care platforms do not have equally viable in-person care options, often due to geography or economics. This lack of options constitutes a threat to justice, as they are effectively denied a reasonable set of possibilities to choose from. And although fees for virtual care are often less than the full price of traditional care models, requiring patients to be able to immediately pay for services further threatens the just and equitable dissemination of health services. Furthermore, questions have been raised about the payment practices for practitioners on these platforms as well as whether they can actually meet the demands of their working conditions (e.g., managing large client portfolios, around the clock availability to respond to messages). Virtual care platforms may be yet another area to examine whether the hype aligns with the reality of the available evidence and current practices in eMental health.

Future Directions

The current evidence and state of eMental health interventions demonstrates a considerable amount of both promise and limitations. Such interventions can be effective, but most of this evidence draws from tightly controlled randomized controlled trials that recruit patients that may or may not be representative of the intended end users, operating under conditions which do not adequately replicate their lived experience outside of study conditions. Data on real-world effectiveness has begun to accrue in limited capacities – such as from national efforts like the IAPT initiative in the UK and the MindSpot Clinic in Australia – yet rigorous studies of implementation at scale are rare, and rarer still outside the Global North. Study designs which incorporate measures related to implementation science, cost-effectiveness, and equity would bridge the gap between efficacy and effectiveness. However, two forces make this gap in the creation of knowledge difficult to fill: The lack of incentive for companies to provide rigorous empirical support of their products and services (given the willingness of users to accept promotional materials with a veneer of scientific support), and the rapid movement of technological progress rendering the cutting edge out of date long before the slow work of empirical research can be completed.

The seemingly added value of including human support raises questions about whether the potential benefits of digital mediums can be realized. However, it is possible that better designed persuasive features and technological advances could make future eMental health interventions more engaging without the need for human support. No one-size-fits-all solution exists, but work should consider what treatment approaches and technological features work best for whom. The most useful eMental health tools of the future will likely parallel changes in technology, and psychological theory and interventions need to adapt to these changes as well.

Summary

In this chapter, the possibilities and limitations of eMental health interventions were discussed. Guided interventions, self-guided interventions, and virtual care were presented, and an overview of research, examples of interventions, and ethical considerations was provided. It has become clear that eMental health interventions have a lot of potential to improve the mental health of a broad range of people, but that there still is much work to be done to actualize this potential on a large scale. The take-home messages for this chapter are:

- eMental health interventions are effective for a variety of mental disorders, particularly for depression, anxiety, and posttraumatic stress disorder. When provided along with human support, they can be as effective as face-to-face treatment;
- Most eMental health interventions are based on cognitive-behavioural therapy and include didactic content, interactive tools and human support that mirrors aspects of face-to-face care, such as weekly sessions with homework assignments provided by a therapist;
- Despite overwhelming evidence that eMental health interventions can be beneficial, the majority have not undergone rigorous research evaluations. Despite this, many propose they use evidence-based practices and are research backed in their marketing materials;
- A small, but growing, body of evidence demonstrates the successful implementation and use of eMental health in real-world settings, but these successes have been in narrowly defined use-cases and further work needs to determine how best to disseminate and implement these interventions;
- Although often treated as a mechanism to increase access and improve equity, the use of technology can replicate and reinforce societal inequalities if not appropriately built and deployed.

Key References for Further Reading

Bakker, D., Kazantzis, N., Rickwood, D., & Rickard, N. (2016). Mental health smartphone apps: Review and evidence-based recommendations for future developments. *JMIR Mental Health*, 3(1), e7.

Clarke, A. M., Kuosmanen, T., & Barry, M. M. (2015). A systematic review of online youth mental health promotion and prevention interventions. *Journal of Youth and Adolescence*, 44(1), 90–113.

Mohr, D. C., Azocar, F., Bertagnolli, A., Choudhury, T., Chrisp, P., Frank, R., Harbin, H., Histon, T., Kaysen, D., Nebeker, C., Richards, D., Schueller, S. M., Titov, N., Torous, J., Areán, P. A. (2021). Banbury forum consensus statement on the path forward for digital mental health. *Psychiatric Services*, 72(6), 677–683.

Mohr, D. C., Weingardt, K. R., Reddy, M., & Schueller, S. M. (2017). Three problems with current digital mental health research... And three things we can do about it. *Psychiatric Services*, 68(5), 427–429.

Torous, J., Bucci, S., Bell, I. H., Kessing, L. V., Faurholt-Jepsen, M., Whelan, P., ... & Firth, J. (2021). The growing field of digital psychiatry: current evidence and the future of apps, social media, chatbots, and virtual reality. *World Psychiatry*, 20(3), 318–335.

References

Adashi, E. Y., Walters, L. B., & Menikoff, J. A. (2018). The Belmont report at 40: Reckoning with time. *American Journal of Public Health*, 108(10), 1345–1348.

Alavi, N., Hirji, A., Sutton, C., & Naeem, F. (2016). Online CBT is effective in overcoming cultural and language barriers in patients with depression. *Journal of Psychiatric Practice*, 22(1), 2–8.

Andersson, G. (2018). Internet interventions: Past, present and future. *Internet Interventions*, 12, 181–188.

Andersson, G., Bergström, J., Buhrman, M., Carlbring, P., Holländare, F., Kaldo, V., ... & Waara, J. (2008). Development of a new approach to guided self-help via the internet: The Swedish experience. *Journal of Technology in Human Services*, 26(2–4), 161–181.

Andersson, G., Cuijpers, P., Carlbring, P., Riper, H., & Hedman, E. (2014). Guided Internet-based vs. face-to-face cognitive behavior therapy for psychiatric and somatic disorders: A systematic review and meta-analysis. *World Psychiatry*, 13(3), 288–295.

Andersson, G., Estling, F., Jakobsson, E., Cuijpers, P., & Carlbring, P. (2011). Can the patient decide which modules to endorse? An open trial of tailored Internet treatment of anxiety disorders. *Cognitive Behaviour Therapy*, 40(1), 57–64.

Balaskas, A., Schueller, S. M., Cox, A. L., & Doherty, G. (2021). The functionality of Mobile apps for anxiety: Systematic search and analysis of engagement and tailoring features. *JMIR mHealth and uHealth*, 9(10), e26712.

Balaskas, A., Schueller, S. M., Cox, A. L., & Doherty, G. (2022). Understanding users' perspectives on mobile apps for anxiety management. *Frontiers in Digital Health*, 4, 854263.

Barnett, I., & Torous, J. (2019). Ethics, transparency, and public health at the intersection of innovation and Facebook's suicide prevention efforts. *Annals of Internal Medicine*, 170(8), 565–566.

Baumeister, H., Reichler, L., Munzinger, M., & Lin, J. (2014). The impact of guidance on Internet-based mental health interventions – A systematic review. *Internet Interventions*, 1(4), 205–215.

Baumel, A., Edan, S., & Kane, J. M. (2019a). Is there a trial bias impacting user engagement with unguided e-mental health interventions? A systematic comparison of published reports and real-world usage of the same programs. *Translational Behavioral Medicine*, 9(6), 1020–1033.

Baumel, A., & Kane, J. M. (2018). Examining predictors of real-world user engagement with self-guided eHealth interventions: Analysis of mobile apps and websites using a novel dataset. *Journal of Medical Internet Research*, 20(12), e11491.

Baumel, A., Muench, F., Edan, S., and Kane, J. M. (2019b). Objective user engagement with mental health apps: Systematic search and panel-based usage analysis. *Journal of Medical Internet Research*, 21, e14567.

Burgoyne, N., & Cohn, A. S. (2020). Lessons from the transition to relational teletherapy during COVID-19. *Family Process*, 59(3), 974–988.

Carlbring, P., Andersson, G, Cuijpers, P., Riper, H., & Hedman-Lagerlöf, E. (2018). Internet vs. face-to-face cognitive behavior therapy for psychiatric and somatic disorders: An updated systematic review and meta-analysis. *Cognitive Behaviour Therapy*, 47(1), 1–18.

Consumer Health Apps and Digital Health Tools Proliferate, Improving Quality and Health Outcomes for Patients, Says New Report from IQVIA Institute. (2021). IQVIA. https://www.iqvia.com/newsroom/2021/07/consumer-health-apps-and-digital-health-tools-proliferate-improving-quality-and-health-outcomes-for

Eysenbach, G. (2005). The law of attrition. *Journal of Medical Internet Research*, 7(1), e11.

Fitzpatrick, K. K., Darcy, A., & Vierhile, M. (2017). Delivering cognitive behavior therapy to young adults with symptoms of depression and anxiety using a fully automated conversational agent (Woebot): A randomized controlled trial. *JMIR Mental Health*, 4(2), e7785.

Fleming T., Bavin L., Lucassen M., Stasiak K., Hopkins S., Merry S. (2018). Beyond the trial: Systematic review of real-world uptake and engagement with digital self-help interventions for depression, low mood, or anxiety. *Journal of Medical Internet Research*, 20(6), e199.

Gellatly, J., Bower, P., Hennessy, S., Richards, D., Gilbody, S., & Lovell, K. (2007). What makes self-help interventions effective in the management of depressive symptoms? Meta-analysis and meta-regression. *Psychological Medicine*, 37(9), 1217–1228.

Hilty, D. M., Ferrer, D. C., Parish, M. B., Johnston, B., Callahan, E. J., & Yellowlees, P. M. (2013). The effectiveness of telemental health: A 2013 Review. *Telemedicine and E-Health*, 19(6), 444–454.

Inkster, B., Sarda, S., & Subramanian, V. (2018). An empathy-driven, conversational artificial intelligence agent (Wysa) for digital mental well-being: Real-world data evaluation mixed-methods study. *JMIR mHealth and uHealth*, 6(11), e12106.

Kelders, S. M., Bohlmeijer, E. T., Pots, W. T., & van Gemert-Pijnen, J. E. (2015). Comparing human and automated support for depression: Fractional factorial randomized controlled trial. *Behaviour Research and Therapy*, 72, 72–80.

Ku, B. S., Li, J., Lally, C., Compton, M. T., & Druss, B. G. (2021). Associations between mental health shortage areas and county-level suicide rates among adults aged 25 and older in the USA, 2010 to 2018. *General Hospital Psychiatry*, 70, 44–50.

Larsen, M. E., Huckvale, K., Nicholas, J., Torous, J., Birrell, L., Li, E., & Reda, B. (2019). Using science to sell apps: Evaluation of mental health app store quality claims. *Npj Digital Medicine*, 2, 18.

Larsen, M. E., Nicholas, J., & Christensen, H. (2016). Quantifying app store dynamics: Longitudinal tracking of mental health apps. *JMIR mHealth and uHealth*, 4(3), e96.

Lattie, E. G., Schueller, S. M., Sargent, E., Stiles-Shields, C., Tomasino, K. N., Corden, M. E., … & Mohr, D. C. (2016). Uptake and usage of IntelliCare: A publicly available suite of mental health and well-being apps. *Internet Interventions*, 4(2), 152–158.

Linardon, J., Cuijpers, P., Carlbring, P., Messer, M., & Fuller-Tyszkiewicz, M. (2019). The efficacy of app-supported smartphone interventions for mental health problems: A meta-analysis of randomized controlled trials. *World Psychiatry*, 18(3), 325–336.

March, S., Donovan, C. L., Baldwin, S., Ford, M., & Spence, S. H. (2019). Using stepped-care approaches within internet-based interventions for youth anxiety: Three case studies. *Internet Interventions*, 18, 100281.

Miner, A. S., Milstein, A., Schueller, S., Hegde, R., Mangurian, C., & Linos, E. (2016). Smartphone-based conversational agents and responses to questions about mental health, interpersonal violence, and physical health. *JAMA Internal Medicine*, 176(5), 619–625.

Mohr, D. C., Azocar, F., Bertagnolli, A., Choudhury, T., Chrisp, P., Frank, R., Harbin, H., Histon, T., Kaysen, D., Nebeker, C., Richards, D., Schueller, S. M., Titov, N., Torous, J., & Areán, P. A. (2021). Banbury forum consensus statement on the path forward for digital mental health treatment. *Psychiatric Services*, 72(6), 677–683.

Mohr, D. C., Lattie, E. G., Tomasino, K. N., Kwasny, M. J., Kaiser, S. M., Gray, E. L., ... & Schueller, S. M. (2019). A randomized noninferiority trial evaluating remotely-delivered stepped care for depression using internet cognitive behavioral therapy (CBT) and telephone CBT. *Behaviour Research and Therapy*, 123, 103485.

Mohr, D. C., Tomasino, N., Lattie, E. G., Palac, H. L., Kwasny, M. J., Weingardt, K., … & Schueller, S. M. (2017). IntelliCare: An eclectic, skills-based app suite for the treatment of depression and anxiety. *Journal of Medical Internet Research*, 19(1), e10.

Muñoz, R. F. (2010). Using evidence-based internet interventions to reduce health disparities worldwide. *Journal of Medical Internet Research*, 12(5), e60.

National Institute for Health and Care Excellence. (2020). Space from depression for treating adults with depression. www.nice.org.uk/guidance/mib215

Newman, M. G., Szkodny, L. E., Llera, S. J., & Przeworski, A. (2011). A review of technology-assisted self-help and minimal contact therapies for anxiety and depression: Is human contact necessary for therapeutic efficacy? *Clinical Psychology Review*, 31(1), 89–103.

Nguyen, J., McNulty, N., Grant, N., Martland, N., Dowling, D., King, S., … & Dom, G. (2022). The effectiveness of remote therapy in two London IAPT services. *The Cognitive Behaviour Therapist*, 15, e23.

O'Loughlin, K., Neary, M., Adkins, E. C., & Schueller, S. M. (2019). Reviewing the data security and privacy policies of mobile apps for depression. *Internet Interventions*, 15, 110–115.

Owen, J. E., Jaworski, B. K., Kuhn, E., Makin-Byrd, K. N., Ramsey, K. M., & Hoffman, J. E. (2015). mHealth in the wild: Using novel data to examine the reach, use, and impact of PTSD coach. *JMIR Mental Health*, 2(1), e7.

Peipert, A., Krendl, A. C., & Lorenzo-Luaces, L. (2022). Waiting lists for psychotherapy and provider attitudes toward low-intensity treatments as potential interventions: Survey study. *JMIR Formative Research*, 6(9), e39787.

Powell, A. C., Bowman, M. B., & Harbin, H. T. (2019). Reimbursement of apps for mental health: Findings from interviews. *JMIR Mental Health*, 6(8), e14724.

Powell, A., Singh, P., & Torous, J. (2018). The complexity of mental health app privacy policies: a potential barrier to privacy. *JMIR mHealth and uHealth*, 6(7), e9871.

Schueller, S. M., Tomasino, K. N., & Mohr, D. C. (2017). Integrating human support into behavioral intervention technologies: The efficiency model of support. *Clinical Psychology: Science and Practice*, 24(1), 27–45.

Simon, G. E., Shortreed, S. M., Rossom, R. C., Beck, A., Clarke, G. N., Whiteside, U., ... & Smith, J. (2022). Effect of offering care management or online dialectical behavior therapy skills training vs usual care on self-harm among adult outpatients with suicidal ideation: A randomized clinical trial. *JAMA*, 327(7), 630–638.

Titov, N., Dear, B. F., Staples, L. G., Bennett-Levy, J., Klein, B., Rapee, R. M., … & Nielssen, O. B. (2015). MindSpot clinic: An accessible, efficient, and effective online treatment service for anxiety and depression. *Psychiatric Services*, 66(10), 1043–1050.

Titov, N., Dear, B. F., Nielssen, O., Wootton, B., Kayrouz, R., Karin, E., ... & Staples, L. G. (2020). User characteristics and outcomes from a national digital mental health service: An observational study of registrants of the Australian MindSpot Clinic. *The Lancet Digital Health*, 2(11), e582–e593.

Torous, J., Wisniewski, H., Liu, G., & Keshavan, M. (2018). Mental health mobile phone app usage, concerns, and benefits among psychiatric outpatients: C,omparative survey study. *JMIR Mental Health*, 5(4), e11715.

Vaish, R., Wyngarden, K., Chen, J., Cheung, B., & Bernstein, M. S. (2014). Twitch crowdsourcing: Crowd contributions in short bursts of time. In *Proceedings of the 32nd annual ACM conference on human factors in computing systems* (pp. 3645–3654). New York: ACM.

Van der Vaart, R., Witting, M., Riper, H., Kooistra, L., Bohlmeijer, E. T., & van Gemert-Pijnen, L. (2014). Blending online therapy into regular face-to-face therapy for depression: Content, ratio and preconditions according to patients and therapists using a Delphi study. *BMC Psychiatry*, 14(1), 355.

Wasil, A. R., Venturo-Conerly, K. E., Shingleton, R. M., & Weisz, J. R. (2019). A review of popular smartphone apps for depression and anxiety: Assessing the inclusion of evidence-based content. *Behaviour Research and Therapy*, 123, 103498.

Wentzel, J., van der Vaart, R., Bohlmeijer, E. T., & van Gemert-Pijnen, J. E. (2016). Mixing online and face-to-face therapy: How to benefit from blended care in mental health care. *JMIR Mental Health*, 3(1), e9.

White, B. G. (2018). Child advice chatbots fail to spot sexual abuse. BBC News. https://www.bbc.com/news/technology-46507900.

Wright, J. H., Wright, A. S., Albano, A. M., Basco, M. R., Goldsmith, L. J., Raffield, T., & Otto, M. W. (2005). Computer-assisted cognitive therapy for depression: Maintaining efficacy while reducing therapist time. *American Journal of Psychiatry*, 162(6), 1158–1164.

6 Public Health, Behavioural Medicine, and eHealth Technology

Rik Crutzen, Rosalie van der Vaart, Andrea W.M. Evers, & Christina Bode

Introduction

As was pointed out in previous chapters, eHealth has the potential to improve health and healthcare. However, both are very broad concepts and can refer to many different fields and areas of application that can range from, for example, preventing HIV in teenagers to improving quality of life in elderly with rheumatic arthritis. Due to the broad nature of the concept of somatic health, this chapter zooms in on the fields of public health and behavioural medicine, both important contexts for eHealth. The possibilities and limitations when using eHealth technology within these fields will be discussed. The overall aim of this chapter is to introduce the reader to the applicability and effectiveness of the use of eHealth to improve health and prevent diseases.

This chapter zooms in on the fields of public health and behavioural medicine, both important contexts for eHealth. The possibilities and challenges when using eHealth technology within these fields will be discussed and illustrated by examples from practice. After completing this chapter, you will be able to:

- Explain what public health and behavioural medicine are;
- Connect the challenges of the fields of public health and behavioural medicine to the possibilities of eHealth;
- State the effectiveness of the use of eHealth to stimulate healthy lifestyle behaviours and psychological adjustment;
- Provide examples of the application of eHealth within the fields of public health (focusing on primary and secondary prevention) and behavioural medicine;
- Discuss the specific possibilities and challenges within the fields of public health and behavioural medicine with regard to the use of eHealth.

Public Health and Behavioural Medicine

The aim of public health is to promote and protect the health of people and the communities where they live, learn, work and play (American Public Health Association, 2016). This encompasses activities such as preventing disease, prolonging life, and promoting health on different levels (e.g., community or individual) and in different settings (e.g., schools or companies). Public health activities can be directed to all aspects of prevention. The first activity is called primary prevention, which is the prevention of disease before it ever occurs. Secondary prevention refers to the early

DOI: 10.4324/9781003302049-7

detection, optimal treatment, and reduction of the impact of diseases. Finally, tertiary prevention is the prevention of further invalidation or deterioration from already-diagnosed diseases. In general, public health strives to ensure the conditions in which people can live a healthy life.

Behavioural medicine emphasizes the relationship between biological, psychological, and social factors relevant to health and illness. It focuses on the relationship between these factors with the aim to prevent disease, promote recovery and support patients in adapting to treatment and successfully self-managing their lives with a (chronic) disease. Also, improving care and training of health professionals belongs to the scope of behavioural medicine. In general, behavioural medicine strives for the improvement of health by applying a biopsychosocial perspective to prevention, diagnosis, treatment, and rehabilitation (Davidson et al., 2003; Schirmer & Montegut, 2009; Society of Behavioural Medicine, 2016).

Furthermore, both public health and behavioural medicine are related to and use insights from health psychology. Health psychology can be described as 'the aggregate of the specific educational, scientific and professional contribution of the discipline of psychology to the promotion and maintenance of health, the promotion and treatment of illness and related dysfunction' (Matarazzo, 1980). Health psychology considers both direct and indirect pathways from psychological factors to health status. For example, stress can directly have an impact on disease (e.g., coronary heart disease) but can also have an indirect effect via behaviour (e.g., smoking) that can impact health (Ogden, 2012). So, insights from health psychology are used in both behavioural medicine (e.g., how we can help people to cope with cardiovascular disease) and public health (e.g., how we can help people to quit smoking to reduce the prevalence of cardiovascular disease).

To sum up, both approaches aim at improving somatic health. Prevention, cure and care are relevant in both areas, although public health focuses more on prevention, whereas care and cure are more pronounced in behavioural medicine approaches. The following section focuses on eHealth applications in public health (e.g., lifestyle behaviours) and behavioural medicine (e.g., psychological adjustment to somatic conditions).

Using eHealth in the Field of Public Health: Focus on Lifestyle Behaviour

The use of eHealth in the field of public health has the potential ability to reach large audiences. Additionally, eHealth interventions can also be tailored to the psychosocial profile of the user, as opposed to non-technological 'one size fits all' interventions that aim to reach large and distinct groups of people in the same way despite their differences.

eHealth Interventions in Public Health

In the field of public health, many eHealth interventions have been developed, being 'typically behaviourally or cognitive behaviourally based treatments that have been operationalized and transformed for delivery via the Internet' (Ritterband & Thorndike, 2006). Usually, they have highly structured content; are self- or semi-self-guided; are based on effective face-to-face interventions; are personalized to the user; are interactive in nature; are enhanced by graphics, animations, audio and possibly video; and are tailored to provide follow-up and feedback (Ritterband & Thorndike, 2006). These interventions are based on existing behaviour change methods used offline and adapted to be delivered in an online context. For example, writing therapy is a type of semi-self-guided therapy that can be used offline by using paper-and-pencil exercises as well as online (Van Emmerik, Reijntjes, & Kamphuis, 2013).

Although interpersonal face-to-face communication is more individualized than eHealth interventions, the potential to tailor the intervention (content and system) to individual users and subgroups and still reach large audiences gives this approach major promise (Noar, Benac, &

Harris, 2007). Over 360 computer-tailoring studies have been conducted to date by researchers across health and computer sciences (Kamel Ghalibaf et al., 2019). Psychological constructs (e.g., self-efficacy, attitude) have been measured in approximately 60% of these studies, predominantly via questionnaires (91%), diaries or other written records (8%). These psychological constructs can then also be used for tailoring purposes. Kreuter, Farrell, Olevitch, & Brennan (2000) define tailoring as 'any combination of strategies and information intended to reach one specific person, based on characteristics that are unique to that person, related to the outcome of interest, and derived from an individual assessment' (p. 277). It is a commonly used approach in computer- or smartphone-delivered interventions in which the intervention content is based on the psychosocial profile of the user. Each user gets highly personally relevant content based on the screening of his or her profile, without the need and costs of interpersonal communication to assess this profile – as is done in counselling. For example, a user who believes that a certain behaviour leads to a specific outcome (e.g., high outcome expectancy) but does not believe he or she is able to successfully perform that behaviour (e.g., low self-efficacy) will receive other content than a user who scores high on self-efficacy but low in terms of outcome expectancy. In other words, a large audience could be reached with very individualized content without the need of counsellors being available for each and every individual.

Tailoring can be based on brief assessments at the start of the intervention and during the intervention. This can be done by posing questions, but there are also more innovative ways of achieving this. Wearables can, for example, be used to monitor movement or biomedical parameters like heart rate. This data can serve as input for the feedback provided to the user by the eHealth intervention. An example is an intervention using tailored information to facilitate informed decision-making regarding the use of e-cigarettes during smoking cessation (Elling et al., 2021). During the intervention, participants received tailored advice on the pros and cons of quitting smoking (i.e., attitude), social influence, preparatory plans, self-efficacy, and coping plans concerning smoking cessation. The information needed for the tailoring process is gathered by means of questionnaires that the recipient has to fill in during the intervention. Subsequently, a computerized process, employing if-then rules, selects appropriate feedback messages from a pool of all messages based

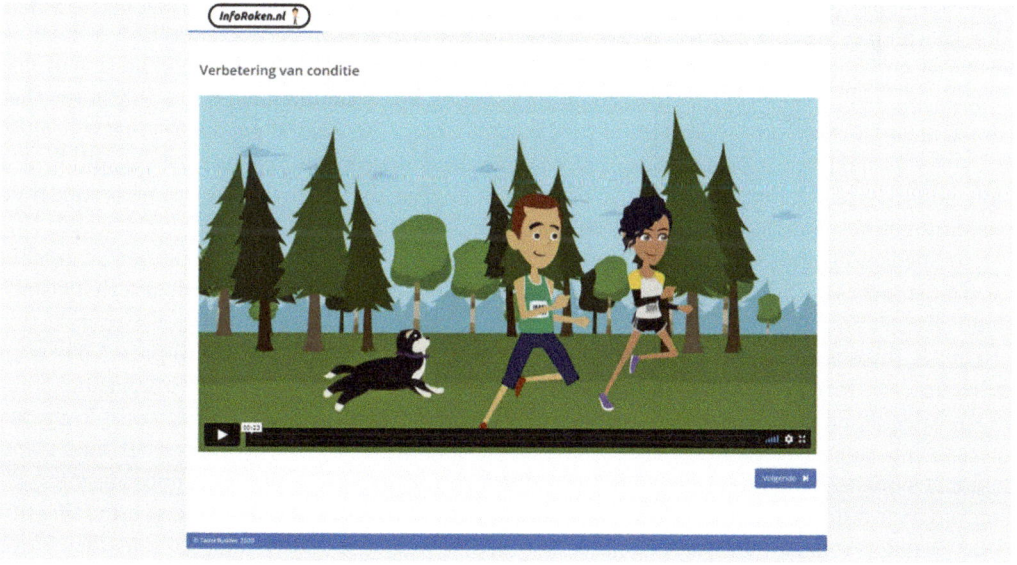

Figure 6.1 Screenshot of a webpage of the intervention showing an animated video advice (Elling et al., 2021).

on the answers that the recipient has given in the questionnaires. All advices are presented in the form of spoken animations with little on-screen text in order to increase user experience and user engagement (Figure 6.1). In the future, both routinely collected data and novel self-assessment methods can be used in tailoring to measure psychological constructs and at the same time reduce participant burden and increase engagement (Short et al., 2022).

Effectiveness of eHealth Interventions in Public Health

Many studies have aimed to provide evidence on the effectiveness of eHealth interventions in the field of public health that are specifically aimed at lifestyle behaviours. Many interventions that have been studied target dietary behaviours, physical activity, alcohol use, smoking, and condom use. The main reason for this is that these behaviours are identified as preventable risk factors contributing to several highly prevalent diseases like diabetes mellitus type 2, several types of cancer, cardiovascular diseases, and sexually transmitted diseases. In this section, the focus lies on primary and secondary prevention. Already in 2013, a total of 41 systematic reviews and meta-analyses were found regarding eHealth interventions targeting these kinds of lifestyle behaviours (Kohl, Crutzen, & De Vries, 2013). Since then, there has been a rapid increase of studies on eHealth interventions focusing on lifestyle behaviours. In 2023, an overview study was published on eHealth interventions for non-communicable disease management in primary healthcare settings of low- and middle-income countries (Xiong et al., 2023). The effectiveness of eHealth interventions was found to be highly mixed for clinical outcomes, more positively inclined for behavioural outcomes, and consistently promising in terms of potential for implementation in practice.

Overall, effect sizes concerning behavioural outcomes were small, rarely moderate. In studies where multiple interventions were compared to each other, eHealth interventions compared to a no-treatment control condition had larger effect sizes than when compared with other interventions (e.g., an intervention delivered face-to-face or on paper). In some cases, eHealth interventions that also included face-to-face elements (also known as blended interventions) were equally or more effective than those without it. Therefore, eHealth interventions have potential to change lifestyle behaviours.

These results are consistent with all types of interventions (not only eHealth interventions) in the field of public health in general, where small-to-moderate effect sizes are commonly reported. This can be partly explained by the prevention paradox: The seemingly contradictory situation where the majority of cases of a disease come from a population at low or moderate risk of that disease, and only a minority of cases come from the high-risk population (Rose, 1985). In other words, most interventions in the field of public health target the general population that is healthy and at low or moderate risk of disease. The changes needed are small in nature but can still have a large impact at population level because of the high number of people that are at low or moderate risk. So small-to-moderate effect sizes can have a large impact if large audiences are reached. This is also relevant in terms of behaviour maintenance. Prevention of obesity, for example, is thought to be most successful when focusing on small changes in dietary intake and physical activity, since small changes are easier to maintain in the long run (Hill, 2009).

Only a fraction of the potential of technology – in terms of public health impact – has been utilized so far. However, using the Internet as the (primary) delivery mode for interventions has expanded substantially. Research has shown that eHealth interventions are efficacious: They can successfully target people's health risk behaviours like sedentary lifestyle, high fat intake and cigarette smoking. Although trials to test the efficacy of interventions provide important information and have a strong internal validity, this paradigm oversimplifies reality in the quest to identify effective interventions (Glasgow, Vogt, & Boles, 1999). Hence, many interventions that prove effective in trials are much less effective when disseminated outside the trial context (Glasgow, Phillips, & Sanchez, 2014). This means that more attention should be paid to the context in which

Box 6.1 Case study: A tailored intervention to improve treatment adherence in patients with type 2 diabetes.

Type 2 diabetes mellitus (T2DM) is on the rise worldwide and is associated with considerable morbidity and mortality rates. Guidelines recommend various behaviours for patients with T2DM. These include healthy lifestyles, that is, improving dietary patterns and increasing physical activity and, if applicable, adequate adherence to medical strategies such as oral hypoglycemic agents (sometimes combined with insulin therapy). Unfortunately, patients' adherence to these separate behaviours is inadequate.

The aim of the intervention My Diabetes Profile (MDP) is to improve patient adherence to these various T2DM-related behaviours (Vluggen et al., 2021). MDP is self-guided and facilitated through periodic prompts and reminders to stimulate program engagement and completion. MDP provides web-based text and video feedback messages, tailored to determinants and underlying salient beliefs of health behaviour change such as attitudes, self-efficacy, goal setting, and action planning [43]. The program is divided into 2 nearly identical blocks, each available to users for 3 months. Each block consists of 3 sessions: (1) health risk appraisal; (2) awareness and motivation; and (3) goal setting, action planning, and self-regulation. The health risk appraisal session provides patients with interactive and tailored content on their health behaviours. Primarily, adherence levels are assessed for all behaviours the patient was involved in. For behaviours where there is room for improvement, the participants' intention to change that behaviour is assessed. The final part of the first session enables patients to select a single improvable behaviour, which will be their focus for the following 3 months while working with MDP. The second session aims to raise patients' awareness of the need to improve their particular behaviour and to increase motivation, with the ultimate purpose of achieving a high intention to change. If a high intention to change is achieved, after either session 1 or session 2, the patient is directed to session 3 on goal setting, action planning, and self-regulation. This session aims to increase the likelihood of a successful translation of the expressed intention into subsequent behaviour. This process is facilitated by setting small and realistic goals; forming action plans on where, when, and how to perform the behaviour; and forming self-regulation strategies to cope with barriers or situations that may impede adherence. In the trial, at six-months follow-up, the overall treatment adherence improved in the intervention group compared with the waiting-list control group.

the intervention will be implemented and used, something that has been acknowledged by the research in the field (Eccles et al., 2009). Also, a shift from efficacy trials towards pragmatic trials and rapid learning studies has been proposed in order to have more rapid public health impact (Kessler & Glasgow, 2011). In the future, to determine what kind of intervention works best for which group of people, and what way of tailoring is most effective, additional evaluation methods like log data analysis and $n = 1$ trials can be used, as will be explained in Chapter 14. This broadening of the evaluation methods fits with the holistic view on eHealth, which states that context, technology, and people are important in development and research.

Using eHealth in the Field of Behavioural Medicine: Focus on Psychological Adjustment

The use of eHealth in the field of behavioural medicine contributes to solving issues such as the lack of trained health professionals, using the time on a waiting list effectively, transferring a part of the self-management training from hospital to home and addressing stigma or hesitation among people to visit a psychologist for a primarily physical problem. In addition, eHealth has been applied to facilitate patient education and self-management for people with chronic somatic diseases. Many patients with (chronic) somatic conditions experience difficulties in daily life, both physically and emotionally.

eHealth Interventions in Behavioural Medicine

In behavioural medicine, eHealth technology can effectively be used for psychological support, to help people increase their self-management and reduce the impact of their disease on their daily life (e.g., tertiary prevention). These eHealth interventions aim, for example, to teach people suffering from pain-related conditions how to cope with their pain (Terpstra et al., 2018), or they target distress by treating moderate mood, anxiety, or fatigue problems, for example, among people with diabetes, cancer, or cardiovascular diseases (Bendig et al., 2018; Paul et al., 2013). Generally, these eHealth interventions are secure websites or mobile applications (e.g., a person logs in from home or on their smartphone, during several weeks or months) and include modules that combine psycho-educational texts, assignments, and relaxation exercises, often supported with video and/or audio files. The content is typically based on treatment methods derived from Cognitive-Behavioural Therapy (CBT) and Acceptance and Commitment Therapy (ACT), in which people learn to alter their behaviour and/or their thoughts in order to decrease the associated negative feelings and problems and to live a meaningful life with the somatic disease (Butler, Chapman, Forman, & Beck, 2006). Next to these approaches which focus on reflective learning, cognitive bias modification (CBM) is a novel technique that targets cognitive biases by directly retraining them by simple computer tasks. CBM showed promising results in helping people with pain, social anxiety, and fear of cancer recurrence. Recently CBM has been tested to modify cognitive fatigue biases (Geerts et al., 2023). Another field of quick eHealth developments in behavioural medicine is Virtual Reality (VR). Especially in the field of pain management VR has been studied as alternative treatment method for pain management (Gupta, Scott, & Dukewich, 2018). Users can immerse themselves in a computer generated 3-D simulation environment which allows to interact with the objects presented in this environment. By combining the virtual environment with a headphone or motion sensor for example, users can receive feedback through multiple sensory modalities which helps them to train beneficial reactions to pain which might have neuromodulating effects in the longer run or help people to distract from pain and learn to relax in an easy and pleasurable way (Mallari, Spaeth, Goh, & Boyd, 2019).

The benefit of delivering these interventions via technology is that it helps overcome typical face-to-face intervention barriers. Especially for self-management support in care for people with chronic diseases, there often is a shortage of trained health professionals and a lack of other financial and organizational resources. Moreover, there is also a stigma or reluctance among people to visit a psychologist for a primarily physical problem. eHealth technology provides a low-key manner to deliver an evidence-based intervention which people carry out in their own time and home environment, with a large focus on their self-efficacy and self-management. Moreover, eHealth interventions can increase access to proper care for people with rarer conditions, since they are more easily reachable through the Internet and are not hindered by distance or limited physical mobility problems in visiting a therapist (Anderson & Klemm, 2008).

Just as the eMental health interventions described in Chapter 5, eHealth interventions in behavioural medicine can be delivered with a broad range of support and guidance, varying from completely unguided – as a self-help intervention – to weekly online feedback from a therapist or coach. Systematic reviews on studies comparing guided and non-guided eHealth interventions overall conclude that offering some form of support increases its effectiveness and is associated with higher levels of completion of therapy modules (Musiat et al., 2021; Newman, Szkodny, Llera, & Przeworski, 2011; Richards & Richardson, 2012; Schubart, Stuckey, Ganeshamoorthy, & Sciamanna, 2011). Studies on the experiences of patients with eHealth interventions also show that personal feedback and support are perceived as positive in order to optimally use the programme and to stay motivated (Beattie, Shaw, Kaur, & Kessler, 2009; Bendelin et al., 2011). Interventions can also be offered as 'blended care', in which the treatment consists of a combination of face-to-face sessions and online modules (Kloek et al., 2017; Wentzel, van der Vaart, Bohlmeijer, & van Gemert-Pijnen, 2016). Another factor affecting the effectiveness of eHealth interventions are the facilities to communicate with other users. Interventions that focused on self-management and which included interaction between participants resulted in better outcomes related to the target behaviour of these interventions. However, research on these kinds of factors is still lacking, especially for people with somatic conditions.

Effectiveness of eHealth Interventions in Behavioural Medicine

The effectiveness of eHealth interventions in the field of behavioural medicine has been studied among a wide range of (chronic) conditions. Systematic reviews have found studies among patients with chronic pain, rheumatic conditions, cardiovascular diseases, headache/migraine, tinnitus, irritable bowel syndrome, diabetes, (breast) cancer, epilepsy, and fatigue (Terpstra et al., 2022; Van Beugen et al., 2014). Especially for eHealth interventions using cognitive behaviour therapies, the reviews showed an overall positive effect on psychosocial outcomes. The main goal of these interventions is generally to support people in coping with their disease and reduce its impact on the patient. The largest effects are, therefore, found on outcome measures related to interference of the condition on daily life (e.g., overcoming barriers to work, execute a hobby or have social interactions) or the disease-specific quality of life of patients (Buhrman et al., 2016; Van Beugen et al., 2014). When looking at psychological outcomes such as depression or anxiety, overall small-to-moderate effects are found (Buhrman et al., 2016; Van Beugen et al., 2014). Concerning the effect that these interventions have on the actual physical symptoms, there is heterogeneity between studies and conditions. A review of Van Beugen et al. (2014) showed, for example, large effects for irritable bowel syndrome, moderate effects for headache and small effects for pain and fatigue.

   To compare the effects of face-to-face interventions and eHealth interventions, Andersson et al. (2014) performed a systematic review on the overall difference in effectiveness between the two. They found that both types of interventions produced equivalent overall effects, which is a positive finding that shows that both types of therapy deserve their place in clinical practice (Andersson et al., 2014). Nevertheless, these results were found on a group level, and an important question that receives growing attention is for whom these interventions are most effective and what parts of the intervention particularly fit which of the intervention groups. It is interesting to know whether there are subgroups or populations for which eHealth interventions would be most suitable, or maybe not suitable at all, for example, based on their age, their socio-economic status, or their health condition. Insight into these moderators could create a better fit between the patient and the offered intervention, possibly resulting in larger treatment effects, as well as better adherence and satisfaction. A factor that is also essential to take into account when it comes to the suitability of eHealth interventions is the level of skill that people have and/or need in order to properly use the interventions; this is defined as their 'eHealth literacy' (van der Vaart, Atema, & Evers, 2016; van der Vaart & Drossaert, 2017; Wentzel et al., 2016). Besides these patient-related moderating factors, a better therapist-patient relationship, which could also be established via technology, has been reported to predict a more favourable outcome in tailored online cognitive-behavioural interventions for patients with psoriasis (Ferwerda et al., 2016; Van Beugen et al., 2016). The therapist-patient relationship is a possible mediator of therapy success, which should receive attention during the course of therapy. Nevertheless, still very little is known about the key moderators and mediators of treatment effects, which are yet insufficiently studied. Therefore, these topics provide challenges for future research in order to gain insight into the proper allocation and application of eHealth interventions in clinical practice.

Box 6.2 Case study: A therapist-guided intervention aimed at patients with chronic somatic conditions.

An example of a therapist-guided eHealth cognitive-behavioural therapy in behavioural medicine is the 'eCoach' programme (Evers, Gieler, Hazes, & Van Middendorp, 2014; Ferwerda et al., 2017b; Van Beugen et al., 2016). This programme consists of several flexible modules that can be generically deployed among a broad range of patients with chronic somatic conditions (see Figure 6.2). The modules focus on themes that chronic patients often experience problems with, such as pain, fatigue, negative mood and problems in social relationships. The main goal is to help people in coping with their disease in daily life by tailoring the programme and the modules to each patient's specific needs and goals. This tailoring is done in two steps; first, illness-specific online screening instruments (regarding disease-related coping, illness cognitions and level of distress) are used to help determine psychological adjustment problems and find out what the essential areas are that should be focused on in therapy. Second, the patient and the therapist meet face-to-face in one or two sessions to discuss the screening outcomes and to set goals to improve the patient's disease-related quality of life. The role of the therapist is essential in this phase, since the therapist monitors that the goals are feasible and that they fit the rationale of the therapy. Based on these goals, specific modules on which the patient will work during the therapy are chosen by the therapist. Typically, a therapy session starts with an introductory module with information on the programme, the rationale of the therapy and goal setting, and ends with a closing module on reflection, long-term goals, and relapse prevention. In between, two or three modules are completed on specific topics that are specifically important for the patient, such as relaxation, mood, (un)helpful thoughts, rest-activity balance, and the social environment.

    These modules are all completed online via a secured therapy environment with log in. As an eCoach, the therapist communicates with the patient via secured email messages in the inbox of the online environment. Approximately once a week the patient receives a message from the eCoach which guides him or her through the modules. The modules contain

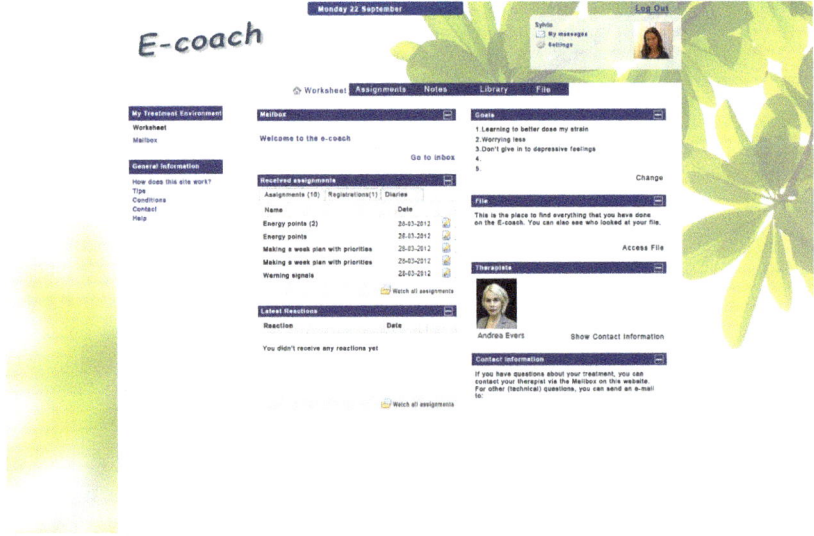

Figure 6.2 Screenshot of the homepage of the eCoach.

psycho-educational texts, assignments, registrations, and relaxation exercises. The patient works on the modules independently and sends the completed assignments to the eCoach at the end of each week, preferably accompanied with a message on how it went and any questions that might have occurred. The eCoach provides individualized feedback based on the completed assignments and answers the patient's additional questions. Therapy duration can vary, based on the patient's goals and accompanying modules (e.g., relaxation exercises or not), but the aim is to complete the intervention in three to six months.

The effectiveness of this programme has been studied among psoriasis and rheumatoid arthritis (RA) patients, with positive results (Ferwerda et al., 2017b; Van Beugen et al., 2016). Both conditions cause chronic complaints, which are known to cause a high disease burden in daily life. In these studies, the eCoach programme affected the disease impact on these patient populations and improved their psychological and/or physical functioning. In addition, evidence was found that both trials were cost-effective for the whole group or subgroups of patients (Ferwerda et al., 2017a; Van Beugen et al., 2017). This intervention shows benefits associated with eHealth interventions for behavioural medicine in general: Patients received support in self-managing their disease and maintaining a good quality of life despite their chronic disease. Using the intervention online makes it accessible to a large number of patients: Time investment is flexible, patients do not have to travel and a therapist can help more patients in the same time span, since it requires less time investment than face-to-face consults. The therapy is also very much presented as a training, which lowers the intensity of participation. In combination with not having to visit a psychologist every (other) week, the intervention helps patients to work on their problems without feeling stigmatized for suffering a mental problem. Applications in other groups of patients with somatic complaints and disorders have further proven the feasibility of the program (Wirken et al., 2018) Nevertheless, there always will be a group of patients for whom this form of therapy is not suitable (e.g., due to lack of skills, motivation, or Internet access). Therefore, future research should focus on what factors are essential to take into account when starting an online therapy and also on improving the usability of and adherence to the online therapy so as to make it suitable for as many patients as possible.

Possibilities and Challenges within the Fields of Public Health and Behavioural Medicine

The Development of eHealth Interventions in Public Health and Behavioural Medicine

Systematic development is as important for the development of eHealth technology as it is for any type of intervention within the field of public health and behavioural medicine. Insights from health psychology are used in the application of systematic approaches regarding development and intervention, such as Intervention Mapping (Bartholomew Eldredge et al., 2016). This means, in short, that after having a clear insight into the problem, outcomes for the intervention have to be determined (e.g., health indicators, behaviour change and environmental outcomes), as well as the determinants/predictors underlying these outcomes. The latter is rather crucial, because the theory-based methods (or behaviour change techniques) used in an intervention are linked to these determinants or predictors. These methods need to be translated into practical applications (Kok et al., 2016). Although this might sound like a very linear approach, the development process is always iterative, and input of the end users and other relevant stakeholders should be included from the beginning of the intervention development (Bartholomew et al., 2016). Especially for eHealth interventions, it is warranted to focus on the technical instantiation (Crutzen, 2014;

Mohr, Schueller, Montague, Burns, & Rashidi, 2014). Moreover, it is important to realize that long-term implementation requires early attention for business modelling, which results in distinctive outcomes (van Gemert-Pijnen et al., 2011). Therefore, also within the domains of public health and behavioural medicine, it is warranted to treat eHealth interventions as technologies or even products that need to be marketed and that require business or service modelling (see also Chapter 9). Moreover, it is important to focus on the content of interventions by means of producing interventions based on theory-based methods that are translated into practical applications (Crutzen, 2012).

As we will elaborate in Chapter 7 on holistic eHealth development, for the development of eHealth interventions in public health and behavioural medicine it is crucial that end users are involved in the process; it is important to consider their needs and characteristics for the integration of theory-based methods in the design of the technology. Within this user-centred design methodology, multiple methods derived from Human Centred Design (see Chapter 11) can be used to involve end users, such as focus groups, interviews, and think-aloud methods. Quick developments in technology and, perhaps even more important the connection of different technologies, will provide improvements for presence, immersion, and embodiment of eHealth applications. The Human Centred Design approach will help to find out which multisensory treatment and artificial self-management environments hold the right balance between simulating day-to day situations realistically for good training results and the effort (e.g., time, money, usability of equipment for patients and professionals) to design and use these.

Previous studies on the development and implementation of eHealth interventions have shown that different patients perceive benefit from different sorts of information and different delivery of that information. As mentioned before, this can depend on personal characteristics, such as age and education level, but also disease characteristics, or the stage of the illness (Keselman et al., 2008; Kontos et al., 2014; Lapsley & Groves, 2004; Nguyen et al., 2004; Pagliari, 2007). These differences can relate to the content of an eHealth intervention (e.g., the level of difficulty of the information or the focus of the information) and to the mode of delivery (e.g., preferences for text-based interventions or the use of video support) and layout. Moreover, the technology that is used (e.g., web-based or mobile-based) and the user interface (look and feel of the intervention, placement of buttons) can cause an essential difference in the usefulness and ease of use for people, which largely affects the acceptance and uptake of interventions (Venkatesh, Morris, Davis, & Davis, 2003). In order to fit an eHealth intervention to the preferences of the end user, and to increase its use, value, and effect, it is crucial to take their needs, skills, and expectations into account during the entire development process (van Gemert-Pijnen et al., 2011).

It is in the translation from theory-based methods to their practical application where technology might offer interesting possibilities. For example, smartphones provide opportunities regarding continuous use of socio-geographical data such as time and location (e.g., to know the location and displacement), accelerometery (e.g., to quantify human movement patterns) and collecting information about heart rate and sleeping patterns (e.g., to determine the balance between activity and rest). The potential lies in the unique opportunities provided by the information gathered from wearable sensors integrated into smartphones. That information can be transformed into usable, personalized and context-specific motivational and skills-centred coaching. For example, Inspirun is a personalized running-application that uses GPS and Bluetooth heart rate monitor support to track a user's progress, which leads to adjustments of the training schedule after each training session (Vos, Janssen, Goudsmit, Lauwerijssen, & Brombacher, 2016). In other words, self-monitoring and feedback are examples of theory-based methods that were used long before eHealth achieved its current status, but nevertheless these can now be meaningfully improved by the opportunities of innovative technology.

The Use and Users of eHealth Interventions in Practice

Reaching the right target group and making sure that they use an intervention as was intended by the developers is a challenge for all types of interventions. However, there are also specific aspects that influence the reach of eHealth interventions, in particular. For example, while anonymity is favourable for interventions regarding behaviours that might involve shame, like condom use or alcohol moderation (Moyer & Finney, 2004), it can also lead to high attrition rates (proportion of users' dropouts) (Eysenbach, 2005). This might affect the public health impact of these interventions. When looking at eHealth interventions targeting lifestyle behaviours, the intended reach is varied, aiming at a diverse population with respect to gender, socio-economic status and ethnic background. However, the actual reach is less diversified; mostly the female, white, middle-aged, highly educated part of the population is reached, who are generally seen as a low-risk population (Kohl et al., 2013). While it is also desirable to reach high-risk users; these are not necessarily attracted at the same rate as low-risk users (Glasgow et al., 2007).

When it comes to eHealth interventions used in healthcare settings, reaching the target population can also be challenging, often related to people's lack of motivation and trust towards starting this type of intervention, or sometimes because it is too generalized and does not fit the specific needs of a patient. For example, when applying for psychological help, people mostly expect a traditional setting, in which they have weekly face-to-face consults with a therapist with whom they discuss their problems, specifically their individual problems and struggles. In that scenario, an eHealth intervention that focused on one's motivation and self-management but is still suitable for a large group of people might seem to be a less attractive alternative. Even though research has found that both modes of delivery can be equally effective, a large group of both patients and therapists still prefers face-to-face treatment (Meurk, Leung, Hall, Head, & Whiteford, 2016; Renn et al., 2019). Therefore, to successfully implement eHealth interventions, health professionals in somatic care and public health play a large role as well. By educating health professionals in 'eTherapy' skills, providing them with the appropriate knowledge and methods, many barriers among themselves, and consequently patients as well, could be overcome. Such a training could involve screening to decide whether an eHealth intervention is suitable for a certain topic or patient group (which of course should also be considered during the development phases), shared decision making to discuss the choice for online treatment with patients and online communication to support and motivate patients using a digital medium (Terspatra et al., 2018; van der Vaart et al., 2016). Taking all these developments together, eHealth technology can have a large impact in the fields of both public health and behavioural medicine.

Summary

This chapter has shown that both the fields of public health and behavioural medicine are important contexts for eHealth. The take-home messages for this chapter are:

- The use of eHealth in the field of public health has the potential ability to reach large audiences and thereby have a big impact in terms of health gains;
- eHealth interventions can be tailored to the psychosocial profile of the user;
- eHealth interventions are used to target a wide range of behaviours and target groups;
- The use of eHealth in the field of behavioural medicine contributes to solving issues such as the lack of trained health professionals, and stigma or hesitation among people to visit a psychologist for a primarily physical problem;
- eHealth interventions can be applied effectively to facilitate patient education and self-management for people with chronic somatic diseases, reducing the impact that their disease has on their daily life.

Key References for Further Reading

Bartholomew Eldredge, L. K., Markham, C. M., Ruiter, R. A. C., Fernández, M. E., Kok, G., & Parcel, G. S. (2016). *Planning health promotion programs: An Intervention Mapping approach* (4th edition). San Francisco, CA: Jossey-Bass.

Eysenbach, G. (2005). The law of attrition. *Journal of Medical Internet Research*, 7(1), e11.

Kamel Ghalibaf, A., Nazari, E., Gholian-Aval, M., & Tara, M. (2019). Comprehensive overview of computer-based health information tailoring: A systematic scoping review. *BMJ Open*, 9(1), e021022.

Kohl, L., Crutzen, R., & De Vries, N. K. (2013). Online prevention aimed at lifestyle behaviours: A systematic review of reviews. *Journal of Medical Internet Research*, 15(7), e146.

Mallari, B., Spaeth, E. K., Goh, H., & Boyd, B. S. (2019). Virtual reality as an analgesic for acute and chronic pain in adults: A systematic review and meta-analysis. *Journal of Pain Research*, 12, 2053–2085. https://doi.org/10.2147/JPR.S200498

Terpstra, J. A., van der Vaart, R., van Beugen, S., van Eersel, R. A., Gkika, I., Erdős, D., Schmidt, J., Radstake, C., Kloppenburg, M., van Middendorp, H., & Evers, A. W. M. (2022). Guided internet-based cognitive-behavioral therapy for patients with chronic pain: A meta-analytic review. *Internet Interventions*, 30, 100587.

References

American Public Health Association. (2016). What is public health? Retrieved from www.apha.org/what-is-public-health

Anderson, A. S., & Klemm, P. (2008). The internet: Friend or foe when providing patient education? *Clinical Journal of Oncology Nursing*, 12, 55–63.

Bartholomew Eldredge, L. K., Markham, C. M., Ruiter, R. A. C., Fernández, M. E., Kok, G., & Parcel, G. S. (2016). *Planning health promotion programs: An Intervention Mapping approach* (4th edition). San Francisco, CA: Jossey-Bass.

Beattie, A., Shaw, A., Kaur, S., & Kessler, D. (2009). Primary-care patients' expectations and experiences of online cognitive-behavioural therapy for depression: A qualitative study. *Health Expectations*, 12, 45–59.

Bendelin, N., Hesser, H., Dahl, J., Carlbring, P., Nelson, K. Z., & Andersson, G. (2011). Experiences of guided Internet-based cognitive-behavioural treatment for depression: A qualitative study. *BMC Psychiatry*, 11, 107.

Bendig, E., Bauereiß, N., Ebert, D. D., Snoek, F., Andersson, G., & Baumeister, H. (2018). Internet-based interventions in chronic somatic disease. *Dtsch Arztebl Int*. Nov 5;115(40), 659–665. doi:10.3238/arztebl.2018.0659. PMID: 30381130; PMCID: PMC6234467.

Butler, A. C., Chapman, J. E., Forman, E. M., & Beck, A. T. (2006). The empirical status of cognitive-behavioral therapy: A review of meta-analyses. *Clinical Psychology Review*, 26(1), 17–31.

Crutzen, R. (2012). From eHealth technologies to interventions. *Journal of Medical Internet Research*, 14(3), e93.

Crutzen, R. (2014). The behavioral intervention technology model and Intervention Mapping: The best of both worlds. *Journal of Medical Internet Research*, 16(8), e188.

Davidson, K. W., Goldstein, M., Kaplan, R. M., Kaufmann, P. G., Knatterud, G. L., Orleans, C. T., … & Whitlock, E. P. (2003). Evidence-based behavioral medicine: What is it and how do we achieve it? *Annals of Behavioral Medicine*, 26, 161–171.

Eccles, M. P., Armstrong, D., Baker, R., Cleary, K., Davies, H., Davies, S., … & Sibbald, B. (2009). An implementation research agenda. *Implementation Science*, 4, 18.

Elling, J. M., Crutzen, R., Talhout, R., & de Vries H. (2021). Effects of providing tailored information about e-Cigarettes in a web-based smoking cessation intervention: Protocol for a randomized controlled trial. *JMIR Res Protoc*. May 14;10(5), e27088. doi:10.2196/27088. PMID: 33988520; PMCID: PMC8164120.

Emmerik van, A. A., Reijntjes, A., & Kamphuis, J. H. (2013). Writing therapy for posttraumatic stress: A meta-analysis. *Psychotherapy & Psychosomatics*, 82, 82–88.

Evers, A. W. M., Gieler, U., Hazes, M., & van Middendorp, H. (2014). Incorporating biopsychosocial characteristics into personalized healthcare: A clinical approach. *Psychotherapy & Psychosomatics*, 83, 148–157.

Eysenbach, G. (2005). The law of attrition. *Journal of Medical Internet Research*, 7(1), e11.

Ferwerda, M., van Beugen, S., van Middendorp, H., Smit, J. V., Zeeuwen-Franssen, M. E. J., Kroft, E. B. M., … & Evers, A. W. M. (2017a). Economic evaluation of a tailored therapist-guided internet-based cognitive behavioral treatment for patients with rheumatoid arthritis. Submitted.

Ferwerda, M., van Beugen, S., van Middendorp, H., Spillekom-van Koulil, S., Donders, A. R. T., Visser, H., … & Evers, A. W. M. (2017b). A tailored guided internet-based cognitive-behavioral intervention for patients with rheumatoid arthritis as an adjunct to standard rheumatological care: Results of a randomized controlled trial. *Pain*, 158(5), 868–878.

Ferwerda, M., van Beugen, S., van Riel, P. C. L. M., van de Kerkhof, P. C. M., De Jong, E. M. G. J., Smit, J. V., … & Evers, A. W. M. (2016). Measuring the therapeutic relationship in Internet-based interventions. *Psychotherapy & Psychosomatics*, 85, 47–49.

Geerts, J., Pieterse, M., Laverman, G., Waanders, F., Oosterom, N., Slegten, J., . . . Bode, C. (2023). Cognitive bias modification training targeting fatigue in patients with kidney disease: Usability study. *JMIR Form Res*, 7, e43636. doi:10.2196/43636

Glasgow, R. E., Nelson, C. C., Kearney, K. A., Reid, R., Ritzwoller, D. P., Strecher, V. J., … & Wildenhaus, K. (2007). Reach, engagement, and retention in an Internet-based weight loss program in a multi-site randomized controlled trial. *Journal of Medical Internet Research,* 9(2), e11.

Glasgow, R. E., Phillips, S., & Sanchez, M. (2014). Implementation science approaches for integrating eHealth research into practice and policy. *International Journal of Medical Informatics*, 83, e1–e11.

Glasgow, R. E., Vogt, T. M., & Boles, S. M. (1999). Evaluating the public health impact of health promotion interventions: The RE-AIM framework. *American Journal of Public Health,* 89, 1322–1327.

Gupta, A., Scott, K., & Dukewich, M. (2018). Innovative technology using virtual reality in the treatment of pain: Does it reduce pain via distraction, or is there more to it? *Pain Medicine*, 19(1), 151–159. doi:10.1093/pm/pnx109

Hill, J. (2009). Can a small-changes approach help address the obesity epidemic? A report of the Joint Task Force of the American Society for Nutrition, Institute of Food Technologists, and International Food Information Council. *American Journal of Clinical Nutrition*, 89, 477–484.

Kamel Ghalibaf, A., Nazari, E., Gholian-Aval, M., & Tara, M. (2019). Comprehensive overview of computer-based health information tailoring: A systematic scoping review. *BMJ Open*, 9(1), e021022. https://doi.org/10.1136/bmjopen-2017-021022

Keselman, A., Logan, R., Smith, C. A., Leroy, G., & Zeng-Treitler, Q. (2008). Developing informatics tools and strategies for consumer-centered health communication. *Journal of the American Medical Informatics Association*, 15, 473–483.

Kessler, R., & Glasgow, R. E. (2011). A proposal to speed translation of healthcare research into practice: Dramatic change is needed. *American Journal of Preventive Medicine*, 40, 637–644.

Kloek, C., Bossen, D., de Bakker, D. H., Veenhof, C., & Dekker, J. (2017). Blended interventions to change behavior in patients with chronic somatic disorders: Systematic review. *Journal of Medical Internet Research*, 19(12), e418. https://doi.org/10.2196/jmir.8108

Kohl, L., Crutzen, R., & De Vries, N. K. (2013). Online prevention aimed at lifestyle behaviours: A systematic review of reviews. *Journal of Medical Internet Research*, 15(7), e146.

Kok, G., Gottlieb, N. H., Peters, G.-J. Y., Mullen, P. D., Parcel, G. S., Ruiter, R. A. C., … & Bartholomew, L. K. (2016). A taxonomy of behavior change methods: An Intervention Mapping approach. *Health Psychology Review*, 10, 297–312.

Kontos, E., Blake, K. D., Chou, W.-Y. S., & Prestin, A. (2014). Predictors of eHealth usage: Insights on the digital divide from the Health Information National Trends Survey 2012. *Journal of Medical Internet Research*, 16(7), e172.

Kreuter, M. W., Farrell, D., Olevitch, L., & Brennan, L. (2000). *Tailoring health messages: Customizing communication with computer technology*. Mahwah, NJ: Erlbaum.

Lapsley, P., & Groves, T. (2004). The patient's journey: Travelling through life with a chronic illness. *BMJ*, 329, 582.

Mallari, B., Spaeth, E. K., Goh, H., & Boyd, B. S. (2019). Virtual reality as an analgesic for acute and chronic pain in adults: A systematic review and meta-analysis. *J Pain Res*, 12, 2053–2085. doi:10.2147/jpr.S200498

Matarazzo, J. D. (1980). Behavioral health and behavioral medicine: Frontiers for a new health psychology. *American Psychologist*, 35, 807–817.

Meurk, C., Leung, J., Hall, W., Head, B. W., & Whiteford, H. (2016). Establishing and governing e-mental health care in Australia: A systematic review of challenges and a call for policy-focussed research. *Journal of Medical Internet Research*, 18(1), e10.

Mohr, D. C., Schueller, S. M., Montague, E., Burns, M. N., & Rashidi, P. (2014). The behavioral intervention technology model: An integrated conceptual and technological framework for eHealth and mHealth interventions. *Journal of Medical Internet Research*, 16(6), e146.

Moyer, A., & Finney, J. W. (2004). Brief interventions for alcohol problems: Factors that facilitate implementation. *Alcohol Research & Health*, 28, 44–50.

Musiat, P., Johnson, C., Atkinson, M., Wilksch, S., & Wade, T. (2022). Impact of guidance on intervention adherence in computerised interventions for mental health problems: A meta-analysis. *Psychological Medicine*, 52(2), 229–240. https://doi.org/10.1017/S0033291721004621

Newman, M. G., Szkodny, L. E., Llera, S. J., & Przeworski, A. (2011). A review of technology-assisted self-help and minimal contact therapies for anxiety and depression: Is human contact necessary for therapeutic efficacy? *Clinical Psychology Review*, 31, 89–103.

Nguyen, H. Q., Carrieri-Kohlman, V., Rankin, S. H., Slaughter, R., & Stulbarg, M. S. (2004). Internet-based patient education and support interventions: A review of evaluation studies and directions for future research. *Computers in Biology and Medicine*, 34, 95–112.

Noar, S. M., Benac, C. N., & Harris, M. S. (2007). Does tailoring matter? Meta-analytic review of tailored print health behavior change interventions. *Psychological Bulletin*, 133, 673–693.

Ogden, J. (2012). *Health psychology: A textbook* (5th edition). Maidenhead, UK: Open University Press.

Pagliari, C. (2007). Design and evaluation in ehealth: Challenges and implications for an interdisciplinary field. *Journal of Medical Internet Research*, 9(2), e15.

Renn, B. N., Hoeft, T. J., Lee, H. S., Bauer, A. M., & Areán, P. A. (2019). Preference for in-person psychotherapy versus digital psychotherapy options for depression: Survey of adults in the U.S. *NPJ Digital Medicine*, 2, 6. https://doi.org/10.1038/s41746-019-0077-1

Richards, D., & Richardson, T. (2012). Computer-based psychological treatments for depression: A systematic review and meta-analysis. *Clinical Psychology Review*, 32, 329–342.

Ritterband, L. M., & Thorndike, F. (2006). Internet interventions or patient education web sites? *Journal of Medical Internet Research*, 8(3), e18.

Rose, G. (1985). Sick individuals and sick populations. *International Journal of Epidemiology*, 14, 32–38.

Schirmer, J. M., & Montegut, A. J. (2009). *Behavioral medicine in primary care: A global perspective*. New York, NY: Radcliffe Publishing.

Schubart, J. R., Stuckey, H. L., Ganeshamoorthy, A., & Sciamanna, C. N. (2011). Chronic health conditions and internet behavioral interventions: A review of factors to enhance user engagement. *Computers, Informatics, Nursing*, 29, TC9–T20.

Short, C. E., Smit, E. S., & Crutzen, R. (2022). Measuring psychological constructs in computer-tailored interventions: Novel possibilities to reduce participant burden and increase engagement. *The European Health Psychologist*, 22, 801–815.

Society of Behavioral Medicine. (2016). What is behavioral medicine? Retrieved from www.sbm.org/about/behavioral-medicine

Terpstra, J. A., van der Vaart, R., Spillekom-van Koulil, S., van Dam, A., Rosmalen, J. G. M., Knoop, H., van Middendorp, H., & Evers, A. W. M. (2018). Becoming an eCoach: Training therapists in online cognitive-behavioral therapy for chronic pain. *Patient Education and Counseling*, 101(9), 1702–1707. https://doi.org/10.1016/j.pec.2018.03.029

Terpstra, J. A., van der Vaart, R., van Beugen, S., van Eersel, R. A., Gkika, I., Erdős, D., Schmidt, J., Radstake, C., Kloppenburg, M., van Middendorp, H., & Evers, A. W. M. (2022). Guided internet-based cognitive-behavioral therapy for patients with chronic pain: A meta-analytic review. *Internet Interventions*, 30, 100587. https://doi.org/10.1016/j.invent.2022.100587

Beugen, S. van, Ferwerda, M., Hoeve, D., Rovers, M. M., Spillekom-van Koulil, S., van Middendorp, H., & Evers, A. W. M. (2014). Internet-based cognitive behavioral therapy for patients with chronic somatic conditions: A meta-analytic review. *Journal of Medical Internet Research*, 16(3), e88.

Van Beugen, S., Ferwerda, M., van Middendorp, H., Smit, J. V., Zeeuwen-Franssen, M. E. J., Kroft, E. B. M., … & Evers, A. W. M. (2019). Economic evaluation of a tailored therapist-guided internet-based cognitive behavioral treatment for patients with psoriasis: A randomized controlled trial. *British Journal of Dermatology*, 181(3), 614–616.

Van Beugen, S., Ferwerda, M., Spillekom-van Koulil, S., Smit, J. V., Zeeuwen-Franssen, M. E. J., Kroft, E. B. M., … & Evers, A. W. M. (2016). Tailored therapist-guided internet-based cognitive-behavioural treatment for psoriasis: A randomised controlled trial. *Psychotherapy & Psychosomatics*, 85, 297–307.

Van der Vaart, R., Atema, V., & Evers, A. W. M. (2016). Guided online self-management interventions in primary care: A survey on use, facilitators, and barriers. *BMC Family Practice*, 17, 27.

Van der Vaart, R., & Drossaert, C. H. C. (2017). Development of the Digital Health Literacy Instrument: Measuring a broad spectrum of Health 1.0 and Health 2.0 skills. *Journal of Medical Internet Research*, 19(1), e27.

Van Gemert-Pijnen, J. E. W. C., Nijland, N., van Limburg, M., Ossebaard, H. C., Eysenbach, G., & Seydel, E. R. (2011). A holistic framework to improve the uptake and impact of eHealth technologies. *Journal of Medical Internet Research*, 13(4), e111.

Venkatesh, V., Morris, M. G., Davis, G. B., & Davis, F. D. (2003). User acceptance of information technology: Toward a unified view. *MIS Quarterly*, 27, 425–478.

Vluggen, S., Candel, M., Hoving, C., Schaper, N. C., & de Vries, H. (2021). A web-based computer-tailored Program to Improve treatment adherence in patients with type 2 diabetes: Randomized controlled trial. *Journal of Medical Internet Research*, 23(2), e18524. https://doi.org/10.2196/18524

Vos, S., Janssen, M., Goudsmit, J., Lauwerijssen, C., & Brombacher, A. (2016). From problem to solution: Developing a personalized smartphone application for recreational runners following a three-step design approach. *Procedia Engineering*, 147, 799–805.

Wentzel, J., van der Vaart, R., Bohlmeijer, E. T., & van Gemert-Pijnen, J. E. W. C. (2016). Mixing online and face-to-face therapy: How to benefit from blended care in mental health care. *JMIR Mental Health*, 3(1), e9.

Wirken, L., van Middendorp, H., Hooghof, C. W., Bremer, T. E., Hopman, S. P. F., van der Pant, K. A. M. I., Hoitsma, A. J., Hilbrands, L. B., & Evers, A. W. M. (2018). Development and feasibility of a guided and tailored internet-based cognitive-behavioural intervention for kidney donors and kidney donor candidates. *BMJ Open*, 8(6), e020906. https://doi.org/10.1136/bmjopen-2017-020906

Xiong, S., Lu, H., Peoples, N., Duman, E. K., Najarro, A., Ni, Z., Gong, E., Yin, R., Ostbye, T., Palileo-Villanueva, L. M., Doma, R., Kafle, S., Tian, M., & Yan, L. L. (2023). Digital health interventions for non-communicable disease management in primary health care in low-and middle-income countries. *NPJ Digital Medicine*, 6(1), 12. https://doi.org/10.1038/s41746-023-00764-4

Part 2

eHealth Development, Implementation, and Evaluation

7 The CeHRes Roadmap

*Hanneke Kip, Nienke Beerlage-de Jong, Saskia M. Kelders, &
Lisette (J.E.W.C.) van Gemert-Pijnen*

Introduction

eHealth technologies are being used in different kinds of settings, for example in public, somatic, consumer, and mental health. There are often high expectations of these technologies. However, these expectations are often not met in practice – a lot of them stop being used because they are, for example, hard to understand for the user, require too much effort or time, do not have clear added value for users, or are simply too expensive. One explanation for these issues can be found in suboptimal development, implementation, and evaluation processes, in which insufficient attention is paid to the interrelationships between people, context, and technology. Even though more research is necessary, findings point to the fact that a holistic development, implementation, and evaluation process increases the chances of successful sustained use of effective eHealth technologies, thus increasing the likelihood of achieving the desired impact on health and healthcare. These processes are complex and multifaceted and are thus ideally guided by specific frameworks or models. This chapter is specifically focused on one of such models, which is especially suitable due to its focus on eHealth, interdisciplinary nature, and holistic, iterative approach towards development, implementation, and evaluation: The CeHRes Roadmap.

In this chapter, the CeHRes Roadmap – a framework for eHealth development, implementation, and evaluation – is explained. The Roadmap consists of six main phases: The contextual inquiry, value specification, design, operationalization, summative evaluation, and formative evaluation. The chapter starts with an explanation of the rationale behind the Roadmap. After that, each phase is explained, its objectives are stated, relevant concepts, methods, and activities are explained, and the types of outcomes one might expect from each phase are given. Furthermore, references to other chapters that provide more in-depth information and cases are provided. After reading this chapter, you will be able to:

- Explain the need for a holistic, iterative, and interdisciplinary development, implementation, and evaluation approach for eHealth technology;
- Describe and explain the pillars that underpin holistic eHealth development, implementation, and evaluation;
- Describe and define the six main phases of the CeHRes Roadmap, state their main objectives, and explain the rationale behind each phase;
- Explain how the phases of the CeHRes Roadmap are interrelated and why an iterative, agile development approach is important;

DOI: 10.4324/9781003302049-9

- List several suitable models and methods for eHealth development, implementation, and evaluation and explain the added value of a multi-method, interdisciplinary approach for each phase.

Holistic eHealth Development, Implementation, and Evaluation

Pillars Underpinning eHealth Development, Implementation, and Evaluation

Before presenting the different phases of the CeHRes Roadmap, we will first present the five pillars that underpin it (Figure 7.1). They are based on a review about existing eHealth frameworks (van Gemert-Pijnen et al., 2011), and updated with over a decade of experience with eHealth research guided by the CeHRes Roadmap (Kip et al., 2022), and frameworks, models and insights from different relevant disciplines such as human-centred design, implementation science, and psychology. Given this broad foundation, the methodologies, approaches, and underlying principles of these pillars are not just relevant for those working with the CeHRes Roadmap, but for any eHealth-related process, regardless of the specific framework that is used. An overview of the five pillars is provided below, after which they are explained in more detail.

eHealth development, implementation, and evaluation processes:

- Are ongoing and intertwined rather than phases containing separate and sequential activities;
- Require a holistic approach, focused on a fit between technology, people, and context;
- Require a multi-method, iterative approach with continuous evaluation cycles;
- Require constant active involvement of stakeholders;
- Are based on an interdisciplinary approach.

eHealth development, implementation and evaluation processes are ongoing and intertwined rather than phases containing separate and sequential activities

While it might sound like development, implementation, and evaluation are separate, consecutive stages, this is not the case: They are intertwined, interrelated activities that are all relevant from the start (Mohr, Lyon, Lattie, Reddy, & Schueller, 2017). The same goes for the phases of the CeHRes Roadmap: While, for overview purposes, they are visualized as separate activities, in reality the development, implementation, and evaluation are all intertwined (van Gemert-Pijnen et al., 2011). To illustrate: Too often, implementation is seen as a post-design activity, while attention should be paid to it from the start, for example by identifying potential implementation issues as early as possible to ensure that they can be accounted for during development. Furthermore, development activities of eHealth can also take place during evaluation, for example when new insights and points of improvement arise. Additionally, the evaluation process can already be initiated during

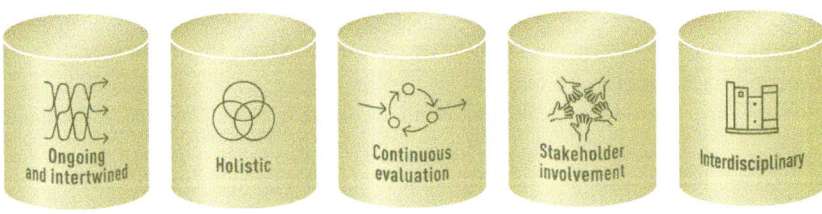

Figure 7.1 Pillars of the CeHRes Roadmap.

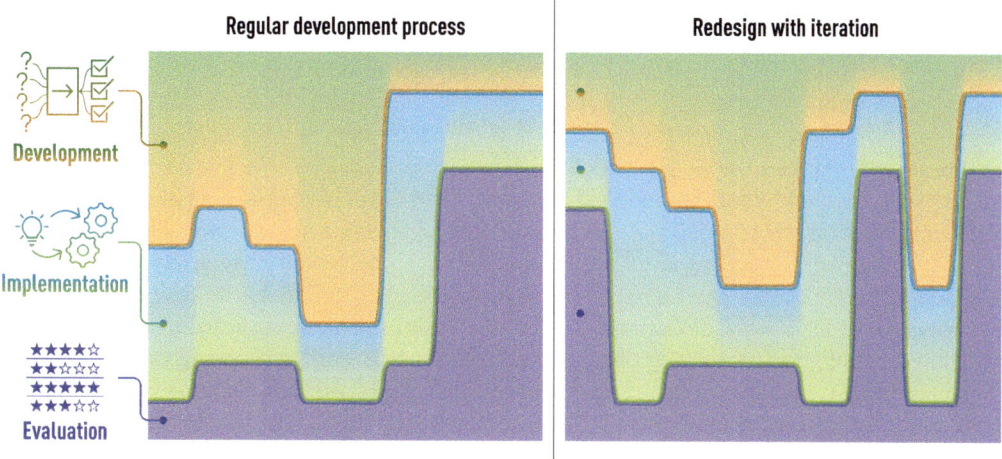

Figure 7.2 Illustration of two different ways of how development, implementation, and evaluation are ongoing and intertwined.

development, for example when a functioning prototype is used to first evaluate its underlying working mechanisms with a different target group, such as students, before it is further developed to optimally fit the intended (and more vulnerable or hard to reach) target group, e.g., psychiatric patients. Furthermore, goals that evaluation research should focus on are ideally specified during development. It is also possible to first conduct thorough evaluation studies to prove effectiveness before fully diving into implementation. During the entire process, a different process will be predominant, but activities from other stages will also be relevant to a lesser extent, as is visualized in Figure 7.2.

As the explanation above already illustrates, it is important to note that eHealth development, implementation, and evaluation processes are never really finished: There will always be room for improvement or updates of the content or design of a technology, there will almost always be a need for more and better implementation strategies, and new questions for evaluating the impact and uptake of a technology will always keep arising. However, this does describe an ideal situation. In practice this is often difficult because of limited resources such as time or money, because a (research) project ends, or because a technology is not of added value and further investments are not considered worthwhile.

eHealth development, implementation, and evaluation processes require a holistic approach, focused on a fit between technology, people, and context

Regardless of the type or goal of an eHealth intervention, there are interrelationships between the design and content of a technology, the needs and preferences of the people involved, and the context in which it is used. While more research is necessary, it seems that a good fit between technology, people, and context increases the chances of successful adoption and sustained use (Nielsen & Mathiassen, 2013 Kip et al., 2019). These interrelationships warrant a holistic approach, in which different elements are all interdependent and part of one whole instead of separate constructs. Because individual elements in a complex system are determined by the relation they have to other elements, separate analysis of its parts should be avoided (James, 1984).

With regard to eHealth, technology, context, and people are interrelated and should not be viewed (and studied) as separate elements. First, technology and the behaviour of people are interrelated. The introduction and sustained use of technology ideally influences the way end-users behave, resulting in, for example, better health outcomes or increased well-being. To enable this behaviour change, users should be adherent, which means that eHealth should be used as intended – this can be viewed as usage behaviour. In order to promote the successful use of eHealth, it is important to investigate and improve the way in which people use and interact with – in other words, behave within – a technology. Concepts such as engagement – the extent to which someone is involved or occupied with an eHealth technology from an emotional, behavioural, and cognitive perspective – are important to account for to ensure adherence and behaviour change (Kelders, Van Zyl, & Ludden, 2020). Second, the use of eHealth is never isolated, but influences and is influenced by the context in which it is used. The introduction of eHealth creates novel structures and processes for healthcare delivery; an adapted or new ecosystem for healthcare emerges (Eysenbach, 2001). Examples of these changes are a shift from hospital- to home-based care enabled by remote patient monitoring systems, or the emergence of shared decision making in healthcare enabled by the rise of personal health records. Furthermore, since a technology is never finished, its design and content ideally change over time to increase the fit with the context and/or incorporate changes (Mohr, Weingardt, Reddy, & Schueller, 2017). To illustrate: After introduction in practice, the content of Internet-based interventions can be rephrased and shortened to better fit the cognitive skills of users, or content can be adapted to be in line with revised treatment guidelines.

eHealth development, implementation, and evaluation processes require a multi-method, iterative approach with continuous evaluation cycles

In order to do justice to the holistic, multifaceted, and complex nature of eHealth, its development, implementation, and evaluation should not be viewed as linear processes with consecutive steps: They are iterative, flexible, and dynamic, with constant changes to the process and products (Hekler et al., 2016; Patrick et al., 2016). This is in line with an agile approach, which currently is common practice in software development. Such an approach is characterized by the division of large tasks into rapid, shorter phases and constant adaptations of plans based on the outcomes of evaluations. Core values are close collaboration, a 'lean' mentality to minimize unnecessary work, active stakeholder involvement, and the acceptance of uncertainty (Dingsøyr, Nerur, Balijepally, & Moe, 2012). In order to apply an agile approach to eHealth, a multi-method approach is key. Researchers need to be able to draw from a broad toolkit of both qualitative and quantitative research methods and products, and select the method that best fits their research objective, the practical demands from the context, and the characteristics and needs and wishes of the participants (Kip et al., 2022). It is important to ensure that the selected methods fit within the entire process and are related to each other. To ensure such a coherent approach and to prevent the project team from 'getting lost', there is a need for continuous formative evaluations in which outcomes of activities are critically analyzed, evaluated, and adapted (Michie, Yardley, West, Patrick, & Greaves, 2017). Constant evaluation in which stakeholders are actively involved can also ensure a good fit with the stakeholders and their context. Within each method, the project team should always strive to gain insight into the perspective and characteristics of the context and users. Moreover, it is important to carefully consider the combination of different methods and to check if and how findings from different methods are consistent with and build upon each other. This can take on different forms, for example, verifying outcomes of a phase with users, checking if outcomes still match the outcomes of previous phases, or gathering stakeholders' opinions on a specific idea for a next phase.

An agile approach might seem like a contradiction to a rigorous scientific approach in which all research activities are meticulously planned (and sometimes even published) in advance. While agile science can indeed be challenging and complex, it is not a synonym for unstructured or messy: It is a way to shape systematic, structured yet dynamic high-quality research processes that are able to deal with changes and new insights (Dingsøyr et al., 2012). Consequently, while a broad research plan with potentially suitable methods can of course be developed, it might be necessary to deviate from this plan based on outcomes of specific methods or new insights regarding the needs of stakeholders or possibilities of a technology. However, as is the case for any scientific activity, it is important to remain transparent: The project team should carefully map all steps, choices, and reasons for that, also to ensure that others can learn from their experiences (Kip et al., 2022).

eHealth development, implementation, and evaluation processes require constant active involvement of stakeholders

In order to create eHealth that meets the needs and wishes of users and other stakeholders, a participatory approach is recommended, in which stakeholders are actively involved throughout the entire process (Bartholomew et al., 2006; Beerlage-de Jong, Wentzel, Hendrix, & van Gemert-Pijnen, 2017; Wentzel et al., 2014; Yardley, Morrison, Bradbury, & Muller, 2015). Participatory development goes beyond merely involving end-users such as patients or healthcare providers, because this might cause a dominance of the user perspective and might lead to overlooking the needs of other stakeholders (Bødker, Kensing, & Simonsen, 2009). Stakeholders such as managers, healthcare insurers, and technology developers should be involved as well to ensure a holistic approach (van Woezik, Braakman-Jansen, Kulyk, Siemons, & van Gemert-Pijnen, 2016). Amongst other things, stakeholders can provide input when identifying problems where technology can be of added value, improving the design of a technology, or identifying boundary conditions for integration in existing healthcare systems. In participatory development, the roles of a stakeholder can range from an informant that mostly provides input on products when invited by researchers, to a co-creator that is actively involved in creating ideas and products (Scaife, Rogers, Aldrich, & Davies, 1997). Stakeholders can (or should) also be part of an interdisciplinary project team that coordinates the entire eHealth process.

A participatory approach is not just important for development: Stakeholders should also be actively involved in implementation processes, for example in setting implementation objectives, identifying strategies, designing implementation material, and evaluating the progress and outcomes of an implementation. Additionally, different groups of stakeholders should also be actively involved in evaluation: To ensure a value-based approach in which technology is aligned with the needs of stakeholders, it is important to evaluate with instead of for the target group (O'Cathain et al., 2019). This means for example that the values that were formulated in close collaboration with stakeholders during the development process should be evaluated. Finally, participatory development does not always have to be about creating new technologies, since existing technologies can be redesigned and reused in different contexts as well, which also requires active stakeholder involvement. As a final note, it is important to emphasize that stakeholders should only be involved when it is necessary: Merely involving end-users for the sake of involving end-users is not of added value and takes up valuable time of participants and researchers (van Velsen et al., 2022). This requires careful consideration and clearly set objectives by the project team.

eHealth development, implementation, and evaluation processes are based on an interdisciplinary approach

In order to capture the complexity of eHealth, an interdisciplinary approach towards research and development is required (Michie et al., 2017). In such an approach, theories, methods, and models from different disciplines are combined and ideally merged, resulting in new approaches, concepts, and models. It is important to make the distinction with a multidisciplinary approach. In a multidisciplinary approach, input is provided by different disciplines, but this is done independently from each other – there is not much integration of different methods, approaches, or theories and people remain working within the boundaries of their discipline. In an interdisciplinary approach, input from different disciplines is actively integrated, aiming to create a synergy that goes beyond the sum of individual contributions. To achieve this, interdisciplinary teams actively work together and aim to blend their approaches. Ideally, eHealth development, implementation, and evaluation are interdisciplinary since their holistic nature requires an integrated approach.

There are multiple paradigms that are relevant for an interdisciplinary approach towards eHealth, a (not exhaustive) overview of which is given in Table 7.1.

Table 7.1 An overview of (some of the) disciplines that are relevant for eHealth development, implementation, and evaluation.

Discipline	Importance	Example contribution	Further reading
Psychology	Accounting for the behaviour, emotions, and cognitions of end-users and other stakeholders.	Theories from, for example, health psychology can be used to explain the behaviour that needs to be changed and support behaviour change (Michie et al., 2013); research methods grounded in psychology such as interviews can be used as well (Bonten et al., 2020).	Chapter 2, Chapter 16
Human-centred design	Ensuring that the eHealth technology fits with the needs, skills, and characteristics of its end-users and other stakeholders.	Methods (e.g., usability tests) and products (e.g. prototypes) from human-centred design can be used to design and evaluate a technology that has the best user experience and usability, which will increase the chances of implementation and impact in practice (Giacomin, 2014; Göttgens & Oertelt-Prigione, 2021).	Chapter 11
Persuasive technology	Developing a technology that increases chances of behaviour change.	Specific persuasive features (e.g. feedback, personalization) can be integrated into a design to increase the chances of adherence and resulting attitude- and behaviour change (Fogg, 2002; Kelders, Kok, Ossebaard, & van Gemert-Pijnen, 2012; Oinas-Kukkonen & Harjumaa, 2009).	Chapter 12
Engineering	Designing and evaluating eHealth with methods and approaches that account for the characteristics of technology.	Methods such as agile science, requirement engineering, and log data analysis can be used to develop and evaluate eHealth technologies (van Velsen, Wentzel, & van Gemert-Pijnen, 2013). It is recommended that behavioural scientists understand the basics of these models and other technology-related aspects (e.g., coding) to ensure that they speak the language of developers.	Chapter 3, Chapter 9
Implementation science	Systematic planning and evaluating implementation of eHealth to ensure integration in practice.	Implementation frameworks such as the CFIR and NASSS, that account for implementation factors in different levels – the intervention, the people involved, and the inner and outer contexts (Damschroder, Reardon, Widerquist, & Lowery, 2022; Greenhalgh et al., 2017), can be used to shape implementation processes.	Chapter 13
Business modelling	Ensuring that a technology is financially feasible and of added value for its context.	Business models such as the Business Model Canvas can be used to determine a value proposition early on and ensure that it is operationalized during implementation (Osterwalder & Pigneur, 2010; van Limburg, Wentzel, Sanderman, & van Gemert-Pijnen, 2015).	Chapter 10
Domain-specific theories	Making sure that the eHealth technology is consistent with guidelines and up-to-date knowledge of the specific domain.	Domain-specific theories and models such as guidelines for cognitive behavioural therapy (CBT) in mental healthcare and knowledge about risk factors for disorders such as depression can be used when developing interventions for that specific context.	Not applicable – depends on domain

The interdisciplinary nature of eHealth is also important when composing the project team that coordinates the development process. Putting together a team with members from different disciplines is deemed essential to ensure that all relevant perspectives are actively involved in the development, implementation, and evaluation and to prevent tunnel vision (Feldman, Schooley, & Bhavsar, 2014; O'Cathain et al., 2019). Two different types of people can be involved: Professionals with knowledge on eHealth development, such as designers, project managers, researchers, and engineers, and people who are expert on the domain in which the eHealth intervention will be used, such as patients, healthcare professionals, or managers (Kip, Kelders, Bouman, & van Gemert-Pijnen, 2019).

The CeHRes Roadmap

eHealth has multiple proven and potential benefits, but there are still many barriers. As mentioned before, thorough development, implementation, and evaluation of eHealth can (partly) help to overcome these barriers. In 2011, a review on the potential and limitations of existing eHealth frameworks was conducted to investigate their value in overcoming these barriers (van Gemert-Pijnen et al., 2011). An important outcome was that it was assumed that barriers can mostly be avoided by applying a participatory development process that creates a good fit between technological, human, and contextual factors. However, most existing frameworks were found to have a rather conceptual approach instead of practical guidelines, were sequential as opposed to iterative, and lacked the stakeholder-driven approach. Consequently, based on this review, the pillars and phases of the CeHRes Roadmap were developed.

The CeHRes Roadmap (Figure 7.3) serves as a guideline for the development, implementation, and evaluation of eHealth technology that fits the people and their context. It assists the project team in planning, coordinating, and executing the sustainable creation of eHealth technologies (van Gemert-Pijnen et al., 2011). This can refer not only to 'new' technologies that are developed from scratch, but also to the improvement of existing technologies – or even the critical analysis of an already conducted development, implementation, and/or evaluation process. The Roadmap consists of five interrelated phases and connecting cycles. These phases are the *contextual inquiry, value specification, design, operationalization,* and *summative evaluation.* Connecting all these phases are continuous *formative evaluation* cycles which can also be viewed as a phase in itself. It ensures that activities during a phase are related to the stakeholder perspective, the context, and outcomes of previous phases. In this chapter, an updated version of the Roadmap is presented. The

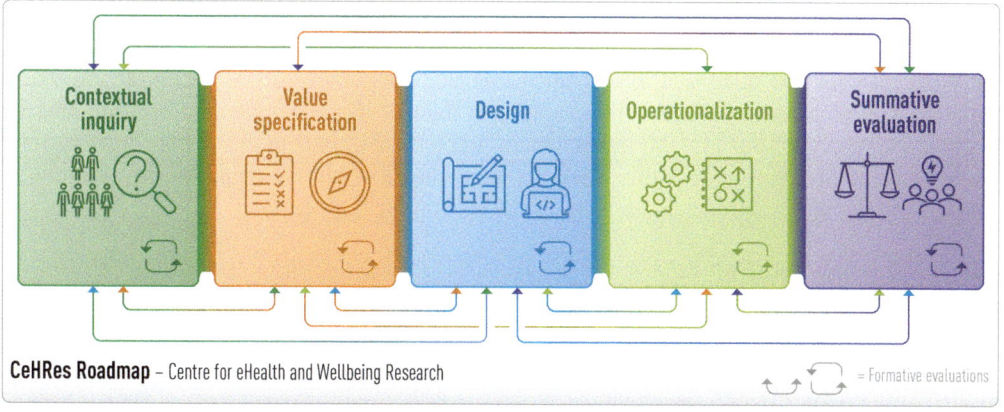

Figure 7.3 The CeHRes Roadmap.

phases have remained the same as in the original version, but their main objectives and accompanying methods and frameworks are revised and updated based on new insights from research and over a decade of experience with working with the CeHRes Roadmap.

Strictly speaking, the first three phases of the Roadmap are related to development of eHealth, operationalization fits best with implementation, and summative and formative evaluation are most aligned with the evaluation phase. However, this distinction is made for visualization and overview purposes – in reality the phases overlap and are intertwined. Furthermore, as is the case with any roadmap, the CeHRes Roadmap is not a checklist or step-by-step approach for developing, implementing, and evaluating eHealth technologies. It is a visualization of an approach and a tool to help researchers and practitioners in shaping their own, unique processes. Finally, the CeHRes Roadmap is not the only model that can be used for eHealth development. There are different types of these models, such as Intervention Mapping (Bartholomew et al., 2006), the person-based approach (Yardley et al., 2015), and the Accelerated Creation-to-Sustainment model (Mohr et al., 2017). These models have some differences, but also many similarities with the Roadmap. Depending on the skills and preferences of the project team, other models can be used, partly supplemented with elements of the Roadmap, or a combination of both models can be generated.

Organization of this Chapter

The upcoming sections of this chapter are focused on the phases of the CeHRes Roadmap. For each phase, the following aspects will be described in separate sections:

- **Description of the phase**
  In this section, a brief description of the phase, its background, and its relation with the entire development process is provided;
- **Objectives**
  This paragraph briefly states the objectives of that phase, which logically arise from the description of the phase;
- **Concepts, methods, and activities**
  This paragraph is structured by the previously stated objectives. For each objective, relevant concepts, methods, and/or activities are described to give an idea of how the objectives of the phase can be reached. Concepts can be models, theories, or approaches. They have to be understood to get a good idea of the rationale behind the methods and activities that can be used.

How Should this Chapter be Read?

The methods presented in this chapter are not an exhaustive list: Other methods might also be used if they are relevant and suitable. Consequently, this chapter's main goal is to provide the reader with insight into the main objectives of the phases of the CeHRes Roadmap and does not provide a step-by-step approach for eHealth development, implementation, and evaluation. In case more in-depth information is required, this book contains chapters that elaborate on the disciplines, methods, and principles introduced here, as can be seen in the table below.

Contextual Inquiry

What is the Contextual Inquiry Phase?

The first step in any eHealth development project is a thorough investigation of the context in which it will be used. In order for an eHealth technology to be successful, it should provide a solution for relevant issues, it should be accepted by (groups of) people such as the users, funders,

Table 7.2 Phases of the CeHRes Roadmap and accompanying chapters.

Phase	Chapter(s)
Contextual inquiry	8 – The Contextual Inquiry
Value specification	9 – Activities for Value Sensitive eHealth Design
	10 – Business Modelling
Design	11 – Human-centred design
	12 – Persuasive Health Technology
Operationalization	13 – Innovation, Improvement, and Implementation – Conceptual Frameworks for Thinking through Complex Change
	14 – Sustainable eHealth Implementation: A Practical Perspective
Summative evaluation	15 – Engagement
	16 – eHealth Evaluation

and policy makers, and it should fit the physical, social, and cultural environment in which it will be used (Glasgow, Phillips, & Sanchez, 2014; Michie et al., 2017). Consequently, a contextual inquiry is necessary to paint a complete picture of the current situation and to pinpoint the most relevant points of improvement that could potentially be addressed with an eHealth technology. A contextual inquiry assists in keeping a focus on the people and their environment from the start (Holtzblatt & Jones, 2017; Wentzel, 2015). In order to achieve this, first an identification and analysis of relevant stakeholders – i.e. (groups of) people who affect or are affected by the potential eHealth technology – has to be conducted.

When an initial list of stakeholders is completed, an overview of the current situation and points of improvement must be created. This overview is created by means of multiple methods, allowing the project team to gain a good understanding of prospective users' daily lives or work routines, the perspectives and ideas of other involved stakeholders, their environments, and any practical organizational constraints such as rules and regulations (Sjöström, von Essen, & Grönqvist, 2014). Besides merely describing a situation, points of improvement for which an eHealth technology could be of added value have to be mapped as well. The outcomes of the contextual inquiry serve as the foundation for the rest of the development, implementation, and evaluation process.

Objectives of the Contextual Inquiry Phase

The contextual inquiry has several main objectives:

1. To identify and gain insight into the roles and activities of relevant stakeholders;
2. To analyze the current situation regarding the involved people's daily lives and behaviour, organizational characteristics and structures, relevant policies and legislation, and potentially useful existing technologies;
3. To identify the main point(s) of improvement for which an eHealth technology could be a solution.

Concepts, Methods, and Activities in the Contextual Inquiry Phase

1. Stakeholder identification and analysis

During every phase of eHealth development, stakeholders should be actively involved. That is why one of the first activities that should be undertaken is a stakeholder identification. There are many different kinds of stakeholders, for example, users, researchers, policy makers, funders, insurance companies, and designers. To make sure every stakeholder is identified, multiple methods can be used and combined (van Woezik et al., 2016). Some commonly used methods are:

- *Literature study*. Stakeholders can be identified by systematically reviewing or rapidly scanning the literature, for example, about stakeholder theories or involved stakeholders in development of similar eHealth technologies;
- *Expert recommendations*. Experts from the field can be asked to nominate stakeholders they consider relevant;
- *Snowball sampling with stakeholders*. Once a preliminary list of stakeholders is created, it is valuable to ask them to supplement the list.

Once an initial overview is created, the stakeholders should be analyzed. There are several ways to conduct a stakeholder analysis (van Woezik et al., 2016). One frequently used framework is that of stakeholder salience (Mitchell, Agle, & Wood, 1997). In this approach, stakeholders can be mapped based on their power, legitimacy, and urgency. They can be ranked by both the project team and other stakeholders (also see Chapter 8). Based on this analysis and – if necessary – other methods, *key stakeholders* can be selected. The main reason for this is that not every stakeholder will be equally important for the eHealth technology, and intensively involving each stakeholder requires too many resources. The selection of key stakeholders can be made solely by the project team (which should of course include stakeholders), but also by letting a group of stakeholders who are not part of the team decide on who the key stakeholders are (van Woezik et al., 2016). It is important to keep in mind that the initial overview of stakeholders is definitely not final, since it should be updated throughout the remainder of the process.

2. Analysis of the current situation

To ensure that the project team knows for whom and for what context they are creating eHealth, a thorough understanding of the current situation is essential. The exact context is part of the contextual inquiry as well. Besides the perspectives and opinions of the stakeholders on the current situation, the context can include the rules, regulations, organizational culture, ethical issues, and other important matters that have to be considered during the development (Sjöström et al., 2014). Examples of broad research questions related to people, the context, and technology are:

- What is (and is not) part of the context within this project?
- What does the delivered care look like? What is the patient journey, and what (treatment) protocols are used by healthcare providers?
- What rules, regulations, guidelines, and ethical themes play a role within the relevant organizations?
- What does the behaviour of the intended end-users look like? What are the determinants of their behaviour, and what theories can be used to analyse and explain their behaviour?
- What are important domain-specific theories, frameworks, or models?
- What technologies are used within the context and what are the users' experiences?
- What is known about potentially useful technologies in terms of technological possibilities, working mechanisms, and experiences in other contexts?

Throughout this entire process, it is important to integrate scientific and grey literature, theories and frameworks, and the perspective of the involved people because combining multiple sources results in a more comprehensive overview. An overview of potentially useful methods is provided in the next section.

3. Identification of points of improvement

Merely describing a context does not suffice: The project team needs to gain insight into points of improvement that can be addressed by the to-be-developed eHealth technology. When doing this, it is important to specifically describe the behaviour that needs to be improved and identify accompanying determinants that can be targeted with an intervention (also see Chapter 2). A (simplified) example of a behaviour is the prescription of antibiotics, and accompanying determinants that arise from literature and theories might be knowledge and attitudes of healthcare providers. Besides using research and theory, it is essential to thoroughly involve the stakeholders. By combining methods, insight can be gained into what needs to be changed from an individual and organizational perspective. This also helps in identifying the initial conditions for implementation, which shows that implementation is relevant from the start of a development process. Implementation barriers such as limited financial resources or low literacy skills of prospective end users can be identified in the contextual inquiry to ensure that they are accounted for in upcoming phases. Examples of methods that can be used in the contextual inquiry are (Kip et al., 2022):

- *Desk research.* This method is useful to map existing, non-scientific documents such as protocols, news articles, or internal communication about relevant topics, such as a specific situation, regulations, or technology;*Systematic literature review.* A systematic search of scientific literature can be conducted to find out about the current state of affairs of a specific topic from a scientific point of view. Examples are determinants for the behaviour that has to be changed, an overview of eHealth interventions within a specific field, or possibilities and working mechanisms of a specific eHealth technology that is considered to be developed;
- *Focus groups.* Structured group discussions with one or multiple groups of stakeholders can be organized to, for example, identify problems and strong points of the current way of delivering care;
- *Interviews.* Interviews, guided by an interview scheme, can be conducted with stakeholders to identify their individual perspectives on a certain situation, for example about problems with current use of technology;
- *Observation.* Observing daily practice within a context can reveal relevant, ecologically valid information about the designated end users of the eHealth technology and their daily tasks, issues, and preferences.

It is important to note that these methods are often combined and complement each other, and are often also used for both this and the previous phase (i.e., to analyze the situation and immediately also identify points of improvement). As is the case for any part of eHealth development, there is not one correct way to conduct this process. The selected methods should fit the research questions, skills, and needs of the participants (e.g., lower cognitive skills, stigma regarding the disorder), and practical limitations of the context (e.g., shortage of staff, geographical distances). The better the researcher understands their stakeholders, the better they can select suitable methods, which is another advantage of paying much attention to getting to know the context (Schouten et al., 2022).

Outcomes of the Contextual Inquiry Phase

In line with the three objectives, a well-performed contextual inquiry has three main outcomes. The first is an overview of stakeholders, which can be visualized in a stakeholder map. In this map, similar stakeholders can be grouped together, key-stakeholders can be pointed out, and relationships can be visualized. Second, an overview of the current situation should be created. The way this is documented, presented, and summarized will differ per project, one example of this is a patient journey. Third, the main points of improvement for which a technology might be of added value should be described. This can range from one to multiple relevant issues. The identified points of improvement can be related to, for example, *efficiency*, *effectiveness*, timely delivery of care, or safety of healthcare.

The contextual inquiry lays the groundwork for the remainder of the development, implementation, and evaluation processes. The choices that are made in the contextual inquiry regarding the issue(s) that a technology should address will be elaborated on and made more specific and concrete in the value specification. The design phase is also grounded in the contextual inquiry, since the technology should address the problem(s) and accompanying behaviour that were described in the contextual inquiry, it has to fit within the organizational structures, and should be in line with the needs of the identified stakeholders. In the operationalization phase, implementation strategies should be designed with and for the stakeholders and with a keen eye on their fit within the specific context. For example, the foundation for an implementation plan can already be created in the contextual inquiry by identifying elements that need to be accounted for when using a technology within a specific organization – i.e., an initial identification of implementation factors such as limited resources or the importance of integration in treatment protocols (Kip et al., 2019). Finally, in the summative evaluation phase, it should be determined whether the identified point(s) of improvement(s) were actually improved, again by involving relevant stakeholders. While it is often overlooked or underestimated, a contextual inquiry provides the foundation for any eHealth development process by ensuring insight into what is needed to enable a good fit between the people, organization, and technology.

Value Specification

What is the Value Specification Phase?

The outcomes of the contextual inquiry provide a broad, general idea of the added value that a certain technology might have. However, these outcomes are not concrete enough to specify what is needed from or asked of an actual technology. In the value specification, the identified topics are narrowed down and translated into specific requirements for a technology. This is again done in close cooperation with stakeholders that were identified in the contextual inquiry – but in addition to that new stakeholders might pop up in this phase. The value specification supports the project team in becoming as precise and concrete as possible in terms of what a technology should do and look like. In order to achieve this, several activities have to be performed. As is almost always the case, these activities are often performed in parallel to each other, can be combined, and are related to activities of earlier or later phases.

The name of this phase already indicates that values have to be formulated to summarize the needs, ideals, and interests of all key-stakeholders. Besides the stakeholder perspective, it is also important to consider evidence-based elements that can be added to a technology to support behaviour change. In addition to that, in this stage the identified values are used to formulate requirements to specify what the technology should do, look like, and how it should be delivered. Furthermore, the project team needs to initiate the development of a business model to plan and operationalize the integration of an eHealth technology in practice. In the value specification, first versions of these products are generated to gain insight into the added value of the technology. The value specification phase is quite complex, but also essential for good eHealth development, since the goals and scope of the technology should be clear before it is actually designed and used in practice.

A comprehensive overview of values is pivotal for further stages since they support the project team in constantly checking whether the technology is still in line with these values.

Objectives of the Value Specification Phase

The value specification has several objectives:

1. To formulate and prioritize values from all identified key-stakeholders and set concrete goals based on these values;
2. To select initial behaviour change techniques (BCTs) and persuasive features that fit with the values and needs of the key-stakeholders features;
3. To translate the values into specific requirements to describe the to-be-developed eHealth technology;
4. To create a first version of a business model for the eHealth technology.

Concepts, Methods, and Activities in the Value Specification Phase

1. Formulate and prioritize values and objectives

While there are many definitions of values, in relation to value-sensitive design, values can be viewed as things that are important to people in their personal lives, related to for example ethics and morality (also see Chapter 9). Relating this to eHealth, values also incorporate what stakeholders find important regarding the technology from their own, personal perspective. In other words: Values represent ideals or interests of stakeholders and summarize what they find important on an abstract level (van Velsen et al., 2013). They assist the project team in specifying what stakeholders want to achieve or improve via a technology, which implies that values are aligned with the point(s) of improvement that were identified in the contextual inquiry. Values can be related to social, behavioural, cognitive, emotional, economic, or healthcare issues. Examples are saving costs, personalized care, increasing efficiency of care, increasing access to healthcare, improved decision-support for healthcare professionals, autonomy, improving specific health-outcomes, or improved self-image (Asbjørnsen et al., 2020; Kip, Kelders, & van Gemert-Pijnen, 2019). Since values can remain quite abstract, it is important to add specific definitions to ensure a shared understanding (Kip, Kelders, & van Gemert-Pijnen, 2019).

Values can be uncovered through several methods, such as interviews or focus groups. Combining multiple methods can be helpful to paint a complete picture of the values of all key-stakeholders. When collecting data, it can be helpful to discuss concrete examples of existing or potential technologies, since discussing values in an abstract way can be very complex. This is also an illustration of overlap with the design phase, because prototypes of potential eHealth technologies are often used in both phases (Kip, Kelders, & van Gemert-Pijnen, 2019). Since multiple stakeholders should be involved in this process, conflicting values might arise. For example, managers might have different interests than patients: They might emphasize cost-saving, while patients require a very personalized approach that could be quite expensive. Such conflicting values should be identified as early as possible and can be discussed with an interdisciplinary project team to make a decision on what to prioritize.

Values can be used as a foundation for specific objectives that should be reached by the eHealth technology. These objectives are ideally formulated in a SMART way (specific, measurable, achievable, realistic, and timely) and serve as the basis for the evaluation of the technology. Connecting values to objectives helps to ensure that the stakeholder perspectives are involved in the goals of the project and the accompanying evaluation studies. Of course, these objectives can (and should) be further defined throughout the process, but explicitly formulating them early on helps to keep the process focused.

2. Select behaviour change techniques and persuasive features

eHealth interventions almost always aim to support behaviour change. However, this has appeared to be very difficult to achieve, not just because changing behaviour in itself is difficult, but also because it is challenging to ensure that users remain engaged and adhere to the intervention. In order to increase the chances of adherence, engagement, and behaviour change, behaviour change techniques (BCTs) and persuasive features can be integrated in the technology. BCTs are derived from behaviour change theories from psychology and can be defined as a general technique to influence or create changes in the predictors of specific behaviour (Michie et al., 2013), also see Chapter 2. In the free BCT taxonomy app, 93 evidence-based BCTs are described, which are divided into multiple overarching categories, such as Goals and planning, Social support, Feedback and Monitoring, and Reward and Threat. Persuasive features are part of the Persuasive System Design (PSD) model and are divided into four categories (Oinas-Kukkonen & Harjumaa, 2009), also see Chapter 12: Primary task support, Dialogue support, Credibility support, and Social support. Furthermore, it might be relevant to also use domain-specific theories that were identified in the contextual inquiry. To illustrate: According to existing models on risk assessment and management for treatment of offenders, risk factors such as impulsiveness or intoxication play an important role in treatment of delinquent behaviour, which means that they could be integrated into eHealth interventions that target that specific behaviour.

BCTs partly overlap with persuasive techniques since they both target behaviour change, but the main difference is that the PSD is specifically aimed at technology, while BCTs are applicable to any kind of behaviour change intervention. Furthermore, BCTs are explicitly linked to psychological behaviour change theories. BCTs and persuasive features can be combined since they can complement each other. For example, the BCT 'feedback and monitoring' can be combined with the PSD 'tunnelling', in which the user is guided through a system/process, to facilitate the user experience.

To be able to select the most appropriate BCTs, persuasive techniques, and other features based on domain-specific theories, it is important to clearly identify the main objectives of a technology and the values of its user. Getting from these values to specific behaviour change mechanisms is an iterative process that will also play an important part in the design and evaluation phases of the Roadmap. However, the foundation for this is laid in the value specification phase. An important reason for this is that behaviour change mechanisms should be aligned with user needs, and not just be selected by researchers, as is often the case (Asbjørnsen et al., 2019). For example, the identified values can rule out some BCTs or persuasive features, e.g., a value related to cooperation might rule out the persuasive feature competition. Additionally, values can also provide insight into how to apply specific BCTs or features to a technology. For example, if 'privacy' is an important value and comparison of behaviour seems to be an effective BCT, it is important to do this without sharing personal information. The identified values can be connected to an initial set of suitable BCTs and persuasive features. For example, the value 'Feeling supported' can be identified in focus groups, via quotes such as '*It is really important that the technology motivates and supports me to keep up*'. Based on this value and accompanying quotes, the BCT 'feedback and monitoring' can be used, as well as the persuasive feature 'praise', to ensure a positive, motivating approach (Asbjørnsen et al., 2020). Previously collected data on values, e.g., quotes from interviews, can help the project team in selecting and operationalizing suitable BCTs. Consequently, identifying values, connecting them to BCTs and persuasive features, operationalizing them in a prototype, and updating and fine-tuning them is an iterative process. The project team has to be aware of the fact that the initially identified BCTs and persuasive features will probably change throughout the remainder of the process: It is possible that some techniques are not feasible to integrate in a technology, new ideas for features might arise during the design process, or something might not be technically feasible.

3. Formulate specific requirements

Requirements describe what an eHealth technology should do, what data it should store or retrieve, what content it should display, and what kind of user experience it should provide. In other words, they are the instructions for developers that tell them how to create a technology that provides value to the end-user (also see Chapter 9). The following types of requirements can be identified: Functional and modality; Service; Organizational; Content; and Usability and user experience requirements.

As is the case with most eHealth activities, there is no clear step-by-step approach that can be followed to develop requirements. Usually, requirements are formulated by the project team, based on, for example, previously or newly conducted focus groups, interviews, questionnaires, literature reviews, card sorting, or comparable studies. Regardless of the methodology, it is always necessary to thoroughly involve the stakeholders, build upon earlier identified outcomes, and add at least one source to show on what data the requirement is based. Since values are more abstract, they can be used to group specific requirements to verify whether all important values are represented in the requirements. The other way around, groups of requirements can also be used to formulate values. As is the case with most eHealth-products, this is an iterative, dynamic process for which no step-by-step guideline is available.

A specific product that can help to design for the end-users and facilitate requirement formulation, is a persona. Personas are 'hypothetical archetypes of actual users' and are presented by means of a short biography with a photo and the goals they have in life or with regard to their work or medical condition (LeRouge et al., 2013; Ten Klooster et al., 2022). Personas can also include the previously identified values. One or more personas can be created to offer a concrete way to keep the end-user in mind when formulating requirements – but they are of course also useful for further steps. However, personas only describe end-users, but do not link them to the technology. This is where scenarios can be useful. Scenarios describe the potential, envisioned use of an eHealth technology by the end-users. Scenarios can contain information about how the end-user uses a technology in relation to their characteristics and values, what activities are supported by a technology, which steps a user follows, in which context this happens, and what the main functionalities that a technology offers are (Rosson & Carroll, 2002). There are of course other types of products that can support developers in formulating requirements, such as use cases or card sorting, depending on the skills and preferences of the project team.

4. Create a first version of a business model

Many eHealth projects suffer from the 'field of dreams' syndrome, in which a project team simply presupposes that users will show up spontaneously as soon as the technology is made available (van Limburg, Wentzel, Sanderman, & van Gemert-Pijnen, 2015). This shows a lack of understanding of important implementation issues like reimbursement dynamics, how much money to ask for the technology, or consumers' willingness to pay for the service (Miron-Shatz, Shatz, Becker, Patel, & Eysenbach, 2014). To prevent this, it is important to start developing a business model as soon as possible. A business model can be defined as 'the rationale of how an organization creates, delivers, and captures value' (Osterwalder & Pigneur, 2010). It can guide the implementation processes and clarifies the costs and benefits (values) for stakeholders. It is important to note that values in relation to a business model often have a narrower (and monetary) definition than those used during value specification activities, which again highlights the importance of using clear definitions and reaching a shared understanding about what values are, amongst the project team.

A frequently used method to create a business model is the business model canvas (Osterwalder & Pigneur, 2010). A business model consists of nine blocks. One block is focused on the value proposition – which is the eHealth technology. The three blocks on the left side (key partners, key activities, and key resources) show the required organizational aspects that are necessary to deliver the value to practice. Three other blocks help the team to identify who the main customers or users are, and what the best way of interacting with them is (customers, customer relationships, and channels). Finally, two blocks represent the financial aspects of the product and help to explain how to account for the costs that are related to offering the intended value (costs and revenues).

Because the project team has to account for implementation from the start, the creation of the business model should also start early in the development process, so it will be relevant in the value specification phase. Of course, it can (and should) be adapted throughout the entire process to ensure that it is in line with recent insights from the stakeholders and context. Multiple methods should be used to create the business model (e.g., interviews, focus groups, desk research), and information from the contextual inquiry and value specification is used to ensure consistency with earlier activities. Since a business model provides a more generic overview instead of a set of predetermined activities, the way it is filled in depends on the skills and preferences of the project team.

Design

What is the Design Phase?

The output of the contextual inquiry and the value specification serves as the blueprint for the eHealth technology, which is actually developed in the design phase. This is again not a hard transition: Often, activities of these phases overlap. The design phase is an extremely dynamic, iterative, creative, and collaborative phase during which there is an active collaboration between end-users, other stakeholders, researchers, designers, behaviour change experts, content experts, and perhaps even funders.

The final technology should not be developed all at once, since chances are that if that does happen, a lot of important problems may be missed and arise only after it has been introduced in practice and thus wasting a lot of time and effort. That is why multiple prototypes – visual representations of the to-be-developed technology – have to be developed based on the requirements. Prototypes are used to visualize and elaborate on initial ideas, using an iterative approach in which changes to the prototype are being constantly made, based on stakeholder input (Beerlage-de Jong et al., 2017; Wentzel et al., 2014). These prototypes have to be based on the requirements and thus also incorporate behaviour change techniques and persuasive features (see also Chapter 12). By creating prototypes and evaluating them with users, the project team can remove any critical issues, add elements that are thought of by the stakeholders, identify potential factors that need to be taken into account during implementation, and adapt the design to preferences and new insights.

Objectives of the Design Phase

The design phase has several main objectives.

1. Both low-fidelity (lo-fi) and high-fidelity (hi-fi) prototypes of the eHealth technology are developed;
2. Persuasive elements, behaviour change techniques, and/or domain-specific theories are operationalized and integrated into the design of the eHealth technology;
3. Usability tests of the prototypes have to be conducted with end users, experts, and other stakeholders.

Concepts, Methods, and Activities in the Design Phase

1. Developing low- and high-fidelity prototypes

When developing prototypes, it is especially important for every member of the project team to have a good understanding of the end users. For starters, the products from the value specification, such as requirements, personas, and values, should be used throughout the entire prototyping process to structurally incorporate the end-user perspective. Ideally, a first step in the prototyping process is to come up with initial ideas by means of ideation. However, in practice, a project team often already has some ideas of what they want to design, based on the earlier phases. These ideas are being constantly specified throughout the prototyping process. It can also be beneficial to involve a professional design company in the prototyping process since user experience (UX) designers have specific expertise and skills to translate requirements into prototypes.

A rough distinction can be made between low-fidelity (lo-fi) and high-fidelity (hi-fi) prototyping. The design process usually starts with very lo-fi prototypes: Prototypes that do not have to resemble the final technology but are mostly used to communicate about the overall goal and most important elements. An advantage of lo-fi prototypes is that they can be drawn up relatively quickly by people with little to no technical skills. There are several methods to create lo-fi prototypes, of which some examples are:

- *Paper-based prototyping/sketching.* Paper prototypes can be created with different kinds of materials such as pencils, paper, paint, sticky notes, cards, or paint. This can range from very basic sketches to more detailed drawings;
- *Digital prototyping.* Computer programmes like PowerPoint or Figma can be used. These programmes can be used to make clickable, interactive lo-fi prototypes;
- *Storyboarding.* Storyboards are sequences of images that clarify how the technology can be used by the user;
- *3D prototyping.* This method uses materials such as cardboard, foam, wood, plastic, clay, and building blocks.

Of course, other methods are possible as well. In addition, these methods are not solely used for lo-fi prototyping, but can also be used for hi-fi prototypes. While the distinction isn't that black-and-white, hi-fi prototypes have a higher resemblance to the final version of the eHealth technology, enable the user (to some extent) interact with it and are suitable for testing specific details of the technology. Developing them requires more technical expertise. The method to develop the hi-fi prototype depends on the technology that is being developed and the skills of the designer. More information on prototypes can be found in Chapter 11.

Often, the project team should also know which kind of information should be provided and how this has to be structured. This can be achieved in multiple ways, for example by using existing (treatment) protocols as the foundation for the content of a technology. Furthermore, Delphi studies can be conducted with experts to gain insight into which information a technology should contain (Yap et al., 2017). Furthermore, experts can be asked to create a first version of the technology's content. A way to structure the content of technologies that contain much information and to gain insight into the desired information structure, is by means of a card-sorting study. Participants are invited to cluster cards with information in whatever way they consider it to be logical. By analyzing these 'card clusters', the information or the menu structure of a certain website can be structured in a way that fits the end users' needs (Wentzel, Müller, Beerlage-de Jong, & van Gemert-Pijnen, 2016).

2. Integrating behaviour change theories and persuasive features in the design

In the value specification phase, initial choices for relevant behaviour change techniques, persuasive features, and possibly also features based on domain-specific theories were made and integrated into the requirements. However, since behaviour change is extremely complex, the set of behaviour change techniques will most likely be adapted throughout the process. Consequently, in the design phase, attention should again be paid to behaviour change. This can be done by collecting new data via interviews, focus groups, or questionnaires, and by using scientific literature on behaviour change techniques or features that are specifically relevant for a certain target group or behaviour (Asbjørnsen et al., 2020). Furthermore, these behaviour change techniques should be operationalized and integrated into prototypes. There is not a single, straightforward way to do this. On the contrary, it requires an iterative and creative approach. Techniques can be integrated in a prototype in multiple ways, amongst other things through brainstorming sessions with stakeholders, by involving experts on design and behaviour change, by investigating working mechanisms in similar technologies, and via co-creation sessions with end-users. Once these mechanisms are integrated into prototypes, they should be presented to stakeholders and experts to investigate if they are potentially effective and fit the skills and preferences of end-users. Again, this is an iterative process, which means that it will probably take some time to identify the most suitable techniques and integrate them in the most optimal way.

3. Conducting usability tests with stakeholders and experts

Prototypes have to be tested with stakeholders to gain insight into overall opinions, points of improvement, and recommendations. This can be done by means of *usability testing*. Usability tests can be used to study how someone interacts with the system, to test the ease of use and user-friendliness of the technology, or to assess whether behaviour change mechanisms and requirements are correctly translated into the design. Very broadly speaking, there are two ways of testing usability: Involving usability experts or involving users.

Some studies indicate that the best results occur when both kinds of usability testing are combined. Some examples of methods for usability testing are (Jaspers, 2009):

- *Think-aloud method.* In this method, intended end-users are provided with a scenario in which they have to use a prototype, and while doing this, they are asked to think aloud, i.e., verbalizing their thoughts about the system while using it;
- *Heuristic evaluation.* In this method, design experts assess the usability of the system by exploring it using a set of recognized usability principles, called heuristics. Examples of heuristics are visibility of system status, recognition rather than recall, and aesthetic and minimalist design (Nielsen, 1995);
- *Cognitive walk-through.* In this type of usability testing, experts are asked to execute tasks that a user would want to perform to identify usability issues (Wharton, Rieman, Lewis, & Polson, 1994). This method can also be used by experts on content.

Operationalization

What is the Operationalization Phase?

Operationalization refers to the planning and actions for the introduction, dissemination, adoption, and internalization of the technology in the intended context. In this phase, the technology is launched, marketing is set into motion, and organizational working procedures are put into practice. This phase is part of implementation, but the main difference between operationalization and implementation is that implementation is more overarching and already begins in the contextual inquiry, while operationalization is mostly focused on the actual rollout of plans that are necessary for the use of a technology within a specific context.

In this phase, the business model should be completed and applied to practice using the input from earlier phases, but also by collecting new data. Additionally, previously collected data and new research has to be combined into a concrete implementation plan with specific activities, ideally structured by means of an implementation framework. This plan needs to be holistic, i.e., it should pay attention to the involved people, the organizational and wider context, and the eHealth technology that has to be implemented. Operationalization is very complex and should not be underestimated. A participatory approach is also necessary in the operationalization phase, to iden-tify relevant implementation factors and set obtainable objectives, and the input of stakeholders is also needed for the development of implementation strategies and accompanying materials.

Objectives of the Operationalization Phase

The operationalization phase has three main objectives.

1. Finalize the business model with input of the stakeholders and put it into practice;
2. Create an overview of implementation barriers and facilitators, using input from the previous phases, new data, and implementation frameworks;
3. Developing a concrete implementation plan based on the previously identified implementation factors, including implementation outcomes, objectives, strategies, and materials, and apply it to practice.

Concepts, Methods, and Activities in the Operationalization Phase

1. Complete the business model

In the value specification, a start was made with the development of a business model by, for example, filling in the business model canvas or a similar method (also see Chapter 10). A business model was further specified alongside the development process and should be finalized and rolled out in the operationalization phase. Concrete plans on how to deal with the nine blocks of the business model canvas have to be created, again in close cooperation with stakeholders (Osterwalder & Pigneur, 2010). By means of methods like desk research, focus groups or interviews with stakeholders, a plan to implement the business model should be drawn up. Documented infor-mation from the scientific or grey literature on comparable operationalization processes might be used as well. Again, there are no step-by-step guidelines, since the way to do this depends on the context, the technology, and the preferences and competences of the team. This implies that the project team has to make deliberate, well-substantiated decisions and should of course constantly cooperate with stakeholders. It is important to determine whether the business model will focus on one organization, or if it will be organization-overarching, e.g., focusing on a network of different hospitals. While the business model should be as complete as possible, this does not mean that the model is finished: Chances are that it will have to be updated constantly, in line with, for example, new insights, policy changes, new customers, or new ways of financing.

2. Create an overview of implementation barriers and facilitators

Too often, implementation is underestimated or seen as a post-design activity. As became apparent in the pillars and previous phases, implementation starts alongside the development process. Consequently, throughout the process, insight will already have been gained into factors that are important for implementation. In the operationalization phase, additional attention needs to be paid to such implementation factors. Examples of studies that can be conducted are systematic reviews on similar implementation processes, interviews or focus groups with stakeholders, or questionnaires to ask a larger group of people about their perceived implementation barriers. Previous and new research should lead to a clear and comprehensive overview of implementation factors that may bolster or hinder implementation success.

Implementation frameworks are useful tools for identifying and structuring these barriers and facilitators – and thus are also broader and more comprehensive than business models. These frameworks can also be used to evaluate existing implementation processes and learn from them for future implementation processes for to-be-developed technologies (Kip, Sieverink, van Gemert-Pijnen, Bouman, & Kelders, 2020). Examples of much-used models in eHealth research, are the Consolidated Framework for Implementation Research (CFIR) and the Nonadoption, Abandonment, Scale-up, Spread, and Sustainability (NASSS) frameworks. The CFIR is a comprehensive implementation model that is based on an exhaustive review of literature on multiple existing implementation theories (Damschroder et al., 2022). To take the different levels of implementation into account, the CFIR incorporates different domains with several accompanying constructs: (1) the Innovation domain (e.g., evidence base, relative advantage); (2) Outer Setting domain (local attitudes, policies, and laws); (3) Inner Setting domain (e.g., tension for change, available resources); (4) Individuals domain (e.g., implementation facilitators, characteristics); and (5) Implementation Process domain (e.g., planning, tailoring strategies). The NASSS framework is specifically focused on value-based technology in healthcare (Greenhalgh et al., 2017). This model incorporates elements related to the seven main domains and includes several sub-categories: (1) Condition (e.g., nature of condition or illness, comorbidities); (2) Technology (e.g., material features, knowledge needed to use); (3) Value proposition (supply-side value, demand-side value); (4) Adopters (e.g., staff and patient); (5) Organisation (e.g., capacity to innovate, extent of change needed to routines); (6) Wider system (political, socio-cultural); and (7) Embedding and adaptation over time (e.g., scope for adaptation over time, organizational resilience). While there are differences between these models, they both pay attention to the people involved, the characteristics of the intervention, and the context in which a technology is used, in line with a holistic approach.

A final note is that there are of course other frameworks that might be suitable and the choice for the framework depends on different elements, such as the preferences and skills of the involved researchers. Often, models such as the Technology Acceptance Model (TAM) model are used (Venkatesh & Bala, 2008). Individual differences, system characteristics, social influence, and facilitating conditions are part of the model, but most emphasis lies on perceived usefulness and perceived ease of use, which are viewed as predictors for intention, which in turn is considered to directly influence usage behaviour. While these types of models can be relevant for specific research questions, it is important to note that most focus lies on the individual implementation factors, and less attention is paid to the wider context and characteristics of the eHealth intervention. Furthermore, intention is viewed to be a direct predictor of actual usage behaviour, while there is a huge intention-behaviour gap in implementation behaviour (Kip et al., 2020). Too often, implementation research focuses only on one aspect of implementation, so when using these models, it is essential to carefully ensure that all levels of implementation are taken into account – i.e., the people, the organization, wider context, and the technology.

3. Developing and rolling out an implementation plan with objectives and strategies

Based on the previously identified factors (i.e., barriers and facilitators), a concrete plan on how to implement the eHealth technology in a sustainable way should be developed. Based on the factors, specific objectives can be set. These objectives help the team in ensuring that the implementation plan remains focused and allows for evaluation of the success of the implementation process.

These objectives can also be related to implementation outcomes, again to ensure that all relevant elements of implementation are accounted for. Proctor et al. (2011) identified the following implementation outcomes: Acceptability, adoption, appropriateness, cost, feasibility, fidelity, penetration, and sustainability.

Besides the factors, outcomes, and objectives, there is also a need for specific strategies that are drawn up to reach the set objectives and thus address the identified factors (Kouijzer et al., 2023). Implementation strategies are activities that are undertaken to realize the adoption, dissemination, and sustainable integration of eHealth in healthcare (Powell et al., 2012). Examples are training of healthcare providers, changes in an organization's infrastructure, management support, development of technology-enhanced protocols, practical support of clinicians in using the intervention, or information flyers for patients (Varsi et al., 2019). It can be difficult to translate objectives into specific strategies that fit within the context. This requires creativity, but also active stakeholder involvement and highlights the importance of a participatory approach in which implementation materials and activities are co-created. Service modelling can be used to support this process. Such a model describes how an end-user will receive and use a technology in context and can be used to specify what is needed to achieve this (also see Chapter 9). Furthermore, since implementation often requires behaviour change from the involved stakeholders, the aforementioned BCTs might be useful when designing implementation strategies as well (Kouijzer, Kip, Bouman, & Kelders, 2023).

Finally, when designing implementation processes, it is important to be aware of the different types of adopters. The Diffusion of Innovation theory makes a distinction between innovators, early adopters, early majority, late majority, and laggards (Rogers, 2010). While this distinction may primarily be a paper truth and isn't black-and-white, it does help in understanding that not all stakeholders will be very enthusiastic about adopting a new eHealth technology. This implies that when designing implementation, one has to take these differences into account. To illustrate: Innovators might serve as project champions and can take on an active role from the start of the implementation process, while the late majority and laggards first need to see that an innovation works for their peers before using it. This shows that different groups of people require different, tailored implementation approaches.

Summative Evaluation

What is the Summative Evaluation Phase?

A holistic vision on eHealth in which technology, context, and people are intertwined, is essential for the entire process, including evaluation. However, often, a monodisciplinary view is applied, and attention is paid to only one type of outcome measure, using only one type of research method. Thorough eHealth evaluation should not be viewed as a post-development or -implementation activity, but as an iterative, multi-method process that is focused on a broad range of objectives, in line with the holistic view on eHealth. In evaluation processes, the project team has to check whether the eHealth technology succeeds in addressing the objectives formulated in previous phases, and during evaluation, development, and implementation activities can also still take place.

For overview purposes, a rough distinction can be made between three aspects of eHealth evaluation – even though they overlap. First, the impact of eHealth on its users, other stakeholders and their context should be investigated. This type of evaluation aims to measure the effects on different types of outcomes, e.g., clinical, organizational, and behavioural. However, evaluation should not only be focused on *if* a technology works; it also should provide insight into how, for whom, when and why it is of added value. Consequently, a second focal point of eHealth evaluation is related to the uptake, in other words: How was the technology used? To illustrate: If an impact evaluation shows no effects, a reason might be that a technology was hardly used, or not in the right way. This does not become apparent if no attention is paid to the way in which the users navigated through the technology. Third, evaluation methods can be used to provide insight into working mechanisms – why does an eHealth technology work? This can relate to constructs such as engagement, but also to effective persuasive features or BCTs such as personalization. These types of evaluations do not just provide insight into why eHealth works, but also provide valuable points of improvement for design and implementation.

These three elements of eHealth evaluation are not separate but should be viewed as aspects of a larger evaluation process. An example of a suitable framework for this approach is the Multiphase Optimization Strategy (MOST) framework, that consists of three phases: Preparation, Optimization, and Evaluation (Collins, Murphy, & Strecher, 2007). In the Preparation phase, the groundwork is laid: A conceptual model for the intervention – including pilot testing, identification of 'core components', and determining the main outcomes – is developed. As you may notice, this overlaps with multiple phases of the CeHRes Roadmap. In the Optimization phase, different types of research designs are used to investigate which components of the intervention are effective. In the Evaluation phase, studies are conducted to determine the effectiveness of the eHealth technology and reach consensus about which components have to be incorporated. While there are other useful approaches for eHealth evaluation, the example of the MOST framework shows that evaluation is a multi-method, iterative process.

Objectives of the Summative Evaluation Phase

The summative evaluation phase has three main objectives:

1. Determining the impact of an eHealth technology on the users, other stakeholders, and their context, based on the predetermined values;
2. Analyzing the uptake of an eHealth technology in terms of adoption or use of the technology by its intended users;
3. Investigating relevant working mechanisms that explain why an eHealth intervention is (not) effective for its users.

Concepts, Methods, and Activities in the Summative Evaluation Phase

1. Determining the impact of an eHealth technology

Since there are many different types of technologies with a broad range of goals, there is not one set of research questions that should be answered. In any case, they should be closely related to the values of the stakeholders. Examples of research questions for evaluating the impact of an eHealth technology are provided below.

- To what extent does the eHealth technology influence patient or consumer health and well-being?
  - Clinical values (e.g., blood pressure, depression)
  - Quality of life (e.g., general well-being, mental health)
  - Lifestyle behaviours (e.g., alcoholic beverages, steps per day)
  - Cognitions (e.g., attitudes, knowledge, intentions)
  - Treatment fidelity (e.g., treatment adherence, therapeutic relationship)
- To what extent does the eHealth technology influence the delivery of healthcare?
  - Accessibility (e.g., availability of healthcare, independent of place and time)
  - Efficiency (e.g., utilization of healthcare services, time savings, cost savings)
  - Safety (e.g., errors by healthcare professionals, increased privacy)

- Communication (e.g., contact moments, improved communication)
- Quality of care (e.g., patient and healthcare professional satisfaction).

In order to assess the impact of eHealth, multiple methods should be used to paint a broad, comprehensive picture of the influence that the technology has on the context and stakeholders (Bonten et al., 2020). It is important to note that there is not one gold standard for evaluating eHealth: The suitability of the method always depends on the fit with the research question, target group, and practical considerations such as the available time of participants and the budget of the study. Some commonly used examples are provided below.

- *Randomized controlled trials (RCTs)*. RCTs can be used to evaluate the outcomes of an eHealth technology in an experimental way. RCTs are used to assess whether the experimental group of patients who used the eHealth technology had better health outcomes after using the intervention, compared to a control group that did not use the technology;
- *Interviews/focus groups*. Interviews or focus groups with stakeholders can be conducted to gather qualitative data on their perspective on the technology, for example, on the experienced benefits and influence on their context. Often, qualitative data is combined with quantitative data in a mixed- or multiple-method approach to paint a broader picture of the impact of a technology;
- *Single-case experimental designs (SCEDs)*. SCEDs are experimental research designs in which individual participants are monitored for a longer period of time, for example with experience sampling apps. In SCEDs, the eHealth intervention is systematically introduced after a baseline and withdrawn. There can be one or more intervention phases;
- *Health Technology Assessment (HTA)*. HTA is a broad form of evaluation and refers to the evaluation of properties, effects, or impacts of health technology. It is a multidisciplinary process to evaluate several issues of an eHealth technology, such as social, economic, or ethical.

2. Analysing the uptake of an eHealth technology

Just as for impact, uptake also can be measured in multiple ways, using different types of research methods. The following types of questions can be answered when studying the way in which an eHealth technology is used:

- How often did the users log in and for how long did they use the technology?
- How often was the technology used by different organizations/teams?
- How often was the technology used over time?
- What features of the system were used and in what combination?
- Who are the 'hardcore' users and who are the dropouts?
- Are there differences in usage between adherent and non-adherent users?

There are multiple ways to investigate uptake, yet log data analysis is a commonly used method for doing so (Sieverink, Kelders, Poel, & van Gemert-Pijnen, 2017). Log data represents the actual use of the different elements of the technology. Examples of log data are the number of website visitors, the times during which users log in, or the frequency of use of the functionalities used.

3. Investigating working mechanisms of an eHealth technology

Most outcomes of impact- or uptake-related studies are not very generalizable: They mostly give insight into the effectiveness and usage of a single eHealth technology within a specific context. Understanding why an eHealth technology achieves a certain effect, can provide insight into how behaviour change can be achieved, thus contributing to creating (health) impact. Therefore, investigating *why* an eHealth technology is (not) effective provides relevant knowledge for other researchers and eHealth developers as well, and can be used to make future interventions more effective. Examples of questions that can be answered are:

- Is the level of a user's adherence (the extent to which a technology is used as intended) related to effectiveness?
- To what extent is engagement a predictor of adherence and effectiveness?
- Which persuasive features/BCTs are related to effectiveness?
- Are certain usage patterns related to the success of the eHealth technology?

Important for all these questions is that they attempt to take on a broader perspective relating the effectiveness of an intervention to a certain concept (or working mechanism) that may play a similar role in other interventions. Therefore, it is important to check the validity of these outcomes in various studies with various eHealth technologies. Questions like these can be integrated in different study designs such as RCTs or factorial designs (also see Chapter 16). Factorial designs are a specific method that can be used to investigate the effectiveness of elements such as persuasive features or BCTs (Collins et al., 2007). In such a design, every user is exposed to different variations of an intervention, e.g., a version with or without personalization, and with or without feedback. By means of this, the researcher can screen for the effects of specific features of an intervention by searching for differences in effects between variations of an intervention. Furthermore, a combination of interviews with log-data or a larger-scale RCT can be used to acquire qualitative in-depth understanding of certain outcomes, in close cooperation with stakeholders. In addition to that, interviews can help to identify subjectively experienced working mechanisms.

Formative Evaluation

What is the Formative Evaluation Phase?

Formative evaluation is not a separate development phase, but a principle that is intertwined throughout all stages of the eHealth development process. It is very important to note that its place at the end of this chapter does not mean that it is the final phase. Within the CeHRes Roadmap, it is visualized as the cycles that are connected to all five phases, and thus is relevant within each phase. As was emphasized in the third pillar and throughout this chapter, eHealth development, implementation, and evaluation processes are not linear, but iterative and dynamic. Formative evaluation cycles are a good example of this proposition. The basic presumption of formative evaluation is that ongoing information on how to improve the process and eHealth technology is collected. This information assists the project team in ensuring that there is a constant focus on the context and people involved. In this way, formative evaluation can be seen as creating by evaluating.

Formative evaluation is twofold: It can be used within and between phases of the Roadmap. First, formative evaluation within phase refers to activities that support the project team in ensuring that there is a fit between their activities or output and the perspective of the stakeholders and context, for example by actively involving and verifying results with stakeholders. These kinds of activities should be conducted in every phase of eHealth development, and thus are the activities that were described for each of the previous phases. Second, formative evaluation between phases refers to ensuring that outcomes of phases are consistent with each other. At the 'end' of a phase, the team has to check whether the outcomes of a previous phase have been accounted for and haven't been forgotten along the way. Besides this, decisions also have to be made on whether changes in the outcomes of previous phase are required.

Objectives of the Formative Evaluation Phase

The formative evaluation has two main goals, both related to the development process:

1. Using methods to gather information from the stakeholders and context to continuously include their perspectives within the phases of the CeHRes Roadmap (within phase);
2. Checking whether the outcomes of previous phases of the CeHRes Roadmap have been accounted for in the current phase and ensuring that the outcomes of all phases are related to each other (between phases).

Concepts, Methods, and Activities in the Formative Evaluation Phase

1. Evaluation within phases by gathering input from the stakeholders and context

The formative evaluation does not entail separate methods since it is an overarching approach that refers to principles behind eHealth development, implementation, and evaluation. However, to illustrate and further clarify this, some practical examples of methods that convey the principles from formative evaluation within a phase are provided below.

- In the *contextual inquiry* phase, snowball sampling is used to ask existing stakeholders to identify missing stakeholders. This is an example of formative evaluation, since it assists in validating whether the list of stakeholders is complete and reflects the actual context;
- In the *value specification* phase, lists of *requirements* are often verified by stakeholders once they are drawn up. This supports the team in ensuring that the requirements they derived from focus groups and interviews make sense to the stakeholders;
- In the *design phase* of the technology, a straightforward example of formative evaluation is usability testing among end-users via the think-aloud method. This method aims to make sure the technology fits the user's needs;
- During the *operationalization* phase, the involvement of stakeholders in completing the *business model* and making a plan on how to operationalize the model is an example of formative evaluation;
- The *summative evaluation* phase also contains formative evaluation cycles, for example by asking users to explain the outcomes of a randomized controlled trial or log data analysis in a mixed-methods approach.

2. Evaluation between phases by checking whether phases are related to each other

This element of formative evaluation mainly focuses on ensuring that there is a clear relationship between the content and output of the separate phases. For example, in the design phase, the project team has to make sure that the designed technology incorporates the requirements and addresses the values. No concrete methods are prescribed for this; the approach used depends on the nature of the project and the preferences of the project team. However, it is essential for team members to be aware of the decisions that are being made and to, if necessary, involve external stakeholders. Another requirement is that thorough, transparent documentation of the activities and outcomes of each phase in an eHealth development project are created. If the documentation isn't clear, it is hard to retrieve what the main outcomes of previous phases were, and what the grounds for specific decisions were. Deciding on whether the outcomes of the current phase match those of previous phases can be achieved by means of, for example, meetings with the project team or focus groups with stakeholders.

Summary

As can be seen in this chapter, the CeHRes Roadmap is a framework – consisting of five phases, underpinned by pillars – that can be used to shape the development, implementation, and evaluation of eHealth technologies (see Figure 7.4). While the Roadmap provides a broad overview, it should not be seen as a step-by-step template: A tailored process that fits the context, technology, and users is essential. This highlights the importance of an experienced, interdisciplinary project team that can set clear objectives, use suitable research methods, and ensure a coherent process. While each eHealth development, implementation, and evaluation processes are unique, a systematic, iterative approach is key. Ultimately, a good fit between the eHealth technology, the involved people, and their context should be reached to increase the chances of making an impact with eHealth. The take-home messages for this chapter are:

- The CeHRes Roadmap is a set of principles that are combined in a framework for overview purposes, so in practice, the different phases overlap and the way in which they are executed will differ per project;
- In line with a holistic view, attention should constantly be paid to the interrelationship between the behaviour and preferences of stakeholders, the healthcare context, and the features of a technology;
- eHealth development, implementation, and evaluation are all iterative, highly interdisciplinary processes, which require active collaboration between researchers with flexible and creative mindsets;
- During each development phase, multiple methods should be used. Which methods are used should depend on the research question that was posed by the project team, the skills and preferences of the participants, and the practical preconditions from the context;

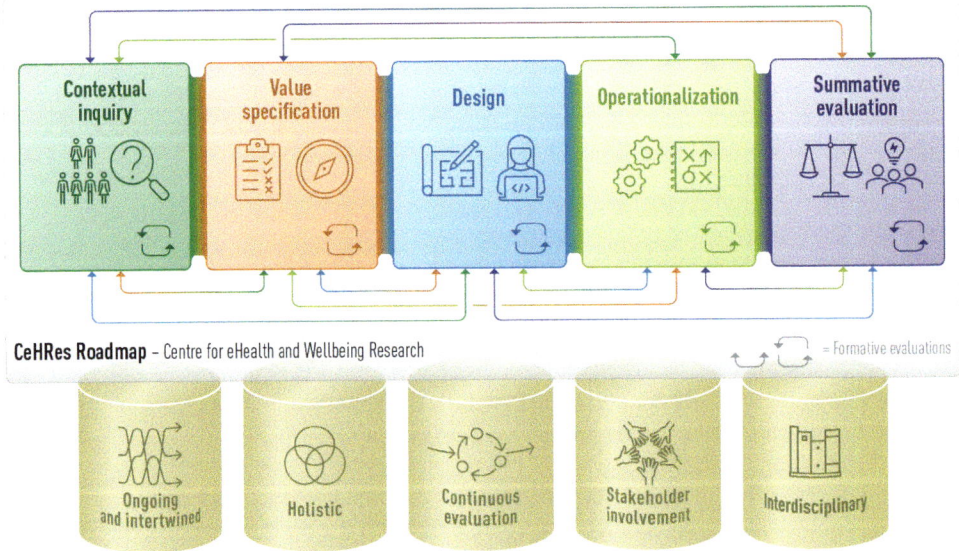

Figure 7.4 The CeHRes Roadmap.

- eHealth development, implementation, and evaluation are never finished: There is always a need for improvements of or additions to the technology, new or improved implementation strategies, and further evaluation.

Key References for Further Reading

Van Gemert-Pijnen, J. E. W. C., Nijland, N., van Limburg, M., Ossebaard, H. C., Kelders, S. M., Eysenbach, G., & Seydel, E. R. (2011). A holistic framework to improve the uptake and impact of eHealth technologies. *Journal of Medical Internet Research*, 13(4), e111.

Asbjørnsen, R. A., Wentzel, J., Smedsrød, M. L., Hjelmesæth, J., Clark, M.M., Solberg Nes, L., & van Gemert-Pijnen, J. E. W. C. (2020). Identifying persuasive design principles and behavior change techniques supporting end user values and needs in eHealth interventions for long-term weight loss mainten-ance: Qualitative study. *Journal of Medical Internet Research, 22*(11), e22598.

Kip, H., Kelders, S. M., Bouman, Y. H., & van Gemert-Pijnen, J. E. W. C. (2019). The importance of system-atically reporting and reflecting on eHealth development: Participatory development process of a virtual reality application for forensic mental health care. *Journal of Medical Internet Research*, 21(8), e12972.

Kip, H., Keizer, J., da Silva, M. C., Beerlage-de Jong, N., Köhle, N., & Kelders, S. M. (2022). Methods for human-centered eHealth development: Narrative scoping review. *Journal of Medical Internet Research*, 24(1), e31858.

Kouijzer, M. M., Kip, H., Bouman, Y. H. A., & Kelders, S. M. (2023). Implementation of virtual reality in healthcare: A scoping review on the implementation process of virtual reality in various healthcare settings. *Implementation Science Communications*, 4(1), 1–29.

References

Asbjørnsen, R. A., Smedsrød, M. L., Nes, L. S., Wentzel, J., Varsi, C., Hjelmesæth, J., & van Gemert-Pijnen, J. E. (2019). Persuasive system design principles and behavior change techniques to stimulate motivation and adherence in electronic health interventions to support weight loss maintenance: Scoping review. *Journal of Medical Internet Research*, 21(6), e14265.

Asbjørnsen, R. A., Wentzel, J., Smedsrød, M. L., Hjelmesæth, J., Clark, M. M., Solberg Nes, L., & van Gemert-Pijnen, J. E. (2020). Identifying persuasive design principles and behavior change techniques supporting end user values and needs in eHealth interventions for long-term weight loss maintenance: Qualitative study. *Journal of Medical Internet Research*, 22(11), e22598.

Bartholomew, L. K., Parcel, G. S., Kok, G., Gottlieb, N. H., Schaalma, H. C., Markham, C. C., . . . Mullen, P. D. C. (2006). *Planning health promotion programs: An intervention mapping approach*. Hoboken, NJ: Jossey-Bass.

Beerlage-de Jong, N., Wentzel, J., Hendrix, R., & van Gemert-Pijnen, L. (2017). The value of participa-tory development to support antimicrobial stewardship with a clinical decision support system. *American Journal of Infection Control*, 45(4), 365–371.

Bødker, K., Kensing, F., & Simonsen, J. (2009). *Participatory IT design: Designing for business and work-place realities*. MIT Press.

Bonten, T. N., Rauwerdink, A., Wyatt, J. C., Kasteleyn, M. J., Witkamp, L., Riper, H., . . . Schijven, M. P. (2020). Online guide for electronic health evaluation approaches: Systematic scoping review and concept mapping study. *Journal of Medical Internet Research*, 22(8), e17774.

Collins, L. M., Murphy, S. A., & Strecher, V. (2007). The multiphase optimization strategy (MOST) and the sequential multiple assignment randomized trial (SMART): New methods for more potent eHealth interventions. *American Journal of Preventive Medicine*, 32(5), S112–S118.

Damschroder, L. J., Reardon, C. M., Widerquist, M. A. O., & Lowery, J. (2022). The updated Consolidated Framework for Implementation Research based on user feedback. *Implementation Science*, 17(1), 1–16.

Dingsøyr, T., Nerur, S., Balijepally, V., & Moe, N. B. (2012). A decade of agile methodologies: Towards explaining agile software development. *The Journal of Systems & Software*, 6(85), 1213–1221.

Eysenbach, G. (2001). What is e-health? *Journal of Medical Internet Research*, 3(2), e20.

Feldman, S. S., Schooley, B. L., & Bhavsar, G. P. (2014). Health information exchange implementa-tion: Lessons learned and critical success factors from a case study. *JMIR Medical Informatics*, 2(2), e19.

Fogg, B. J. (2002). Persuasive technology: Using computers to change what we think and do. *Ubiquity*, 2002(December), 2.

Giacomin, J. (2014). What is human centred design? *The Design Journal*, 17(4), 606–623. https://doi.org/10.2752/175630614X14056185480186

Glasgow, R. E., Phillips, S. M., & Sanchez, M. A. (2014). Implementation science approaches for integrating eHealth research into practice and policy. *International Journal of Medical Informatics*, 83(7), e1–e11.

Göttgens, I., & Oertelt-Prigione, S. (2021). The application of human-centered design approaches in health research and innovation: A narrative review of current practices. *JMIR mHealth and uHealth*, 9(12), e28102.

Greenhalgh, T., Wherton, J., Papoutsi, C., Lynch, J., Hughes, G., Hinder, S., . . . Shaw, S. (2017). Beyond adoption: A new framework for theorizing and evaluating nonadoption, abandonment, and challenges to the scale-up, spread, and sustainability of health and care technologies. *Journal of Medical Internet Research*, 19(11), e367.

Hekler, E. B., Klasnja, P., Riley, W. T., Buman, M. P., Huberty, J., Rivera, D. E., & Martin, C. A. (2016). Agile science: Creating useful products for behavior change in the real world. *Translational Behavioral Medicine*, 6(2), 317–328.

Holtzblatt, K., & Jones, S. (2017). Contextual inquiry: A participatory technique for system design. In *Participatory design* (pp. 177–210). CRC Press.

James, S. (1984). The content of social explanation: CUP Archive.

Jaspers, M. W. (2009). A comparison of usability methods for testing interactive health technologies: Methodological aspects and empirical evidence. *International Journal of Medical Informatics*, 78(5), 340–353.

Kelders, S. M., Kok, R. N., Ossebaard, H. C., & van Gemert-Pijnen, J. E. (2012). Persuasive system design does matter: A systematic review of adherence to web-based interventions. *Journal of Medical Internet Research*, 14(6), e152.

Kelders, S. M., Van Zyl, L. E., & Ludden, G. D. (2020). The concept and components of engagement in different domains applied to eHealth: A systematic scoping review. *Frontiers in Psychology*, 11, 926.

Kip, H., Keizer, J., da Silva, M. C., Beerlage-de Jong, N., Köhle, N., & Kelders, S. M. (2022). Methods for human-centered eHealth development: Narrative scoping review. *Journal of Medical Internet Research*, 24(1), e31858.

Kip, H., Kelders, S. M., Bouman, Y. H., & van Gemert-Pijnen, L. J. (2019). The importance of systematically reporting and reflecting on eHealth development: Participatory development process of a virtual reality application for forensic mental health care. *Journal of Medical Internet Research*, 21(8), e12972.

Kip, H., Kelders, S. M., & van Gemert-Pijnen, L. J. (2019). Putting the value in VR: How to systematically and iteratively develop a value-based VR application with a complex target group. Paper presented at the Proceedings of the 2019 CHI Conference on Human Factors in Computing Systems.

Kip, H., Sieverink, F., van Gemert-Pijnen, L. J., Bouman, Y. H., & Kelders, S. M. (2020). Integrating people, context, and technology in the implementation of a web-based intervention in forensic mental health care: Mixed-methods study. *Journal of Medical Internet Research*, 22(5), e16906.

Kouijzer, M. M. T. E., Kip, H., Bouman, Y. H. A., & Kelders, S. M. (2023). Implementation of virtual reality in healthcare: A scoping review on the implementation process of virtual reality in various healthcare settings. *Implementation Science Communications*, 4(1), 67. doi:10.1186/s43058-023-00442-2

LeRouge, C., Ma, J., Sneha, S., & Tolle, K. (2013). User profiles and personas in the design and development of consumer health technologies. *International Journal of Medical Informatics*, 82(11), e251–e268.

Michie, S., Richardson, M., Johnston, M., Abraham, C., Francis, J., Hardeman, W., . . . Wood, C. E. (2013). The behavior change technique taxonomy (v1) of 93 hierarchically clustered techniques: Building an international consensus for the reporting of behavior change interventions. *Annals of Behavioral Medicine*, 46(1), 81–95.

Michie, S., Yardley, L., West, R., Patrick, K., & Greaves, F. (2017). Developing and evaluating digital interventions to promote behavior change in health and health care: Recommendations resulting from an international workshop. *Journal of Medical Internet Research*, 19(6), e232.

Miron-Shatz, T., Shatz, I., Becker, S., Patel, J., & Eysenbach, G. (2014). Promoting business and entrepreneurial awareness in health care professionals: Lessons from Venture Capital Panels at Medicine 2.0 Conferences. *Journal of Medical Internet Research*, 16(8), e184. doi:10.2196/jmir.3390

Mitchell, R. K., Agle, B. R., & Wood, D. J. (1997). Toward a theory of stakeholder identification and salience: Defining the principle of who and what really counts. *Academy of Management Review*, 22(4), 853–886.

Mohr, D. C., Lyon, A. R., Lattie, E. G., Reddy, M., & Schueller, S. M. (2017). Accelerating digital mental health research from early design and creation to successful implementation and sustainment. *Journal of Medical Internet Research*, 19(5), e153.

Mohr, D. C., Weingardt, K. R., Reddy, M., & Schueller, S. M. (2017). Three problems with current digital mental health research... and three things we can do about them. *Psychiatric Services*, 68(5), 427–429.

Nielsen, J. (1995). How to conduct a heuristic evaluation. Nielsen Norman Group, 1(1), 8.

Nielsen, J. A., & Mathiassen, L. (2013). Interpretive flexibility in mobile health: Lessons from a government-sponsored home care program. *Journal of Medical Internet Research*, 15(10), e236.

O'Cathain, A., Croot, L., Sworn, K., Duncan, E., Rousseau, N., Turner, K., . . . Hoddinott, P. (2019). Taxonomy of approaches to developing interventions to improve health: A systematic methods overview. *Pilot and Feasibility Studies*, 5(1), 1–27.

Oinas-Kukkonen, H., & Harjumaa, M. (2009). Persuasive systems design: Key issues, process model, and system features. *Communications of the Association for Information Systems*, 24(1), 28.

Osterwalder, A., & Pigneur, Y. (2010). *Business model generation: A handbook for visionaries, game changers, and challengers* (Vol. 1): John Wiley & Sons.

Patrick, K., Hekler, E. B., Estrin, D., Mohr, D. C., Riper, H., Crane, D., . . . Riley, W. T. (2016). The pace of technologic change: Implications for digital health behavior intervention research. In *American Journal of Preventive Medicine*, 51(5), 816–824.

Powell, B. J., McMillen, J. C., Proctor, E. K., Carpenter, C. R., Griffey, R. T., Bunger, A. C., . . . York, J. L. (2012). A compilation of strategies for implementing clinical innovations in health and mental health. *Medical Care Research and Review*, 69(2), 123–157.

Proctor, E., Silmere, H., Raghavan, R., Hovmand, P., Aarons, G., Bunger, A., . . . Hensley, M. (2011). Outcomes for implementation research: Conceptual distinctions, measurement challenges, and research agenda. *Administration and Policy in Mental Health and Mental Health Services Research*, 38(2), 65–76.

Rogers, E. M. (2010). *Diffusion of innovations*. Simon and Schuster.

Rosson, M. B., & Carroll, J. M. (2002). Scenario-based design. In *The human-computer interaction handbook: Fundamentals, evolving technologies and emerging applications*. (pp. 1032–1050): L. Erlbaum Associates Inc.

Scaife, M., Rogers, Y., Aldrich, F., & Davies, M. (1997). Designing for or designing with? Informant design for interactive learning environments. Paper presented at the Proceedings of the ACM SIGCHI Conference on Human Factors in Computing Systems.

Schouten, S. E., Kip, H., Dekkers, T., Deenik, J., Beerlage-de Jong, N., Ludden, G. D., & Kelders, S. M. (2022). Best-practices for co-design processes involving people with severe mental illness for eMental health interventions: A qualitative multi-method approach. *Design for Health*, 6(3), 316–344.

Sieverink, F., Kelders, S., Poel, M., & van Gemert-Pijnen, L. (2017). Opening the black box of electronic health: Collecting, analyzing, and interpreting log data. *JMIR Research Protocols*, 6(8), e6452.

Sjöström, J., von Essen, L., & Grönqvist, H. (2014). The origin and impact of ideals in eHealth research: Experiences from the U-CARE research environment. *JMIR Research Protocols*, 3(2), e3202.

Ten Klooster, I., Wentzel, J., Sieverink, F., Linssen, G., Wesselink, R., & van Gemert-Pijnen, L. (2022). Personas for better targeted eHealth technologies: User-centered design approach. *JMIR Human Factors*, 9(1), e24172.

Van Gemert-Pijnen, J. E., Nijland, N., van Limburg, M., Ossebaard, H. C., Kelders, S. M., Eysenbach, G., & Seydel, E. R. (2011). A holistic framework to improve the uptake and impact of eHealth technologies. *Journal of Medical Internet Research*, 13(4), e111.

Van Limburg, M., Wentzel, J., Sanderman, R., & van Gemert-Pijnen, L. (2015). Business modeling to implement an eHealth portal for infection control: A reflection on co-creation with stakeholders. *JMIR Research Protocols*, 4(3), e104–e104. doi:10.2196/resprot.4519

Van Velsen., Wentzel, J., & van Gemert-Pijnen, J. E. (2013). Designing eHealth that matters via a multidisciplinary requirements development approach. *JMIR Research Protocols*, 2(1), e21.

Van Velsen, L., Ludden, G., & Grünloh, C. (2022). The limitations of user- and human-centered design in an eHealth context and how to move beyond them. *Journal of Medical Internet Research*, 24(10), e37341. doi:10.2196/37341.

Varsi, C., Solberg Nes, L., Kristjansdottir, O. B., Kelders, S. M., Stenberg, U., Zangi, H. A., . . . Asbjørnsen, R. A. (2019). Implementation strategies to enhance the implementation of eHealth programs for patients with chronic illnesses: Realist systematic review. *Journal of Medical Internet Research,* 21(9), e14255.

Venkatesh, V., & Bala, H. (2008). Technology acceptance model 3 and a research agenda on interventions. *Decision Sciences*, 39(2), 273–315.

Wentzel, J., Müller, F., Beerlage-de Jong, N., & van Gemert-Pijnen, J. E. W. C. (2016). Card sorting to evaluate the robustness of the information architecture of a protocol website. *International Journal of Medical Informatics*, 86, 71–81.

Wentzel, J., Van Velsen, L., Van Limburg, M., De Jong, N., Karreman, J., Hendrix, R., & van Gemert-Pijnen, J. E. W. C. (2014). Participatory eHealth development to support nurses in antimicrobial stewardship. *BMC Medical Informatics and Decision Making*, 14(1). doi:10.1186/1472-6947-14-45

Wentzel, M. J. (2015). Keeping an eye on the context: Participatory development of eHealth to support clinical practice.

Wharton, C., Rieman, J., Lewis, C., & Polson, P. (1994). The cognitive walkthrough model: A practitioners guide. In: J. Nielsen & R. L. Mack (Eds). *Usability inspection methods*. New York: John Wiley & Sons.

Van Woezik, A. F. G., Braakman-Jansen, L. M. A., Kulyk, O., Siemons, L., & van Gemert-Pijnen, J. E. W. C. (2016). Tackling wicked problems in infection prevention and control: A guideline for co-creation with stakeholders. *Antimicrobial Resistance and Infection Control*, 5(1). doi:10.1186/s13756-016-0119-2

Yap, M. B., Lawrence, K. A., Rapee, R. M., Cardamone-Breen, M. C., Green, J., & Jorm, A. F. (2017). Partners in parenting: A multi-level web-based approach to support parents in prevention and early intervention for adolescent depression and anxiety. *JMIR Mental Health*, 4(4), e8492.

Yardley, L., Morrison, L., Bradbury, K., & Muller, I. (2015). The person-based approach to intervention development: Application to digital health-related behavior change interventions. *Journal of Medical Internet Research*, 17(1), e30.

8   The Contextual Inquiry

Hanneke Kip, Jobke Wentzel, & Nienke Beerlage-de Jong

Introduction

As was explained in Chapter 1, eHealth has many potential benefits for health, healthcare, and well-being. However, in order to reach that potential, it is essential to ensure a good fit between the technology, its users, other stakeholders, and their context. A thorough understanding of the people and context in which a technology will be used is a prerequisite for achieving this fit. For example, the involved stakeholders need to be identified, it should be clear what the main problems within the specific context are, and the roles, tasks, activities, and protocols in a context need to be identified. These findings serve as the foundation for all subsequent activities within development, implementation, and evaluation processes. They also ensure that a technology fits within its context and is aligned with the characteristics and needs of stakeholders. Consequently, the CeHRes Roadmap prescribes that a thorough, iterative, multi-method contextual inquiry should be the first step in eHealth development (see Chapter 7).

In this chapter, the relevance of the contextual inquiry is explained. A non-exhaustive overview of relevant research methods is provided and illustrated by cases from practice. After completing this chapter, you will be able to:

- Explain why and in what way the contextual inquiry is an essential part of eHealth development;
- Provide concrete examples from practice to illustrate the relevance of conducting a contextual inquiry for the development of suitable eHealth technologies;
- Name and explain goals, benefits, and barriers of multiple research methods that can be used in the contextual inquiry;
- Explain the identification, analysis, and added value of stakeholders during the contextual inquiry and connect this to the entire process of eHealth development, implementation, and evaluation;
- Explain the role of the contextual inquiry within the entire process of developing, implementing, and evaluating eHealth.

DOI: 10.4324/9781003302049-10

Contextual Inquiry: The First Step in any eHealth Project

What is the Aim of the Contextual Inquiry?

A contextual inquiry involves activities aimed at gaining a thorough understanding of problems or points of improvement within a specific context, the ways in which technology can contribute to resolving these issues, and the people who might benefit from the technology. A contextual inquiry can be used as part of the development of a new technology, or it can serve as the first step in adapting existing technology to novel contexts. The contextual inquiry was first introduced as a phenomenological research method in which many qualitative methods are used to study a specific phenomenon within a context (Whiteside, Bennett, & Holtzblatt, 1988). It is part of contextual design, in which researchers aim to aggregate data from stakeholders in the context in which they are living and working and apply these findings into a final product (Beyer & Holtzblatt, 1998). Consequently, the goal of the contextual inquiry in eHealth development is to get a thorough understanding of the prospective users, other important stakeholders, and their environment. An in-depth contextual inquiry is needed to ensure that a new or existing technology fits with its intended users, other stakeholders, and their context. If a fit is achieved, chances improve that the developed technology is going to be used and implemented in a sustainable way (van Gemert-Pijnen et al., 2011). Often, developers immediately start with creating a technology, or only conduct a very short needs assessment, for example by conducting a short interview or questionnaire study. A main pitfall of skipping the contextual inquiry, is that the developed technology does not address the most relevant issues within a context, or that it does not fit the expectations, day-to-day activities, or skills of the intended users.

The specific research questions that could be answered in a contextual inquiry depend on the type of project. For example, the following questions can be relevant during the contextual inquiry:

- Who are the stakeholders that are relevant for the project and its development? Which stakeholders are most important?
- What does the current situation look like? What is going well? What could be improved?
- What problem has to be addressed? What does the problem entail and what are its causes according to stakeholders and the literature?
- What kind of behaviour has to be changed? What are the causes of this behaviour according to stakeholders and literature?
- What rules, regulations, theoretical frameworks, and ethical concerns are relevant for the context the technology has to be used in?
- What kind of eHealth technologies are already being used in the context and what are the experiences of users and other stakeholders?

What is the Added Value of the Contextual Inquiry?

Below are some fictional (but reality-inspired) examples to illustrate the added value of executing a thorough contextual inquiry.

Example: Technology in the home care setting

When nurses distribute medication to patients in a nursing home, they make use of registration and medication check apps. Such apps can assist the nurse by enabling video calls with colleagues to provide the required double check before administering medication and allow the nurse to directly (in real-time) register what medications were administered. This is a convenient solution, because a colleague is often not nearby when the nurse is on his/her round. In addition, good registration is important for medication safety and good record-keeping (and transfer). In one home care organization, tablets with medication-apps were provided to the nurses to take with them on their rounds. However, nurses did not actually use the tablets. The reason? The device was so big, it did not fit into their pockets, and carrying it by hand throughout the round was considered quite cumbersome. This resulted in nurses filling out medication registration after completing their rounds or even at the end of their shift, relying on memory. Needless to say, this was not in line with the intended improvement of quality of care.

Example: An app for depression

An app was developed to assist people, who were treated for depression by a therapist, in writing about negative and positive experiences. The developers acknowledged the importance of accounting for the perspective of, according to them, the most important stakeholders: The patients. They continuously asked for their perspective, input, and feedback on the technology. However, they did not include the therapists in the development process. This resulted in a lot of resistance on the therapists' side once the technology was introduced. They didn't agree with the way some of the exercises were described and indicated that important information on depression was missing. Consequently, they did not recommend the app to any of their clients. Had the developers conducted a comprehensive stakeholder identification and analysis, they would have found out about the important role of the psychologists in time.

How is the Contextual Inquiry Performed?

The what and why of the contextual inquiry have been explained, but it is important to address the how as well. What activities could be undertaken to conduct a thorough and systematic contextual inquiry? There is not one clear answer to this question, since there are many ways to do this, depending on the type of project, the context, and of course practical limitations such as budget and time. However, two things are always advisable, which will be further explained in the following sections. First, it is essential to identify and analyze the different types of people that have a stake in the project – i.e., the stakeholders. Second, it is important to use multiple methods to collect information about the context, since this enables the eHealth developers to paint a good, comprehensive picture. These methods can have different characteristics, ranging from explorative and qualitative methods that can provide an in-depth view on a certain topic or situation, to more fact-checking and quantitative approaches that can assess how 'big' or widespread a problem or situation is. Combining methods decreases the chances of overlooking important information and allows researchers to create a more complete picture of a context. In the following paragraph, the focus lies on the identification and analysis of stakeholders. After that, different methods that can be used in the contextual inquiry are described.

Stakeholder Identification and Analysis

A pivotal part of any contextual inquiry is a thorough stakeholder identification and analysis. After all, for an eHealth technology to be successful, it must fit the various goals as well as the work processes and thinking processes of the people that will be in any way in contact with it. Throughout the entire development, implementation, and evaluation process, stakeholders need to be actively involved. To achieve this, researchers and technology developers need to have a clear overview of who the stakeholders are.

A widely known and accepted definition says that a stakeholder is 'any group or individual who can affect or is affected by [the eHealth technology]' (Freeman, 2010, p. 46). Thus, stakeholders are certainly not just the potential users of the technology. For example, policy makers may have a clear say in whether an eHealth technology fits their organization's vision and whether it will be implemented. ICT experts may have clear ideas about what is needed for them to be able to maintain the eHealth technology or what the possibilities of a technology are. This can mean that policy makers, ICT experts and many others, like doctors, therapists, or funders are stakeholders as well.

First, all possible stakeholders must be identified. After that, their interdependencies (e.g., manager vs. employee), responsibilities, and stakes are evaluated in a stakeholder analysis. While the identification and analysis are initiated in the contextual inquiry, this does not mean that they have to be 'finished' in this phase. Stakeholder identification and analysis activities can (or should) be updated and adapted throughout the entire process, even during implementation and evaluation activities. For example, based on decisions that are made about the design of a technology, a specific technology development company can be added as a stakeholder. In the next two sections, the stakeholder identification and analysis are explained further.

Stakeholder identification

First, researchers need to determine who the relevant stakeholders are during the stakeholder identification (Van Velsen, Wentzel, & van Gemert-Pijnen, 2013; van Woezik, Braakman-Jansen, Kulyk, Siemons, & van Gemert-Pijnen, 2016). A first example is a scoping review of scientific literature. This is a suitable way to gain quick insight into the stakeholders that might be present. Such an overview based on literature is often used as a starting point, from which to further progress towards insight in who the stakeholders for the specific project are. A second approach is to ask known experts in the field to identify who they perceive as being stakeholders, which is called expert recommendation. Third, besides the experts, the stakeholders themselves may also have clear ideas about who other stakeholders are, which is referred to as snowball sampling.

The end result of stakeholder identification is a (long) list and/or visualized map (see Figure 8.1 for an example) of stakeholders. A broad range of stakeholders can be identified: They can be individuals (e.g., nurses), groups of people (e.g., patient associations), or organizations (e.g., hospitals). However, it is often impossible or even undesirable to involve them all in the development process. Therefore, the next step is to determine who the key stakeholders are and what their stakes are by means of a stakeholder analysis.

Stakeholder analysis

Some stakeholders may have a greater influence on or may be more influenced by the technology than others. Such stakeholders are referred to as key stakeholders. Examples are end-users, or decision makers in an organization. To find the key stakeholders among the list of all stakeholders, different frameworks have been developed. One of the most widely used frameworks is that of Mitchell et al. (1997). In this approach, stakeholders can be mapped based on their power, legitimacy, and urgency. Their power reflects the amount of influence their opinions, needs, or wishes will have. Legitimacy of a stakeholder reflects whether they should be involved; it shows that stakeholders are the ones who 'really count' because they are relevant for and central to the project (Mitchell et al., 1997; van Woezik et al., 2016). A stakeholder's urgency concerns to what extend the stakeholders' needs and wishes would require immediate action. Based on the stakeholder analysis, a substantiated decision can be made about who key stakeholders are and should thus be involved during the entire development process.

Of course, researchers or developers can attempt to determine the stakeholders' power, legitimacy, and urgency themselves. However, it is unlikely that they are able to oversee all interests, relationships, and consequences of all different stakeholders for an eHealth technology. It is therefore advisable to again involve experts in the field and/or the stakeholders themselves in rating the stakeholders and identifying the key stakeholders. Finally, the outcome of a stakeholder analysis is not merely a 'ranking', but also needs to contain a qualitative overview of what the stakes are.

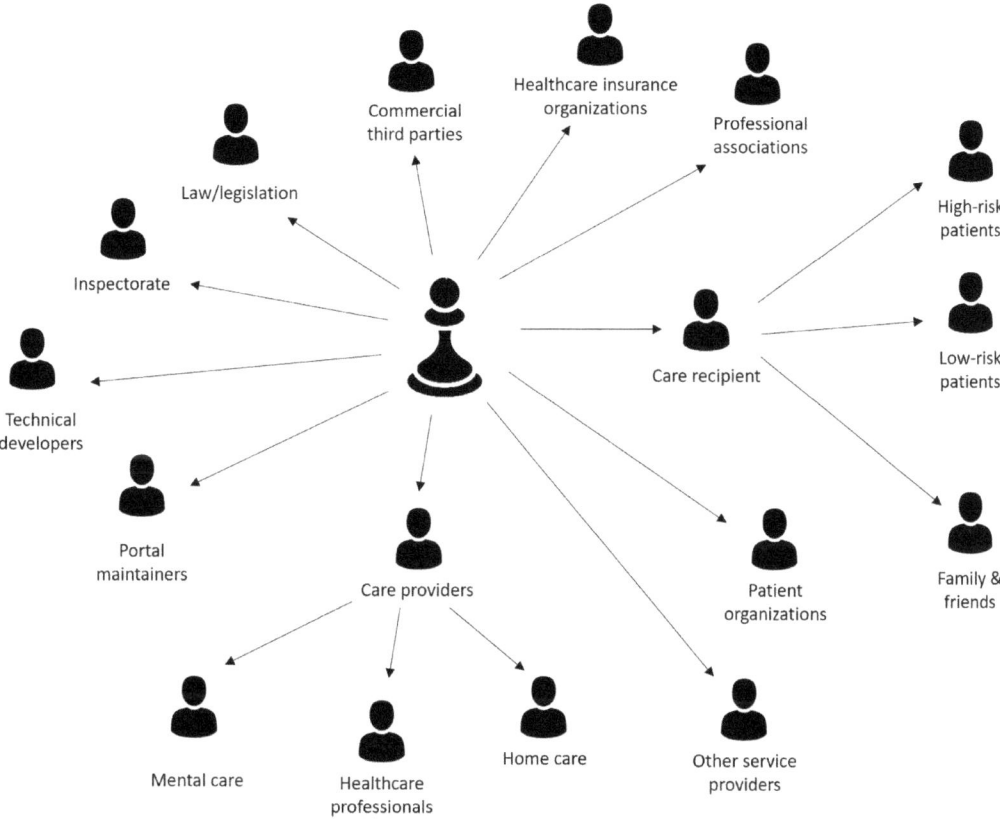

Figure 8.1 An example of a stakeholder map (van Limburg, 2016).

Box 8.1 Case Study: The wicked problem of zoonotic diseases.

Zoonotic diseases are one of the major threats to public health. In fact, over 60% of human pathogens by now are zoonotic in origin (e.g., AIDS, bird flu, SARS-CoV-2). The prevention and control of such infections is challenging and highly complex. It is described as a 'wicked' problem (van Woezik et al., 2016), as many factors contribute to their occurrence, it involves many (often interdependent) stakeholders and there is no single solution that would solve the entire problem. Researchers aimed to develop an online platform to support multidisciplinary collaboration to prevent and control outbreaks of zoonotic infections.

First, researchers needed to investigate who should use the platform and who other stakeholders were (stakeholder identification). They performed a literature scan to formulate an initial list of relevant stakeholders. Then, recommendations from experts in the fields of infectious diseases and public health helped them validate the stakeholder list.

Second, key stakeholders had to be identified to decide who to involve in the further development of the platform. For that purpose, the researchers sent a survey to representatives of their stakeholders and asked them to rate the complete list of stakeholders, according to the approach by Mitchell et al. (1997). Once they were identified, these key stakeholders were actively involved during the further development, implementation, and evaluation of the online platform for risk- and crisis communication.

Insight needs to be provided in – amongst other things – what the needs and wishes of stakeholders are, what their roles and interrelations look like, and why they are important for the project. As mentioned before, a stakeholder analysis is never really finished, and can – or even should – be adapted throughout the entire process, based on new insights.

Research Methods for the Contextual Inquiry

A stakeholder identification and analysis are not the only activities that should be conducted during the contextual inquiry: Many more methods can be used to learn as much as possible about the context. In many of these methods, the identified stakeholders can be involved as participants. Methods in the contextual inquiry do not have to be used sequentially: Several research activities can be performed alongside each other, and their results might even be intertwined. In the next section, a non-exhaustive overview of methods that might be used in the contextual inquiry is presented. Some commonly used methods are discussed more in-depth, while others are presented more briefly. The order in which these methods are presented does of course not imply the order in which they should be applied: This chapter does not serve as a blueprint for a contextual inquiry, since the choice for any method depends on the intended objective, practical preconditions, and fit with the intended participants and their context.

Desk Research

What is desk research?

One of the first exploratory activities that is often conducted during the contextual inquiry phase is *desk research*. Within eHealth development, desk research is the non-systematic collection of material that helps the development team to learn as much as possible about the context (Kip et al., 2022). Examples of relevant materials are scientific and non-scientific literature, policy documents, videos, or readily available reports such as the outcomes of employee satisfaction surveys. Desk research can be conducted in several ways, e.g., using search engines, going through relevant websites, asking stakeholders for material, or using an organization's archive. A prerequisite is that all the collected material should already exist; no primary research activities are carried out.

Table 8.1 Potential methods for the contextual inquiry that are discussed in this chapter.

Method	Definition
Desk research	Collecting material in a non-systematic way in order to help the development team to learn as much as possible about the context.
Literature review	Gaining insight into the current status quo of scientific literature in a certain broad field of study by means of a systematic search of literature.
Focus group	Collecting qualitative data among a small number of stakeholders in a group discussion, 'focused' around a particular topic or set of issues.
Interviews	Asking questions in a structured, semi-structured, or unstructured way to obtain answers from an individual.
Questionnaires	Collecting quantitative or qualitative data by asking participants to fill out open- or closed-ended questions, either online or on paper.
Observations	Observing an event of interest while it occurs by a researcher, direct or technology mediated.
Log data analysis	Using data that log certain behaviour on a system or in daily life to analyze patterns.
Delphi study	Creating consensus among experts on a certain topic through asking questions, reflecting upon the answers of others, and potentially adjusting one's opinion until consensus is reached, in multiple consecutive rounds.

An advantage of desk research is that it can lead to results that are not (yet) available through scientific publications, such as ongoing studies, innovative technologies, or treatment protocols, and provides a better reflection of the actual working place. A pitfall is that while a systematic approach is not a requirement for desk research, it should not be viewed as a synonym for randomly collecting information. Structure can be added, for example by mapping and describing existing apps by means of an evaluation tool (Breeman et al., 2021), or by using frameworks to evaluate the quality of sources. When scientific evaluation instruments such as lists for quality checks, e.g., from Cochrane, are not applicable because sources are not science-based, more generic source evaluation sources such as the CRAAP test can help to assess the value of a source (Blakeslee, 2004)

What kind of results can desk research generate?

Desk research can be used throughout the entire contextual inquiry, but it is often deployed as one of the first steps in a development process (Kip et al., 2022). Desk research can be used for a broad range of goals, for example:

- Gaining insight into existing communication processes by studying existing patient care communication (Gulmans et al., 2009);
- Identifying (ongoing projects on) virtual reality interventions that are used within forensic mental healthcare (Kip et al., 2019).

Literature Review

What is a literature review?

When gaining insight in the status quo of the scientific literature in a certain field, several types of literature reviews are available, such as a meta-analysis, a systematic review, umbrella review, narrative review, and a scoping review. All of these have in common that they are based on a carefully comprised search strategy and that data collection and analysis are conducted in a systematic way. However, with a scoping review, a broad field of study, where research questions are relatively unspecific and various kinds of study designs are used, can be addressed within a relatively short amount of time (Arksey & O'Malley, 2005). In systematic reviews, a quality assessment is often added, and meta-analyses make use of quantitative data from other studies, such as randomized controlled trials.

A main advantage of a literature review is the systematic collection of research centred on a specific topic, which is often valuable for any eHealth project. A pitfall is that usually quite some time has passed between initial data collection and publication of a study, meaning that not all state-of-the-art knowledge can be gathered via literature reviews (Kip et al., 2022). This again underlines the importance of combining different research methods. Furthermore, many literature reviews in the eHealth domain do not contain a quality appraisal because it is time consuming, impossible due to the broad range of included studies, or irrelevant for the goal of the review. This means that results have to be interpreted with care. Literature reviews in very new or quickly evolving fields (such as eHealth) and with exploratory aims may yield narrative results, offering a more qualitative description of the literature. Fields that have already been more established and have more focused aims can yield results that are more quantitative and focused on effectiveness.

What kinds of results can a literature review generate?

The results of a literature review consist of an overview of the literature that is available in a previously defined topic. In eHealth development, literature reviews can be used for a very broad range of goals, such as:

- Gaining insight into existing eHealth interventions on weight loss and the used behaviour change techniques and persuasive features (Asbjørnsen et al., 2019);
- Providing insight into existing development and implementation strategies for audit and feedback systems for antimicrobial resistance (Keizer et al., 2022).

Focus Group

What is a focus group?

Focus groups are a much-used method for the development of technology (Kip et al., 2022). Focus groups can be defined as 'a way of collecting qualitative data, which - essentially - involves engaging a small number of people in an informal group discussion (or discussions), "focused" around a particular topic or set of issues' (Wilkinson, 2003, p. 181). In the contextual inquiry, a homo- or heterogeneous group of stakeholders can be brought together within this discussion group format (Kip et al., 2022). The level of structure can range from unstructured, with the researcher announcing the topic to be discussed and allowing the participants to respond freely to semi-structured, with the researcher using a predetermined scheme to cover questions and topics presented in some order (Krueger & Casey, 2001).

In focus groups, the interaction that takes place between the participants often allows for bouncing ideas off each other, comparing attitudes, identifying new topics of interest, and sharing experiences (Wilkinson, 2003). The interaction between participants can lead to new information that wouldn't have been discovered when using individual methods like interviews, and one can explore a variety of different opinions and visions that wouldn't become apparent in methods like questionnaires (Kip et al., 2022). Focus groups can also be conducted online and anonymously (e.g., using a chat platform), which has been found to be a feasible and valid method for collecting sensitive data on, e.g., sexual health (Wettergren, Eriksson, Nilsson, Jervaeus, & Lampic, 2016). Some drawbacks might be greater planning and recruitment efforts to assemble groups, the disproportionate influence of dominant participants, and potential power differences – which is especially relevant when conducting a focus group with a heterogeneous group of stakeholders, such as managers and therapists. Finally, focus groups with vulnerable participants, such as people with dementia or an intellectual disability, require another approach than those with, e.g., doctors or managers, which requires specific skills from researchers (Kip et al., 2022).

What kind of results can focus groups generate?

Focus groups can be used for several activities of the contextual inquiry, for example, identifying stakeholders and their roles, describing a current situation, finding out about points of improvement, describing relevant behaviour, or uncovering attitudes and other predictors of behaviour. Examples of studies that made use of focus groups in order to learn more about the context are:

- Identifying points of improvement of self-management of patients with chronic obstructive pulmonary disease (COPD; Van de Dijk et al., 2013);
- Finding out about current uses, preferences, facilitators, and barriers to using existing electronic health resources by veterans (Haun et al., 2015).

Interviews

What is an interview?

An interview is a conversation involving a researcher asking an individual questions about the phenomenon/subject of interest. Interviews can be highly structured, semi-structured, or unstructured.

Interviews are often conducted by one researcher and guided by an interview scheme with predetermined questions and topics, often combined with probing questions.

Interviews are considered a suitable method to gather in-depth information in individual experiences and can be used throughout the entire development process (Kip et al., 2022). A potential pitfall is that they can offer a one-sided picture of a topic and that there might be a selection or recollection bias, warranting the need for combining interviews with other methods. Because of the direct interactive setting, participants may be prone to answer questions in a socially desirable way, or in a way they think 'pleases' the researcher. Contrastingly, interviews can be an especially suitable method for hard-to-involve target groups such as people with dementia or a severe psychiatric disorder because of the possibility to tailor questions (Kip et al., 2022). To increase the likelihood of successfully involving people with limited cognitive skills it is advisable to, for example, use concrete examples, such as scenarios or existing interventions, and to have the interviews conducted by skilled researchers (Kip et al., 2019, Noordman et al., 2017).

What kind of results can interviews generate?

The most common aim of an *interview* is obtaining answers to questions of an individual participant (Dooley, 2001). Within the contextual inquiry, interviews can be conducted with, for example, possible users, experts, or project managers. Some examples of the use of interviews during the contextual inquiry are:

- Questioning several kinds of stakeholders working in public health about their personal experience with social media and the context of public health (Hart, Stetten, & Castaneda, 2016);
- Describing current behaviour and its determinants or improving physical activity (Sporrel et al., 2020).

Questionnaires

What are questionnaires?

A *questionnaire* is a method in which participants individually fill out open- or closed-ended questions, either online or on paper. Questionnaires can be administered once (cross-sectional) or multiple times, over a longer period of time (longitudinal). A specific form of questionnaire is experience sampling – a form of Ecological Momentary Assessment (EMA). In these types of questionnaires, participants are asked very short questions on their current state or behaviour, via e.g., their smartphone, often multiple times throughout the day and for a longer period of time. This specific method is characterized by the collection of data in the real world, a focus on individual's current or recent states, and multiple assessments (Trull & Ebner-Priemer, 2009). Questionnaire studies can make use of existing, validated questionnaires, such as the eHealth literacy scale (Norman & Skinner, 2006), or can consist of questions that were created by researchers, specifically tailored to the project.

One of the main advantages of questionnaires is that a relatively large sample can be included, especially when using online questionnaires (Kip et al., 2022). An accompanying challenge is that in-depth information is often lacking because probing questions cannot be asked. Another pitfall of questionnaires are potential biases, such as self-selection bias; when using language-driven questionnaires, target groups with low literacy or little technological skills might be excluded. Recollection biases can be overcome by using the aforementioned experience sampling method, in which participants are asked questions about a situation or feeling in (near) real-time, as opposed to reflecting on it in hindsight.

What kind of results can questionnaires generate?

Questionnaires can be used throughout the entire contextual inquiry and are suitable for a broad range of goals. Examples of objectives are:

- Analyzing how and when people look for information at different points during an infection outbreak, according to a diary study (van Velsen et al., 2012);
- Identifying points of improvement in conceptions and knowledge of stakeholders on antimicrobial resistance (Keizer et al., 2019).

Other Suitable Research Methods for the Contextual Inquiry

In the previous section, several methods that are often used in contextual inquiries were described in-depth. However, there are of course many other methods that can be used as well, some of which will be briefly explained below. Again, it is important to note that the choice to use one of these methods depends on the goal that needs to be reached, the characteristics of participants, and the practical demands and requirements that are relevant within a specific context.

First, in observations, the researcher observes an event of interest while it occurs. This is especially useful in situations that are (1) highly complex and therefore difficult for subjects to adequately report on, (2) prone to social desirability or shame, (3) when the subjects of interest are not able to describe their behaviour, e.g., in case of severe dementia or intellectual disabilities, or (4) are so obvious and routine to the people involved in the situation under study that it would not occur to them to report on it, even though such information can be crucial to the researcher. An example of an objective of an observational study is to investigate how often physicians disinfect their hands during rounds, and whether there are differences in frequency and accuracy of disinfection behaviour between physicians or situations.

A second example is log data: These typically consist of the registration of an event (e.g., logging in, entering a room, sending a message, performing a certain action, and a 'timestamp'). Log data are different from observations in that they are especially relevant for quantifiable events. There are two ways in which log data can be used to learn more about the current situation during the contextual inquiry: System and behaviour log data. With system log data, researchers can check how often, in what way, and when people visited a technology, have used a feature, or logged into the system. Behaviour log data tracks measurable behaviour such as frequency of use of alcohol dispensers for hand hygiene, or routes of healthcare workers through a hospital. An example is the logging of call buttons pressed by nursing home residents who have a request for a nurse (van Eeden, Moeke, & Bekker, 2016).

Finally, instead of studying an event, sometimes it is pivotal to determine what consensus about a certain topic is among stakeholders, for example to determine future directions of a project. For that purpose, a Delphi study is highly suitable. It solicits opinions from groups in an iterative process of answering questions, usually in multiple rounds of (online) questionnaires. Thus, it offers a systematic way to reach consensus on a certain topic among various stakeholders, mostly experts. An example is the use of Delphi studies to gain insight into expert opinions on relevant self-management behaviours for reducing the impact of COPD (Korpershoek et al., 2020).

Using the Results of the Contextual Inquiry

The contextual inquiry is a flexible, multi-method, and iterative process

As became clear in the previous sections, a broad range of methods can be used in the contextual inquiry. However, the methods that are discussed in this chapter, and the order in which they are presented, should not be viewed as a set blueprint for the contextual inquiry. Because eHealth development can take place in many different contexts, with different stakeholders, and with different technologies, a step-by-step approach is not feasible, nor desirable. In fact, a flexible, adaptive approach of choosing the appropriate methods is key (Kip et al., 2019). The choice for the most suitable method should always be made based on the research objective, the characteristics of the intended participants, and the preconditions that arise within a specific context. Furthermore, conclusions about the current situation and points of improvement within a specific context should be drawn based on different kinds of data to prevent a too narrow vision or overlooking important information (Kip et al., 2022). For example, interviews can be used to provide more context and depth to the outcomes of a literature review, and a questionnaire with a large sample can be added to make more generalizable statements. Additionally – as is the case for the entire eHealth development process – the contextual inquiry has an iterative nature (van Gemert-Pijnen et al., 2011). This means that the development team should go back and forth between different methods used, and should be flexible enough to revise decisions when needed at every step of the process. To illustrate: During the design phase, a new stakeholder might arise that wasn't accounted for in the initial stakeholder identification. It might be necessary to include that stakeholder's perspective about points of improvement of the current situation as well, i.e., moving (temporarily) back to the contextual inquiry. To summarize: Any contextual inquiry should be flexible and adaptive, multiple methods should be selected and combined, and the process should be iterative.

Decisions should be made by interdisciplinary groups of stakeholders

Based on the results of the methods used in the contextual inquiry, decisions on the direction of the eHealth development are made. These can be decisions about the target group, the main problem that an intervention should address, or the behaviour that has to be influenced. However, not every decision might be feasible, e.g., because of a lack of funding or specific regulations. Therefore, any decision in a contextual inquiry, ranging from the selection of a research method to conclusions that can be drawn based on data, should ideally be discussed with stakeholders. This can be done in stakeholder meetings, or in interdisciplinary project team meetings that consist of stakeholders. By using the perspective of multiple stakeholders when making decisions, tunnel vision is prevented. To illustrate: Researchers can provide an overview of potentially useful methods for an intended objective, patients can determine the suitability of a research method for the target group, healthcare professionals can think about the content of questions asked in, e.g., interviews, managers can shed light on potential practical barriers, and project leaders can manage the execution of data collection.

Future directions: The importance of transparency and sharing lessons learned

A pitfall of the multi-perspective, multi-method, iterative nature of contextual inquiries can be that it becomes 'messy' and the overview can be lost. This illustrates the importance of a systematic and transparent development process. A well-organized, methodical approach enables the development team to evaluate their process and to figure out where and why certain decisions were made. This makes it easier to go back to a specific point in the development process when decisions need to be revised. In order to do this, it is essential that every activity and every choice that is made within the contextual inquiry is well-documented. This is also important because the team has to be able to retrieve the results of the contextual inquiry during the entire development process, since they constantly have to check if the output of other development activities still matches the stakeholders and their environment. However, researchers often do not publish about the contextual inquiry or only publish about one method used, e.g., a literature review, which implies that an important future direction is to improve documentation and publication of entire contextual inquiry processes, including a reflection on the decisions made. Good documentation and publication of outcomes of the contextual inquiry also has another benefit: It allows researchers to learn from each other and prevents them from having to reinvent the wheel when looking for suitable research methods (Kip et al., 2019). An important future direction for improving contextual inquiries, is to create a comprehensive 'toolkit' with an overview of potentially useful methods, examples of application, and lessons learned about using these methods in different types of contexts and with different target groups. While first steps have been taken (e.g., Kip et al., 2022), there is still work to be done to increase the possibilities for researchers to learn from each other and receive more support when selecting the most suitable and feasible research method. Finally, an important future direction is to explore which other methods can be used in the contextual inquiry. Methods such as eye-tracking, card sorting, or usability testing might be suitable as well, but more research with and on these methods in different stages of eHealth development is necessary.

The Contextual Inquiry and the CeHRes Roadmap

During eHealth development, it is necessary to always keep the context in mind since this ensures the fit with the context of the output of development activities. When looking at the CeHRes Roadmap, as described in Chapter 7 of this book, the results of the contextual inquiry are relevant in multiple ways. In general, the stakeholders that are identified in this phase should be involved throughout all other phases as well. There are also multiple other ways in which the contextual inquiry is intertwined with other phases of the Roadmap, such as:

- The *value specification* builds upon the results from the contextual inquiry about e.g., points of improvement by converting them into concrete, more specific goals, values, and requirements;
- In the *design phase*, the technology that addresses the problem or aims to improve a current situation is developed, in co-creation with key stakeholders. Furthermore, the development team should constantly check if the prototypes still fit with the problems and context as analyzed in the contextual inquiry;
- The *operationalization phase* is focused on the implementation of the technology within the context. Because of the involvement of the stakeholders and analysis of the context, implementation of the technology has already begun at the start during the contextual inquiry;
- *Evaluation* should focus on the technology within the specific context. This means that, relevant stakeholders have to be involved, e.g., by interviewing them or measuring health outcomes. The environment also has to be included in the evaluation, since researchers should make clear what the impact of the technology on the entire context is (also see Chapter 14).

Summary

This chapter has shown that the contextual inquiry serves as the foundation for the entire development, implementation, and evaluation processes of eHealth. A thorough understanding of the stakeholders, the current situation, and points of improvement within a specific context is necessary. It is essential to keep central for whom, what, and where an eHealth technology is being developed. The take-home messages of this chapter are:

- The contextual inquiry is often skipped or conducted partially, while it is pivotal since it serves as the basis for the development process;
- Multiple methods can and should be used iteratively to get a thorough understanding of the context;
- Decisions on what methods to use should be based on research questions, characteristics of participants, and practical considerations;

- Identifying stakeholders and getting a good overview of their main tasks, roles, and perspectives serves as the foundation for any eHealth development process;
- The stakeholders identified during the contextual inquiry continue to play an important role in every stage of development, implementation, and evaluation.

Key References for Further Reading

Beyer, H., & Holtzblatt, K. (1998). *Contextual design: Defining customer-centered systems.* San Francisco: Morgan Kaufmann.

Kip, H., Keizer, J., da Silva, M. C., Beerlage-de Jong, N., Köhle, N., & Kelders, S. M. (2022). Methods for human-centered eHealth development: Narrative scoping review. *Journal of Medical Internet Research,* 24(1), e31858.

Mitchell, R. K., Agle, B. R., & Wood, D. J. (1997). Toward a theory of stakeholder identification and salience: Defining the principle of who and what really counts. *Academy of Management Review,* 22(4), 853–886.

Trull, T. J., & Ebner-Priemer, U. W. (2009). Using experience sampling methods/ecological momentary assessment (ESM/EMA) in clinical assessment and clinical research: Introduction to the special section. *Psychological Assessment,* 21(4), 457–462.

Van Woezik, A. F., Braakman-Jansen, L. M., Kulyk, O., Siemons, L., & van Gemert-Pijnen, J. E. W. C. (2016). Tackling wicked problems in infection prevention and control: A guideline for co-creation with stakeholders. *Antimicrobial Resistance & Infection Control,* 5(1), 20.

References

Arksey, H. & O'Malley, L. (2005). Scoping studies: Towards a methodological framework. *International Journal of Social Research Methodology,* 8(1), 19–32.

Asbjørnsen, R. A., Smedsrød, M. L., Nes, L. S., Wentzel, J., Varsi, C., Hjelmesæth, J., & van Gemert-Pijnen, J. E. W. C. (2019). Persuasive system design principles and behavior change techniques to stimulate motivation and adherence in electronic health interventions to support weight loss maintenance: Scoping review. *JMIR,* 21(6), e14265.

Beyer, H. & Holtzblatt, K. (1998). *Contextual Design: Defining Customer-Centered Systems.* San Francisco: Morgan Kaufmann.

Blakeslee, S. (2004). The CRAAP test. *Loex Quarterly,* 31(3), 4.

Breeman L. D., Keesman, M., Atsma, D. E., Chavannes, N. H., Janssen, V., & van Gemert-Pijnen, J. E. W. C., BENEFIT consortium. (2021). A multi-stakeholder approach to eHealth development: Promoting sustained healthy living among cardiovascular patients. *Int J Med Inform,* 147, 104364.

Dooley, D. (2001). *Social Research Methods* (4th edition). Upper Saddle River, NJ: Prentice-Hall.

Freeman, R. E. (2010). *Strategic management: A stakeholder approach.* Cambridge University Press.

Gulmans, J., Vollenbroek-Hutten, M. M. R., van Gemert-Pijnen, J. E. W. C., & Van Harten, W. H. (2009). Evaluating patient care communication in integrated care settings: Application of a mixed method approach in cerebral palsy programs. *International Journal for Quality in Health Care,* 21(1), 58–65.

Hart, M., Stetten, N., & Castaneda, G. (2016). Considerations for public health organizations attempting to implement a social media presence: A qualitative study. *JMIR Public Health Surveillance,* 2(1), e6.

Haun, J. N., Nazi, K. M., Chavez, M., Lind, J. D., Antinori, N., Gosline, R. M., & Martin, T. L. (2015). A participatory approach to designing and enhancing integrated health information technology systems for veterans: Protocol. *JMIR Research Protocols,* 4(1), e28.

Kip, H., Keizer, J., da Silva, M. C., Beerlage-de Jong, N., Köhle, N., & Kelders, S. M. (2022). Methods for human-centered eHealth development: Narrative scoping review. *JMIR,* 24(1), e31858.

Kip, H., Kelders, S. M., Bouman, Y. H. A., & van Gemert-Pijnen, J. E. W. C. (2019). The importance of systematically reporting and reflecting on eHealth development: Participatory development process of a virtual reality application for forensic mental health care. *JMIR,* 21(8), e12972.

Keizer, J., Bente, B. E., Al Naiemi, N., van Gemert-Pijnen, J. E. W. C., & Beerlage-De Jong, N. (2022). Improving the development and implementation of audit and feedback systems to support health care workers in limiting antimicrobial resistance in the hospital: Scoping review. *JMIR,* 24(3), e33531.

Keizer, J., Braakman-Jansen, L. M. A., Kampmeier, S., Köck, R., Al Naiemi, N., Riet-Warning, T., ... & van Gemert-Pijnen, J. E. W. C. (2019). Cross-border comparison of antimicrobial resistance (AMR) and AMR prevention measures: The healthcare workers' perspective. *Antimicrobial Resistance & Infection Control*, 8(1), 1–13.

Korpershoek, Y. J., Hermsen, S., Schoonhoven, L., Schuurmans, M. J., & Trappenburg, J. C. (2020). User-centered design of a mobile health intervention to enhance exacerbation-related self-management in patients with chronic obstructive pulmonary disease (copilot): Mixed methods study. *JMIR*, 22(6), e15449.

Krueger, R. A., & Casey, M. A. (2001). Designing and conducting focus group interviews. In R. A. Krueger, M. A. Casey, J. Donner, S. Kirsch, & J. N. Maack (Eds.), *Social analysis: Selected tools and techniques* (pp. 4–23). Washington, DC: Social Development Family of the World Bank.

Mitchell, R. K., Agle, B. R., & Wood, D. J. (1997). Toward a theory of stakeholder identification and salience: Defining the principle of who and what really counts. *The Academy of Management Review*, 22(4), 853–886.

Noordman, J., Driesenaar, J. A., van Bruinessen, I. R., & van Dulmen, S. (2017). ListeningTime; participatory development of a web-based preparatory communication tool for elderly cancer patients and their healthcare providers. *Internet Interventions*, 9, 51–56.

Norman, C. D., & Skinner, H. A. (2006). eHEALS: The eHealth literacy scale. *Journal of medical Internet research*, 8(4), e507.

Sporrel, K., De Boer, R. D., Wang, S., Nibbeling, N., Simons, M., Deutekom, M., ... & Kröse, B. (2021). The design and development of a personalized leisure time physical activity application based on behavior change theories, end-user perceptions, and principles from empirical data mining. *Frontiers in Public Health*, 711.

Trull, T. J., & Ebner-Priemer, U. W. (2009). Using experience sampling methods/ecological momentary assessment (ESM/EMA) in clinical assessment and clinical research: Introduction to the special section. *Psychological Assessment*, 21(4), 457–462.

Van de Dijk, M., Te Lintelo, J., Willems, C. G., & van Gemert-Pijnen, J. E. W. C. (2013). eCOPD: User requirements of older people with COPD for eHealth support at home, a user-centred study. In: *Assistive Technology: From Research to Practice* (pp. 1272–1278). IOS Press.

Van Eeden, K., Moeke, D., & Bekker, R. (2014). Care on demand in nursing homes: A queueing theoretic approach. *Health Care Management Science*, 19(3), 227–240.

Van Gemert-Pijnen, J. E. W. C., Nijland, N., Limburg, M. van, Ossebaard, H. C., Kelders, S. M., Eysenbach, G., & Seydel, E. R. (2011). A holistic framework to improve the uptake and impact of eHealth technologies. *Journal of Medical Internet Research*, 13(4), e111.

Van Limburg, A. H. (2016). *Implementing antibiotic stewardship: Involving stakeholders in eHealth*. Enschede, The Netherlands: University of Twente.

Van Velsen, L., van Gemert-Pijnen, J. E., Beaujean, D. J., Wentzel, J., & van Steenbergen, J. E. (2012). Should health organizations use web 2.0 media in times of an infectious disease crisis? An in-depth qualitative study of citizens' information behavior during an EHEC outbreak. *JMIR*, 14(6), e181.

Van Velsen, L., Wentzel, J., & van Gemert-Pijnen, J. E. (2013). Designing eHealth that matters via a multidisciplinary requirements development approach. *JMIR Research Protocols*, 2(1), e21.

Van Woezik, A. F., Braakman-Jansen, L. M., Kulyk, O., Siemons, L., & van Gemert-Pijnen, J. E. (2016). Tackling wicked problems in infection prevention and control: A guideline for co-creation with stakeholders. *Antimicrobial Resistance & Infection Control*, 5, 20.

Wettergren, L., Eriksson, E. L., Nilsson, J., Jervaeus, A., & Lampic, C. (2016). Online focus group discussion is a valid and feasible mode when investigating sensitive topics among young persons with a cancer experience. *JMIR Research Protocols*, 5(2), e86.

Whiteside, J., Bennett, J., & Holtzblatt, K. (1988). Usability engineering: Our experience and evolution. *Handbook of Human-Computer Interaction*, 35.

Wilkinson, S. (2003). Focus groups. In J. A. Smith (Ed.), *Qualitative psychology: A practical guide to research methods* (pp. 181–204). London: Sage.

9   Activities for Value Sensitive eHealth Design

Lex van Velsen & Christiane Grünloh

Introduction

Imagine a technology that offers a self-help programme to support older adults who lost their spouse in dealing with their new life situation. What would such a self-help programme look like; what support does it offer; what kind of safe guards must be implemented to ensure that it is safe; how, when, and why are healthcare professionals involved? In this chapter, concepts and methods from value sensitive design are described. This chapter builds forth on Chapter 3, as technical modalities are chosen during the design phase. But most of all, this chapter takes input from Chapter 8, Contextual Inquiry, as the activities that are conducted in this phase provide the foundation for the different activities that inform eHealth designs. The design phase, in its turn, is also closely related to activities for eHealth implementation and evaluation. The value proposition and service model inform the business model and implementation strategies, while the service model and the requirements are often used as input for evaluation. Here, evaluation must indicate whether the most important requirements are implemented successfully, and whether the service addresses the needs and values of its end-users and has an effect on key performance indicators, such as quality of life, efficiency, or caregiver workload.

In this chapter, the concepts behind and activities that can be used for value sensitive eHealth design are presented, described, and connected to each other. After completing this chapter, you will be able to:

- Explain the goal, nature, and importance of multiple design activities (personas, scenarios, value propositions, service models and requirements);
- Explain the interrelationship of multiple design activities and connect this to the fit of an eHealth technology with its context and its user;
- Create a value proposition for your eHealth service;
- Translate the findings from your Contextual Inquiry into service and technology design of eHealth via multiple design activities;
- Create a design document, including personas, scenarios, and requirements.

DOI: 10.4324/9781003302049-11

Designing an eHealth Technology

The design of an eHealth technology spans many different activities, all with the goal to make clear what the system should do, what it should look like, and how it should be implemented. It is also the time and place where many sources of inspiration somehow need to be merged. Results from the Contextual Inquiry, a market analysis, as well as creativity and even an eHealth technology push (i.e., when an eHealth technology is available first and drives the design of the product) have to be combined into an innovation that has an added value for the end-users (i.e., that responds to their needs and personal values), can be implemented in the existing healthcare context, and also leads to a viable business model.

The design process consists of several activities and the development of a range of accompanying documents that, together, inform the design that will be used in practice. In this chapter, we will discuss the most prominent ones:

1. Personas;
2. Scenarios;
3. Value propositions;
4. Service models; and
5. Requirements.

These activities form an iterative process, where they are intertwined, inform each other, and lead to document updates as new insights are developed. Before we describe these design activities in detail, we will dive into the topic of value sensitive design, a theoretically grounded approach that accounts for human values throughout the design process and informs the aforementioned design activities.

Value Sensitive Design: eHealth that Adds Value by Accounting for Human Values

A successful innovation corresponds well to the needs of end-users and their context of use and creates added value by making it easier for them to perform a certain task or achieve certain goals. The value proposition of the innovation, which will be described in more detail later, specifies which benefits the buyer and/or user of the eHealth technology can expect. Here, we want to emphasize the different meanings when it comes to the term 'value'. When creating a value proposition, 'value' refers to something that is use worthy, valuable, or has an economic value. The value proposition statement therefore concisely describes the benefit an eHealth technology provides. However, the term 'value' within value sensitive design has a broader meaning. While there are different definitions of human values, within this approach, values have been defined as 'what is important to people in their lives, with a focus on ethics and morality' (Friedman & Hendry, 2019). As technology permeates almost all aspects of our personal and professional lives, it also can support other aspects that are important for people and that go beyond user needs: Their personal values. One prominent example are the contact tracing apps, that were hastily developed during the COVID-19 pandemic and created public debate around value tensions such as privacy, freedom of movement, and epidemic control (Hogan, Macedo, Macha, Barman, & Jiang, 2021). Even though technology can sometimes be considered as a tool, there is a growing consensus that eHealth technology is not value-neutral and to the contrary, design as an activity is always value laden (Friedman, 2007; JafariNaimi, Nathan, & Hargraves, 2015; Miller, 2020).

Depending on the design choices, some values are supported while others are hindered. The contact tracing apps followed either a centralized or decentralized architecture, where the latter prioritized privacy and security over access to data by public health authorities. This means that even if a technology is not designed to explicitly support or hinder human values, the resulting product still might. For example, the design of features and information flows in an eHealth technology can significantly impact a patient's self-sufficiency and ability to engage in self-care, even if autonomy and independence were not explicitly considered during the design process. Imagine an eHealth technology that continuously monitors the medical parameters of a patient and immediately notifies the healthcare provider when these are out of range, without giving patients any information. This would enable healthcare professionals to monitor their patients on distance (i.e., supporting their value of 'responsibility' and 'control'), however, it does not support the patient to engage in self-management. In this example, patients are conceptualised as taking a passive role and patients values of independence, control, and autonomy would not be supported. In summary, although the value proposition can encompass human values, this is not guaranteed unless they have been explicitly considered during the design process.

An important part of the development of eHealth is therefore to identify and conceptualize the human values that the different stakeholders hold. Value sensitive design (VSD) provides a methodology to account for human values throughout the development process (Friedman, Kahn, Borning, Zhang, & Galletta, 2006). Innovations in healthcare impact a wide range of stakeholders, each with their own distinct values, which can sometimes lead to conflicts or tensions. For example, in the Swedish eHealth service that gives patients online access to their electronic health records, a log-list was provided that showed who had accessed their records. This feature aimed to increase trust in patients given that healthcare professionals can access the records even without permission. This feature that supports patient privacy and increases trust, was however perceived as a surveillance tool by professionals and thus in tension with their privacy (Grünloh, 2021).

To account for human values in a systematic and comprehensive way, VSD suggests three investigations that can be carried out (Friedman et al., 2006):

- **Conceptual investigations** aim to identify both the direct and indirect stakeholders affected by the eHealth technology, define the values implicated by its use, and prioritize competing values. This process involves systematically identifying those who interact with the technology and are impacted by it. For example: In the case of patient-accessible electronic health records (PAEHR), direct stakeholders encompass patients and informal caregivers who use the service, while indirect stakeholders include healthcare professionals, among others. Healthcare professionals have their own software to view and edit patient records but may be affected by patients reading their records. Furthermore, you should go through that stakeholder list and identify potential harms and benefits for each stakeholder group and map them to values. Personas can be useful to identify those harms and benefits and literature can be helpful to identify corresponding values (Friedman et al., 2006). It is also useful to check your list of stakeholders with the stakeholders (e.g., when conducting empirical investigations, see next point);
- **Empirical investigations** examine stakeholders' understandings, context, and experiences in relation to the eHealth technology and implicated values. For example: Different stakeholders may have different views on what is considered harmful and therefore detrimental to well-being. While healthcare professionals were concerned about potential harms of PAEHR for patients in terms of creating anxiety caused by reading the records; patients described that having to wait for a long time to receive results would cause anxiety and they preferred to read it themselves (Grünloh, 2021). For the empirical investigations you can utilize a variety of methods, for example, interviews and focus groups or also workshops that support co-creation of our understanding. A recent study combined a variety of empirical methods to map patients' experiences and values along the patient journey (Bui, Oberschmidt, & Grünloh, 2023);
- **Technical investigations** are concerned with specific features of technologies and how their properties and mechanisms support human values. Whether you start with the technology,

or values or the empirical, you can go through all the features, functionalities or technical mechanisms and see how these might support or hinder certain values. For example, features in patient portals such as ordering prescriptions and visualizing lab results support patients' autonomy, independence and control, while the function to only show information in the records to patients that have been signed off by a healthcare professional limits patients' autonomy and support professionals' value of control (Grünloh, 2021; Grünloh, Cajander, & Myreteg, 2016). As VSD is an iterative approach and you started with the technical investigation, continuously reflect on the technical solution in terms of values that come to light in the conceptual and empirical investigations.

The three different investigations within the VSD approach are iterative and are supposed to inform each other. Therefore, each of them can form a starting point, they might overlap, happen in different orders or can be partly conducted (Davis & Nathan, 2015). They can be easily combined with the Contextual Inquiry (Chapter 8), the design activities described in this chapter, human-centred design (Chapter 11), and evaluation (Chapter 16). Furthermore, a number of methods have been developed to support the investigation of values in technology and design activities (Friedman, Hendry, & Borning, 2017; Grünloh, 2021). An important theoretical commitment of VSD is to consider the relationship between technology and human values as fundamentally inter-actional (Friedman & Hendry, 2019). Consider the log-list mentioned earlier, that shows patients which professional had logged into their records. A patient who might be worried that their neighbour, who is working as nurse, reads their records would easily recognize that name in the list. Therefore, being able to see the list might increase trust in the system and supports a feeling of control. However, whether this feature indeed increases trust needs to be seen in practice. This means that values are not just inscribed into eHealth technology, but that certain properties and features of a solution might more easily support or hinder certain values. However, the actual usage of the eHealth technology relies on the goals of the individuals interacting with it (Friedman, Kahn, Borning, & Huldtgren, 2013). For instance, some patients checked the log list while waiting to see if anyone had logged in. They used this information to assess whether there were any ongoing activities in the background (Grünloh, 2018). In this way, the log list was utilized not out of distrust but to reinforce values such as control and transparency during its actual use.

In the following sections, several activities will be described that are part of the design process. These activities are designed to gain a deeper understanding of the end-users and the usage context. Given that the VSD investigations also contribute to this understanding, the activities described below can be carried out together with or can be informed by the insights obtained during the VSD investigations.

Personas

When designing a new eHealth service, it might be hard to imagine who you are designing it for. After all, your innovation is supposed to be used by a large group of people, such as patients or caregivers, who each have their own characteristics, wishes and values. In order to envision typical end-users, one can make use of personas. Originally, personas have been defined as 'hypothetical archetypes of actual users' (Cooper, 1999). Personas are a set of fictitious persons, each one typical for a group of people, who will, potentially, use a new technology. Traditionally, personas are presented by means of a short biography with a photo and the goals they have in life or with regard to their work or medical condition. Combined with the VSD approach, the persona description can also include their values and what each specific value means to them. Personas do not describe how the end-user is envisioned to work with the eHealth service. This is done in a scenario. Personas are used by the design team to get a good grasp of the different user groups, as inspiration for design and, finally, to engage the design team (Pruitt & Adlin, 2005). When the team creates personas, they make their own assumptions explicit, help to focus on the target audience and these personas can also serve as communication tools (Grudin & Pruitt, 2002). For example, if a new feature is suggested, the team can discuss concretely how this may help 'Monica' in their daily life. Personas support the creative process as designers imagine how a persona would utilize the eHealth technology, sparking the emergence of new ideas (Nielsen, 2019).

A persona is often created based on desk research and data gathered during the Contextual Inquiry (Baxter, Courage, & Caine, 2015). Therefore, it is important to ensure that the correct data are collected at the beginning of the development process. Typical snippets of information that should be included in a persona for eHealth are the demographics (e.g., age, educational level, physical capabilities, visual limitations), healthcare specifics (e.g., knowledge about the medical condition, patients' attitudes towards care providers), and technical specifics (e.g., digital skills, technology ownership, use context) (LeRouge, Ma, Sneha, & Tolle, 2013). Based on an analysis of these parameters, it should be determined how many personas need to be developed. This choice depends on how many more or less homogeneous groups one cans identify within the total end-user population. Depending on the eHealth solution, there may be just one type of end-user (e.g., professional marathon runners) or different types of end-users (e.g., a patient and a care professional, or patients with either a high or low motivation to change their lifestyle). Within the end-user group, people might have very different characteristics, values, and needs, which would necessitate the creation of several personas. It can also be very useful to create anti-personas or organizational personas (Pruitt & Adlin, 2005). Anti-personas can be used to make explicit to the team who they are *not* targeting. For example, an eHealth service might be specifically targeting people with low computer literacy and an anti-persona might be a patient who is a retired programmer. Organizational personas are useful when the purchase decision is made by someone else than the end-user, such as a manager (see also value proposition section below) and describe the characteristics of the organisation, their objectives, processes, etc. Personas should never replace co-creation with actual end-users; instead, they should be considered complementary. They help the design team to maintain focus and establish a shared understanding of who the users are, which, in turn, enhances communication within the team (Pruitt & Grudin, 2003).

The final persona(s) needs to be shared in the design team and can be used to make design decisions (What would this persona want to do with the eHealth service? Would this feature be something s/he would like to have?). To illustrate: In the LEAVES project (van Velsen et al., 2020), an eMental health service was developed that supports older adults who have lost their spouse. The service offers psychological support during the grieving process and helps older adult mourners to build a new life without the deceased. As part of the design process, older adult mourners were interviewed about their experiences and challenges during this period. This information was subsequently used to draft several personas that represented widows and widowers in The Netherlands, Portugal, and Switzerland. One of them, Monica, can be seen in Figure 9.1 on page 152.

Scenarios

A scenario describes the envisioned use of an eHealth technology by the designated end-user. Where personas limit themselves to describing prospective end-users and their characteristics, scenarios link these personas to the to-be-developed eHealth technology itself. There are different ways to use scenarios in design. For example, the scenario-based design framework by Rosson & Carroll distinguish between problem, activity, information and interaction scenarios (Rosson & Carroll, 2002). In the conceptual phase of the development, scenarios often describe a day in the life of a typical end-user in which it becomes apparent which functions the eHealth service will have. Combined with the VSD approach, the scenarios can also include information on which values the end-user hold and illustrate how the technology supports these values. As such, scenarios can be used as one of the sources from which requirements can be derived. They further specify the to-be-designed eHealth technology and can be handed over to technical developers (Huis in't Veld et al., 2010).

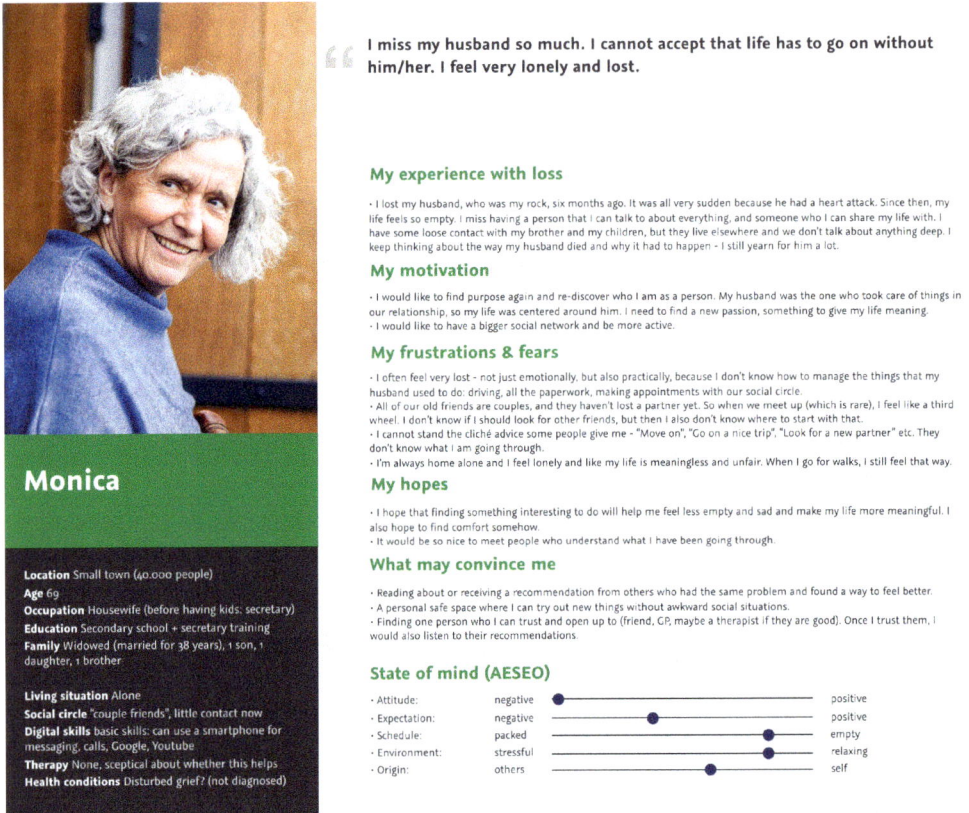

Figure 9.1 One of the LEAVES project personas, 'Monica' (van Velsen et al., 2020).

While there is no set format for writing a scenario, one framework that can be used to ensure that the most important topics are covered is PACT (Benyon & Macaulay, 2002). PACT stands for People, Activities, Context and Technology. According to this framework, a scenario should describe these aspects in relation to the eHealth technology to be used. So, the narrative should describe how and why an end-user (we advise to use the personas here) uses the eHealth technology given their characteristics, goals, and values, what (types of) activities are supported or facilitated by the eHealth technology, and what the steps are that the end-user goes through. It should also describe the context in which the eHealth service is used. Is this in an armchair at home? Or in a crowded and noisy train? And how does this context affect the interaction? Finally, the main functionalities of the eHealth technology itself should be described. Is the service offered via a mobile application? Does it also involve sensors? What type of data is used by the eHealth technology? While it is impossible to cover each and every aspect of an eHealth technology within a scenario (especially as a scenario should not be longer than one page, and because the technology is not developed yet), it should cover and explicate what the most crucial functionalities are that the eHealth service must provide, and the most important goals it must support.

The following excerpt (Box 9.1) is from a scenario developed for a mobile companion called RE-SAMPLE, designed to assist people with COPD in managing their symptoms and detecting exacerbations. In this excerpt, we have underlined the envisioned functionalities, while we put the different types of data that the companion uses in *italic*.

Box 9.1 Example scenario RE-SAMPLE project.

'Bert has been using the RE-SAMPLE companion for some time now and always fills in the questionnaires about his symptoms. One morning, he notices that he does not feel that well, but he thinks this was because the grandkids were around the last days. Maybe that was a bit too much. Or maybe the heater in his living room is set too high – so it might be the temperature. He fills in his <u>daily symptom card</u>, and after a while <u>the companion notifies</u> him that he has a risk of developing an exacerbation. He <u>receives an overview</u> of the pointers for that risk: *He has not moved a lot in the last days, his oxygen level is too low and he had indicated a worsening of symptoms*. Bert was not aware of that, so when the system asks whether it can <u>prompt a review request to his pulmonary nurse</u> Annette, he agrees. Usually he postpones seeking help – and often he waits too long. Maybe it is nothing, but maybe it is a good idea if Annette can have a look.'

The Value Proposition

At this point, after establishing the design foundations through personas and scenarios, commercial interests come into play. And it does not matter whether the service is being developed with the goal of earning money or improving healthcare. In the end, someone needs to cover the costs, and will only do so if the service fits his, her or its (in the case of an organization) needs. Therefore, it is paramount to look at the service from both the end-user's and the buyer's point of view, and to incorporate these views into the design – either of the technology or the service model, which is a schematic representation of how a new technology should be implemented in practice (Broekhuis et al., 2021). Please note that we make a distinction in this section between end-users and buyers. While in many commercial contexts the end-user is the buyer, this is not necessarily the case for eHealth services. For example, a patient with diabetes might use a mobile application that is being paid for by the hospital to monitor potential complications. In cases such as these, you might prefer to develop both an end-user and a buyer or organizational persona and develop a value proposition for each of the stakeholders. This increases the chance that the final product is both purchased and used.

Incorporating the needs and views of end-users and buyers can be achieved by creating the value proposition. A value proposition specifies 'the benefits customers can expect from your products and services' (Pigneur, Osterwalder, Bernada, & Smith, 2014). Value propositions can be used to inform the design and to make clear how the product should be marketed to customers, in this case often end-users and buyers. They should therefore resonate strongly with these groups (i.e., their needs, wishes, and personal values), and explicate both the functional and the experiential elements of the added benefit that is provided (Payne, Frow, & Eggert, 2017). Value propositions can be based upon the data that is collected during the Contextual Inquiry phase of the CeHRes Roadmap, and are mostly executed during the Value Specification phase (Lentferink et al., 2020). This is once you have elicited the end-users' and buyers' needs and requirements regarding the design context.

A practical tool to create a value proposition is a value proposition canvas (Pigneur et al., 2014). By filling in this canvas, you can easily profile the end-user or buyer, and map the added value that your eHealth service provides. A blank value proposition canvas can be found in Figure 9.2 on the next page. On the right side, you profile the end-user or buyer by listing their jobs (What are the tasks that they want to complete with the eHealth service? How do they want to feel?), their pains (What are the things that currently hinder the end-user or buyer from completing the jobs?

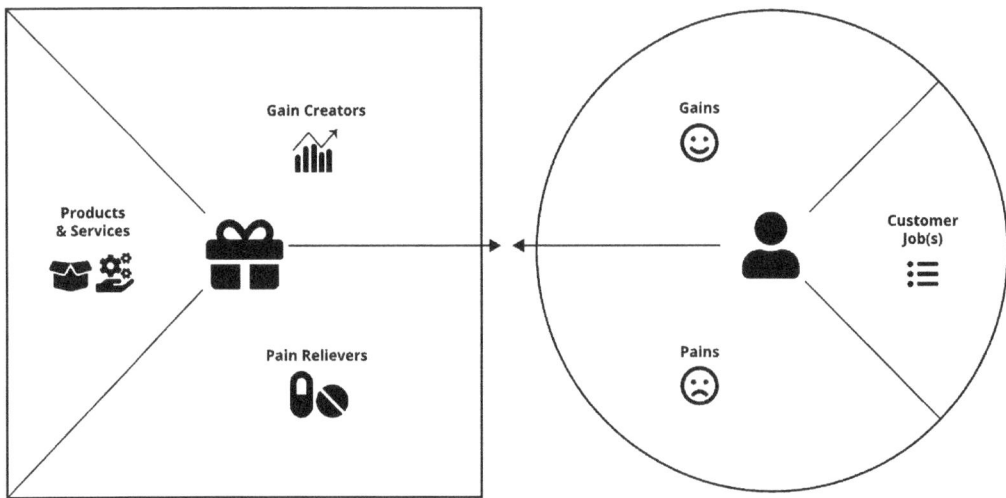

Figure 9.2 A blank value proposition canvas.

What makes them feel bad? What are the risks they have to deal with?), and their gains (What are the positive experiences and emotions that the end-user or buyer wants? What are they looking for? What makes them happy?). It makes sense to complete this part of the value proposition canvas by using your personas and scenarios, given that for writing personas and scenarios, a good understanding of their needs and values was needed and hence can be utilized here. The left side of the canvas describes the to-be-developed eHealth technology. Here, you list the features of your eHealth service and the hardware it uses, how its reliefs the end-users' or buyers' pains (as specified in the profile on the right) and its gain creators (What value does it add for end-users' and buyers? How does it help them complete their jobs? How does it improve the user experience?). The resulting value proposition can then be used to inform the eHealth design and fill out the Business Model Canvas. More detailed information on this can be found in Chapter 10 on Business Modelling.

Service Modelling

The activities that have been introduced so far are related directly to the design of the eHealth technology (i.e., its features, the interaction between human and technology, etc.). However, implementing an eHealth technology into existing work processes, such as care processes, also requires a design activity – specifically, designing the service around the technology. After all, the new eHealth technology not only needs to align with current practices but is also likely to change the way care is provided. A service model is a graphical overview of how an end-user will receive and use a technology in the context of use. For example, how does he or she get into first contact (the onboarding procedure)? What are the tasks that he or she wants to achieve? It also specifies the tasks of secondary end-users. For example, what is the task of the doctor's assistant for a technology that allows patients to make appointments online? Finally, it also specifies how people stop working with the technology (the offboarding procedure). These questions that go beyond the technology design are answered during service modelling. In order to achieve this overview, the service model draws heavily from scenarios and personas.

Service modelling (also referred to as service blueprinting) is a relatively new discipline, especially for the eHealth context. It combines the user experience with the technical design of eHealth and the organizational (re)design that is necessary for implementing the eHealth service. The service model should describe the complete end-user journey, from the moment at which the end-user first gets in contact with the eHealth service, until the point in time where the end-user is expected to stop using it. It can be viewed as part of a larger implementation process, about which there is more information in Chapter 13.

A service model should include these five components (Bitner, Ostrom, & Morgan, 2008):

1. End-user actions (the goals that end-users want to achieve);
2. Interactions with (in)formal care providers and/or the eHealth service (the activities in which the end-user is involved, like entering personal details in a website or talking to a nurse);
3. Backstage actions by (in)formal care providers and/or the eHealth service (the activities that make up the service, but in which the primary end-user is not involved, like doctors discussing a patient);
4. Support actions by other persons or other technologies (other technologies that support the technology you are developing, like a Fitbit that you use for incorporating step data);
5. Physical evidence (all the tangibles that the end-user encounters, like a graphical interface or doctor's office).

Figure 9.3 below shows a part of a service model for the LEAVES project that was introduced before (see the Persona part). It shows the different steps in the (digital) service provision, the steps the end-user has to perform and the possible consequences of each action. Finally, adaptations for the Portuguese version of the service are made explicit.

There are several compelling reasons why you would want to create a service model (Bitner et al., 2008). First, a service model is a focus point that unites different perspectives and is an instrument that provides common ground for people with different backgrounds (e.g., medical, technical, marketing) by visualizing the entire service and its underlying support processes. Second, a service model makes the different roles that people play in the service provision explicit and shows interdependencies among these roles and the technology. Third, it supports tactical and strategic decision making, the service model makes it clear how a technology affects the organization and people using it, and vice versa. By using these insights, organizations can make well-informed decisions. Does this service fit our organization and working routines? Do we need to alter an aspect of the technology or service model? Do we need to embark on an organizational change process in order for this service to work? Fourth, it makes it explicit what the moments of truth are in service provision and enables the design team to create the optimal experience here. Moments of truth are those moments in which end-users interact with a technology or other people. It is these moments at which added value can be created for the end-user. By having these moments clear, one can improve the technology and/or service around it to maximize the value it provides to the end-user.

The service model should be designed with the support of different types of input. When looking at the CeHRes Roadmap, the Contextual Inquiry phase should ensure that all the necessary information is available (especially on working routines), possibly (partly) in the form of personas or scenarios. It is possible that some of the things you decide upon in the service model contradict your persona or scenario. This will be due to the fact that you are now merging the end-user point of view with the organizational and the commercial points of view. It will be up to the interdisciplinary design team to decide when such a conflict arises and to make sure that all three interests are well-balanced. The service model also plays an important role during the operationalization phase since it can be used to facilitate the introduction and integration of a technology in practice and can be used to identify suitable implementation strategies.

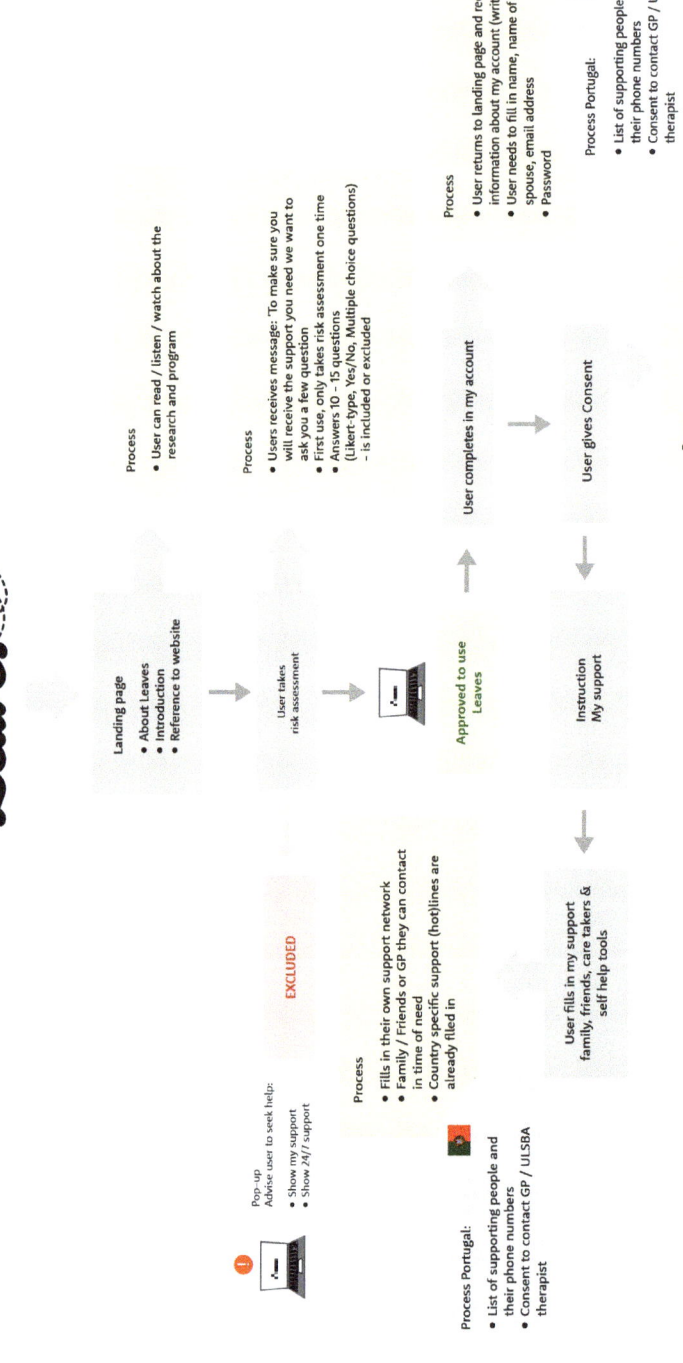

Figure 9.3 Excerpt of the LEAVES service model.

Requirements

Once you are satisfied with the set of design documents that resulted from the previous activities (personas, scenarios, value proposition, and service model), it is time to specify what needs to be developed technically. This is usually done in the form of requirements. Requirements describe what a technology should do, what data it should store or retrieve, what content it should display, and what kind of user experience it should provide. In other words, they are the instructions for developers that tell them how to create a technology that provides value to the end-user. The process of coming to these requirements is fuzzy, as there are no set rules for combining end-user input, the design team's creativity, and (potentially) a technology push. A technology push is the implementation of a technical idea that a potential end-user would never come up with (like using a complicated piece of artificial intelligence). As goes for eHealth development in general, the process of creating requirements is iterative with multiple adaptations throughout.

van Velsen et al. described a requirements development approach for eHealth using a requirements notation template that focuses on values, attributes, and requirements (van Velsen, Wentzel, & van Gemert-Pijnen, 2013). In this particular template, a value is defined as an ideal or interest a (future) end user or stakeholder aspires to or has. Note that this differs from how a 'value' is defined in value sensitive design, which as described above refers to what is important to people in their lives, with a focus on ethics and morality. An attribute is a summary of the need or wish that is spoken out by a (future) end-user or stakeholder. A requirement, finally, is a technical translation of an attribute. Attributes and values can be used to group requirements, which makes it easier to set priorities later on. The design team can start by identifying the different values in all the materials they have. Next, attributes can be determined by enriching the values with the associated wishes that are voiced by the end-user or stakeholders, or that the design team identifies in the value proposition or service model. Finally, requirements are drafted as the technical descriptions that, together, make up this attribute. Every requirement is accompanied by a rationale and a source. Every requirement is accompanied by a rationale and a source. This can be from the empirical work conducted during the contextual inquiry, VSD investigations, or from literature. The rationale description for a certain requirement can also be accompanied by the human values that are supported with this particular requirement. For example, a requirement that specifies that first a patient is notified if their values are out of norm and not the healthcare professional supports the patient value of autonomy.

A question that arises often is 'How do you know that something should be translated into a requirement?' It is impossible to formulate a clear answer to this question. And tempting as it may be, focusing on the frequency with which a problem or desire was voiced by end-users or stakeholders does not guarantee success. If an issue is brought forth only once, it is very well possible that it provides a great contribution to the eHealth service but was simply harder to spot or vocalize. It is suggested that an issue should be translated into a requirement when it captures something important in relation to the overall goal(s) of the eHealth technology, which can be established by an interdisciplinary design team in which multiple perspectives are combined.

Now, each requirement needs to be documented in such a way that it enables programmers to understand what needs to be made and why. There are different ways of writing down requirements. Traditionally, a requirement is written down as a sentence that starts with 'The technology must…' and specifies only one thing to be developed. An example of a requirement would be 'The technology must show the nurse practitioner the disease activity over the past 6 months for each individual patient with COPD'.

You can discern the following types of requirements (van Velsen et al., 2013):

- **Functional and modality requirements**: Technical features and kind of technology (e.g., smartphone, tablet, desktop computer) and operating systems the technology should work with. Example: The mobile application should work on Android and iOS;

- **Service requirements**: How services surrounding the technology (e.g., marketing or user support), need to be organized. Example: The homepage of the site should include a link to a support helpline;
- **Organizational requirements**: How the technology should be integrated in the organizational structure and working routines. Example: A nurse should have five minutes before each consult to check the patient progress in the eHealth service;
- **Content requirements**: The content that needs to be communicated via the technology and, if applicable, language level, persuasive approach, and special accessibility demands. Mostly meant for content managers. Example: The content should be available in Dutch, English, and Arabic;
- **Usability & User experience requirements**: The interface and interaction design of the technology and how user experience factors, such as trust or fun, should be integrated into the technology. Example: Each page on the website should be accessible within four clicks.

When formulating a requirement, it is important to also note its type, as different types of requirements go to different types of people in the development team. For example, functional and modality requirements will go to the technical development team, usability' and user experience (UX) requirements are mostly for interaction designer and human factors specialists, while people from organizational management are responsible for service and organizational requirements.

In Table 9.1 below, an example of a requirement for the LEAVES service is highlighted. The requirement specifies that the technology should monitor the end-user's mental state to identify suicidal ideation. It includes the requirement, its type, the rationale for including the requirement, and a set of fit criteria. The first criterium focuses on end-user acceptance (a delicate matter as personal health data is collected and interpreted). The second criterium (to be tested with a near-ready system) focuses on the quality of the interpretation algorithm, where you do not want to be too many erroneous classifications of suicidal ideation, nor too many misses of these situations.

Another important piece of information for each requirement is its priority. In each development process, there will be limits on time, financial resources, and the available development effort. Therefore, you always have to choose which requirements you will implement first, which ones later, and which ones you will not implement at all. An accessible method to set the priority of a requirement is the MoSCoW method. Following this method, a requirement is either a Must have, a Should have, a Could have, or a Won't have (the latter meaning that a requirement will not be

Table 9.1 Exemplary requirement for the LEAVES service.

Requirement ID: #01	Requirement type: Functional
Value: Mental well-being	**Attribute**: Making sure the end-user is capable of doing online-only therapy.
Requirement: The system should detect, via administering a set of questionnaires every other week, whether an end-user has a suicidal ideation.	
Rationale: When an end-user has a suicidal ideation, s/he should see a professional caregiver and the exit procedure should be triggered.	
Fit Criteria: *Low-fidelity prototype*: The end-user population should find it acceptable that data on his/her mental state is collected and interpreted. *High-fidelity prototype*: The monitoring algorithm should have an acceptable rate of false positives and false negatives.	

implemented in the current version of the eHealth service, but maybe in a later one). When using this method, you also write down the requirement accordingly (The technology must, The technology should, etc.). Determining the priority of a requirement is up to the design and development team and is a decision that is based on many factors: The importance for the end-user, the technical difficulty for implementing the requirement, the scope of the work, dependencies etc.

As is the case with all activities in eHealth development, drafting the requirements is not a job you do once and be done with. It marks the beginning of the technical development process and the start of iterative testing This is part of a larger, human-centred design process (also see Chapter 11). Since requirements are interpretations of what the end-users want or what the market needs, it is very well possible that they are not immediately correct or clearly defined. We therefore advice to formulate a 'fit criterion' for the most important requirements (van Velsen et al., 2013). A fit criterion is a measure which helps you determine whether you implemented your requirement successfully (see Table 9.1). The end-user acceptance of your most crucial functional requirements should be tested as soon as possible, preferably with simple prototypes, like sketches (also called low-fidelity prototypes). If a feature is not liked or should be adapted, you should rephrase, or maybe even remove, the requirement. The other requirements rely on a mature (high-fidelity) prototype of the eHealth service to be tested. In that way, requirements provide the foundation for formative evaluations of prototypes and the functioning version of an eHealth technology. Usability tests, or user experience benchmarks can be of value for assessing how well these requirements have been implemented in the service (see Chapter 11). The collection of requirements should therefore be seen as a living document, to be changed and supplemented throughout the time your eHealth service is being developed and up and running.

Summary

In this chapter, we have discussed the different activities that one needs to undertake in order to specify value sensitive eHealth design, and the associated documentation. We would like to stress here that there is not a single road towards proper design, nor is one road better than the other. Rather, it is an iterative process where results from previous development phases such as the contextual inquiry meet creativity, a technology push, and business interests. Furthermore, the different values identified from different stakeholders might not be perfectly aligned or even be in tension, so that several iterations might be needed to prioritize values. Each design team will therefore come up with a different design. It is of paramount importance here to acknowledge that designing is a process, not a one-time trick. An initial set of requirements should be translated into simple designs, tested, and then the requirements (or maybe the personas and scenarios) should be adapted with the lessons learned. Multiple rounds of design-testing-redesign will be necessary to come to a solution that is acceptable and has added value for all end-users and stakeholders (see Chapter 11 on Human-Centred Design).

The design activities play a pivotal role in the development process of eHealth. It is the time where different interests of different stakeholders, like the end-user, the business manager and the technical developer, meet. It is also the phase in which the subsequent phases have their origin. Business development starts with the value proposition development, implementation starts with service model design, and all subsequent evaluation activities should reflect on proper implementation of the requirements for the eHealth service.

Key References for Further Reading

Baxter, K., Courage, C., & Caine, K. (2015). *Understanding your users: A practical guide to user research methods*. Morgan Kaufmann.

Friedman, B., & Hendry, D. G. (2019). *Value sensitive design: Shaping technology with moral imagination.* MIT Press.

Grünloh, C., Cabrita, M., Dantas, C., & Ortet, S. (2022). Opportunities, ethical challenges, and value implications of pervasive sensing technology for supporting older adults in the work environment. *Australasian Journal of Information Systems*, 26.

Van Velsen, L., Wentzel, J., & van Gemert-Pijnen, J. E. (2013). Designing eHealth that matters via a multidisciplinary requirements development approach. *JMIR Research Protocols*, 2(1), e2547.Article 2.

Van den Hoven, J., Vermaas, P. E., & Van de Poel, I. (Eds.). (2015). *Handbook of ethics, values, and technological design: Sources, theory, values and application domains.* Dordrecht: Springer Netherlands.

References

Baxter, K., Courage, C., & Caine, K. (2015). *Understanding your users: A practical guide to user research methods* (Second edition. ed.). Amsterdam, Netherlands: Morgan Kaufmann.

Benyon, D., & Macaulay, C. (2002). Scenarios and the HCI-SE design problem. *Interacting with Computers*, 14(4), 397–405. doi:10.1016/s0953-5438(02)00007-3

Bitner, M. J., Ostrom, A. L., & Morgan, F. N. (2008). Service blueprinting: A practical technique for service innovation. *California Management Review*, 50(3), 66–94. doi:10.2307/41166446

Broekhuis, M., Weering, M. D.-v., Schuit, C., Schürz, S., & van Velsen, L. (2021). Designing a stakeholder-inclusive service model for an eHealth service to support older adults in an active and social life. *BMC Health Services Research*, 21(1), 654. doi:10.1186/s12913-021-06597-9

Bui, M., Oberschmidt, K., & Grünloh, C. (2023). Patient journey value mapping: Illustrating values and experiences along the patient journey to support eHealth design.

Cooper, A. (1999). *The inmates are running the asylum: Why high tech products drive us crazy and how to restore the sanity.* Pearson Higher Education.

Davis, J., & Nathan, L. P. (2015). Value sensitive design: Applications, adaptations, and critiques. In J. van den Hoven, P. E. Vermaas, & I. van de Poel (Eds.), *Handbook of ethics, values, and technological design: Sources, theory, values and application domains* (pp. 11–40). Dordrecht: Springer Netherlands.

Friedman, B., & Hendry, D. G. (2019). *Value sensitive design: Shaping technology with moral imagination.* The MIT Press.

Friedman, B., Hendry, D., & Borning, A. (2017). A survey of value sensitive design methods. *Foundations and Trends® in human-computer interaction*, 11, 63–125. doi:10.1561/1100000015

Friedman, B., Kahn, P., Borning, A., Zhang, P., & Galletta, D. (2006). Value sensitive design and information systems. *Early engagement and new technnologies: Opening up the laboratory*, 55–95.

Friedman, B., Kahn, P. H., Borning, A., & Huldtgren, A. (2013). Value sensitive design and information systems. In N. Doorn, D. Schuurbiers, I. van de Poel, & M. E. Gorman (Eds.), *Early engagement and new technologies: Opening up the laboratory* (pp. 55–95). Dordrecht: Springer Netherlands.

Friedman, B. P. H. K., Jr. (2007). Human values, ethics, and design. In *The human-computer interaction handbook* (pp. 1241–1266). CRC Press.

Grudin, J. T., & Pruitt, J. S. (2002). Personas, participatory design and product development: An infrastructure for engagement. In: *Proceedings of the Participatory Design Conference; Malmö, Sweden.*

Grünloh, C. (2018). Harmful or empowering? Stakeholders' expectations and experiences of patient accessible electronic health records. [Doctoral dissertation, KTH Royal Institute of Technology].

Grünloh, C. (2021). Using technological frames as an analytic tool in value sensitive design. *Ethics and Information Technology*, 23(1), 53–57. doi:10.1007/s10676-018-9459-3

Grünloh, C., Cajander, Å., & Myreteg, G. (2016). "The Record is Our Work Tool!"—Physicians' framing of a patient portal in Sweden. *J Med Internet Res*, 18(6), e167. doi:10.2196/jmir.5705

Hogan, K., Macedo, B., Macha, V., Barman, A., & Jiang, X. (2021). Contact tracing apps: Lessons learned on privacy, autonomy, and the need for detailed and thoughtful implementation. *JMIR Med Inform*, 9(7), e27449. doi:10.2196/27449

Huis in 't Veld, R. M., Widya, I. A., Bults, R. G., Sandsjö, L., Hermens, H. J., & Vollenbroek-Hutten, M. M. (2010). A scenario guideline for designing new teletreatments: A multidisciplinary approach. *J Telemed Telecare*, 16(6), 302–307. doi:10.1258/jtt.2010.006003

JafariNaimi, N., Nathan, L., & Hargraves, I. (2015). Values as hypotheses: Design, inquiry, and the service of values. *Design Issues*, 31(4), 91–104. Retrieved from http://www.jstor.org/stable/43830434

Lentferink, A., Polstra, L., D'Souza, A., Oldenhuis, H., Velthuijsen, H., & van Gemert-Pijnen, L. (2020). Creating value with eHealth: Identification of the value proposition with key stakeholders for the resilience navigator app. *BMC Medical Informatics and Decision Making*, 20(1), 76. doi:10.1186/s12911-020-1088-1

LeRouge, C., Ma, J., Sneha, S., & Tolle, K. (2013). User profiles and personas in the design and development of consumer health technologies. *Int J Med Inform*, 82(11), e251–268. doi:10.1016/j.ijmedinf.2011.03.006

Miller, B. (2020). Is technology value-neutral? *Science, Technology, & Human Values*, 46(1), 53–80. doi:10.1177/0162243919900965

Nielsen, L. (2019). *Personas – User focused design*. Springer Publishing Company, Incorporated.

Payne, A., Frow, P., & Eggert, A. (2017). The customer value proposition: Evolution, development, and application in marketing. *Journal of the Academy of Marketing Science*, 45(4), 467–489. doi:10.1007/s11747-017-0523-z

Pigneur, Y., Osterwalder, A., Bernada, G., & Smith, A. (2014). Value proposition design: How to create products and services customers want. John Wiley & Sons.

Pruitt, J., & Adlin, T. (2005). *The persona lifecycle: Keeping people in mind throughout product design*. Morgan Kaufmann Publishers Inc.

Pruitt, J., & Grudin, J. (2003). Personas: Practice and theory. Paper presented at the Proceedings of the 2003 Conference on Designing for User Experiences, San Francisco, California.

Rosson, M. B., & Carroll, J. M. (2002). Scenario-based design. In *The human-computer interaction handbook: Fundamentals, evolving technologies and emerging applications* (pp. 1032–1050). L. Erlbaum Associates Inc.

Van Velsen, L., Cabrita, M., Op den Akker, H., Brandl, L., Isaac, J., Suárez, M., . . . Brodbeck, J. (2020). LEAVES (optimizing the mentaL health and resiliencE of older Adults that haVe lost thEir spouSe via blended, online therapy): Proposal for an online service development and evaluation. *JMIR Res Protoc*, 9(9), e19344. doi:10.2196/19344

Van Velsen, L., Wentzel, J., & van Gemert-Pijnen, J. E. (2013). Designing eHealth that matters via a multidisciplinary requirements development approach. *JMIR Res Protoc*, 2(1), e21.

10 Business Modelling

Bart (L.J.M.) Nieuwenhuis

Introduction

In previous chapters, you have learned that the use of eHealth technologies to create new services requires *human-centred design* and *participatory development* processes in order to satisfy the needs of the various stakeholders. This chapter is about the deployment and implementation of these new eHealth services in the day-to-day practice of healthcare organizations. Managers of healthcare organizations (or independent healthcare providers) have to make a number of 'business' decisions before an eHealth technology can be used. They have to select a supplier where they buy the eHealth technologies, get facilities to train employees, set up maintenance, and take care of certificates to allow for the provision of services. The eHealth technology may require new kinds of employees, e.g., for IT and data management. All these decisions come with investments and various operational costs.

These costs need to be counterbalanced by the expected benefits of the eHealth services. For example, eHealth technologies may offer new opportunities to further improve the quality of healthcare, for example with the help of Artificial Intelligence. Further, the eHealth technologies can create cost savings by introducing a more efficient way of working. Finally, eHealth technologies may increase labour productivity through automation. The management of healthcare organizations has to decide whether these potential benefits outweigh the investments and costs. Business modelling can help with this.

In this chapter, the business considerations that play a role in decision making about the services that are provided with eHealth technologies are discussed. This chapter uses the notion of *eHealth services*, which comprises the application of *eHealth technologies*, as well as all the other activities an organization needs to actually provide these services. It starts with introducing the concept of a business model – and specifically, the Business Model Canvas – to investigate whether organizations can provide the desired care, execute the activities, and attract the right resources and partners. The outcomes from activities described in the previous chapters generate relevant input for this. Then, the Value Proposition Canvas is presented, which supports the development of the central element of the business model. The first part of this chapter is completed with a case study where a combination of face-to-face and digital treatment is used for mental healthcare. The last part of this chapter is about Cost Benefit Analysis as a methodology to do some elementary quantitative analysis supporting business and policymaking for eHealth deployment and implementation. This part is finalized with a case study about telemonitoring in heart failure. After completing this chapter, you will be able to:

DOI: 10.4324/9781003302049-12

- Understand the basics of business modelling and explain its importance for eHealth implementation;
- Understand and apply the Business Model Canvas and the Value Proposition Canvas;
- Explain how to analyze the business impact of eHealth implementation;
- Identify the most relevant quantitative variables for eHealth implementation;
- Perform an indicative quantitative analysis for eHealth implementation.

Business Models

Introduction

A business model explains how an enterprise creates and delivers value for customers, and how the business is paid. Business models are used to analyze the viability of a particular organization. The terms business modelling and business models have become popular over the last 30 years, but during that period, the concept of a business model has not received much attention from the academic world. A business model is different from a business case. A business model entails the entire organization, while a business case is about a specific project or investment as part of the organization.

The first time the term business model was used was back in 1957 (Bellman, Clark, Malcolm, Craft, & Ricciardi, 1957; Osterwalder, Gordijn, & Pigneur, 2005; Osterwalder, Pigneur, & Tucci, 2005). The term business modelling originates from the information systems industry and refers to modelling the business in terms of business processes (Wirtz, Pistoia, Ullrich, & Göttel, 2016). In later years, the term has been used only a few times, mostly in the sense of an abstract model of businesses for better understanding how companies operate. However, during the 1990s, the number of papers addressing business models increased significantly, especially in relation to the development of e-commerce (Al-Debei & Avison, 2010). The business model was used to describe how the electronic business works and was used as an instrument for decision making (Wirtz et al., 2016). Later, the notion of business models widened more and more.

Business models were used to describe all sorts of companies, including those not related to the Internet or strongly depending on ICT. Some scholars pointed out that the growth of the number of papers on business modelling shows similarities with growth of the ratings on the stock exchanges. This illustrates the criticism on the lack of grounding of business models during these years. However, since the beginning of this century, scholars accepted this challenge and started to develop a clear concept of business models. One of the difficulties here is that scholars from a wide range of disciplines joined this discussion, using various theoretical models. At this point in time, the theoretical grounding of business models still needs further improvements (DaSilva & Trkman, 2014). Despite these limitations, business modelling is extensively used in practice by consultants and strategists within organizations. The book *Business Model Generation* (Osterwalder & Pigneur, 2010), in which the Business Model Canvas was introduced, and the many worldwide appearances of Alexander Osterwalder have contributed to this. Also, although the origin of business modelling lies in industry, business modelling is also being used in the public sector. That is why eHealth practitioners can benefit from business modelling and the Business Model Canvas.

Business Modelling Literature

There are many overviews in the literature on business modelling and business model innovation, and many case studies have been presented (Al-Debei & Avison, 2010; Casadesus-Masanell & Ricart, 2010; DaSilva & Trkman, 2014; Osterwalder, 2004; Saebi, Lien, & Foss, 2016; Zott, Amit, & Massa, 2011). The literature seems to converge on the definition of business models. Many of the definitions can be related to the definition given by Teece, although other scholars may use different wording (Teece, 2010):

A business model defines how an enterprise creates and delivers value to customers, and then converts payments received to profit.

A business model is essentially a model of an organization. A high-quality business model says something about different aspects of an organization. In spite of the differences among various scholars, we follow Saebi's conclusion (Saebi et al., 2016) that the following elements are necessary parts of a business model:

- Value Proposition. This is the offering from the organization to its customer (another organization or an individual) that can be used to create value, while making use of the offerings. This concept is also being used as part of the CeHRes Roadmap (see Chapter 7). This is, for example, the eHealth service provided by an organization to a patient and of which the organization expects it might contribute to their well-being;
- Market Segments. This is the set of customers with common needs and interests that could benefit from the value proposition. To illustrate, the total of all patients benefiting from an eHealth service is called the eHealth market for that service. A market segment is a part of that entire market for a value proposition, for example a group of diabetes patients;
- The Infrastructure. This is the set of activities and resources of an organization to create and deliver the value proposition. The infrastructure for an organization that provides an eHealth service consists of all facilities required to provide that service. This concerns the people and resources needed, for example, to perform a blood pressure measurement at home;
- The Mechanisms of Value Capturing. This relates to the way in which an organization is being paid by its customers, often called the revenue model. This clarifies, for example, whether patients pay for the service delivery themselves, or if an insurance company is paying the bills on their behalf. It is also about the underlying mechanisms, like, for example, does the eHealth organization receive a fixed amount of money each time a service is delivered, or are they being paid through a monthly or yearly subscription fee?
- The Firm-specific Ways in which these Elements are Linked in an Architecture. This relates to the way the above-mentioned elements of an organization are interrelated and mutually dependent. If, for example, trust is an important aspect of the service provision of telemonitoring, this needs to be reflected in the value proposition, the specific market segments that are served, and the activities and resources that are being made available within the organization.

Business Model Canvas

The *Business Model Canvas* (BMC) is a very popular tool that is used worldwide for creating business models (also see Chapter 7). The BMC includes all of the elements described above. It finds its roots in the research of Alexander Osterwalder (Osterwalder, 2004) and has been popularized in the book *Business Model Generation* (Osterwalder & Pigneur, 2010). They define the business model as follows:

A business model describes the rationale of how an organization creates, delivers, and captures value.

The unit of analysis of a business model is the organization that provides services to its customers. The BMC has been originally developed with commercial companies in mind. However, the model is also being applied successfully for non-profit organizations. As an example, the independent organization can be a hospital, providing care to patients. There is a director who is ultimately responsible for the quality of the health services provided, the costs incurred, and the income that the hospital can generate to cover those costs. In a commercial setting, the hospital wants to make a profit and there must be a positive balance between costs and benefits. In a non-profit setting, the costs and benefits will have to be equal if the hospital is to continue to exist. Hospitals are increasingly replacing traditional healthcare with healthcare based on eHealth technologies. Hospitals do this, for example, to improve the quality of services or to save on costs or human resources. The BMC is very suitable for analyzing the impact of applying eHealth services.

The BMC is a tool to show how the hospital works. On the one hand, the BMC maps out how the hospital works towards its patients. Questions that need to be answered are: Which services does the hospital provide to which patients, what relationships does the hospital want to maintain with its patients, and how is the hospital being paid? On the other hand, the BMC maps what is needed to do this. Questions that need to be answered are: Which activities does the hospital need to carry out, what kind of people and resources are needed, and what does the hospital need to purchase from external suppliers? The BMC (see Figure 10.1) uses nine building blocks that show the logic of how organizations like, for example, the hospital operates. The BMC may be considered a meta-model for business models (Alberts, Meertens, Iacob, & Nieuwenhuis, 2012). Hence, the BMC describes the concepts and rules that apply to creating business models.

The right-hand side of the BMC looks at the external aspects of the organization, the offering to the customers, how the customer pays for the deliveries, and the activities of the organization to maintain a relationship. The left-hand side of the BMC explains what the organization has to do internally to realize its achievements. The business model of the organization comprises descriptions of the following nine aspects of the organization:

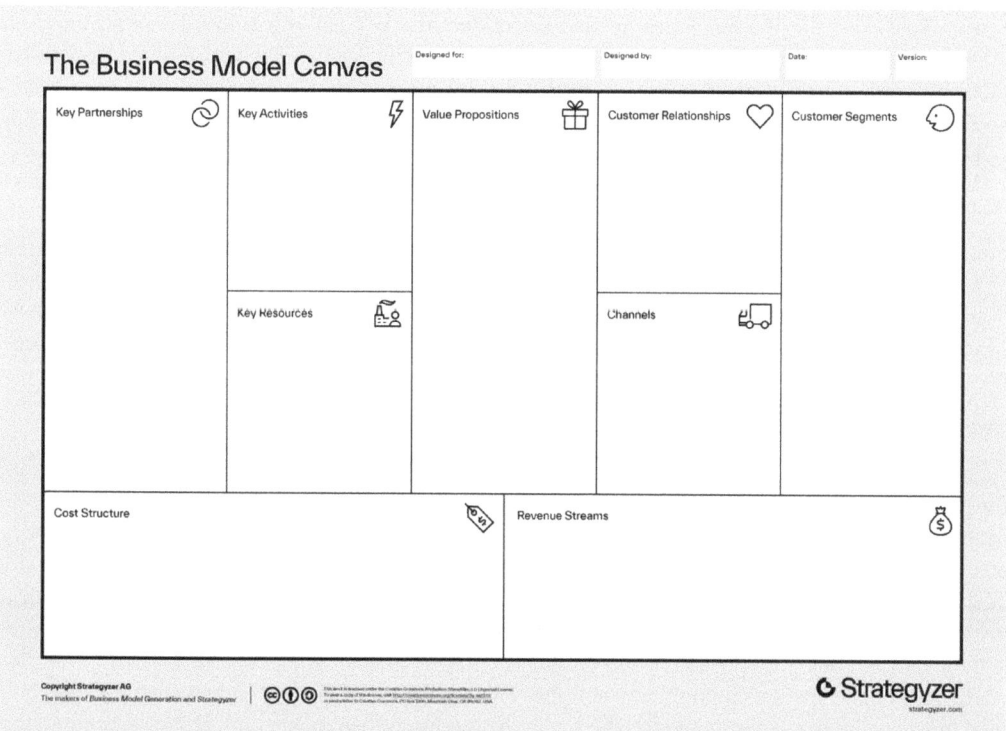

Figure 10.1 Osterwalder's Business Model Canvas (Osterwalder & Pigneur, 2010).

- *Value proposition* consists of the offerings of an organization, targeted to the needs of specific groups of customers. For hospitals, the value propositions are the treatments offered to patients. In Chapter 7, attention is paid to the value specification of companies developing eHealth technologies. In this chapter, the Value Propositions relate to the treatments (possibly eHealth services) provided by hospitals and the value it might create for their patients;
- *Customer Segments* are sets of customers with common characteristics who are supposed to benefit from the same set of value propositions. The terminology originates from a commercial setting. However, the customers are the organizations or persons that should be benefitting from the value proposition of the organization, including organizations providing eHealth services (Kimble, 2015). For hospitals, these are the patient groups benefitting from the same treatments;
- *Customer Relationship* describes the characteristics of the relationship the organization strives to achieve with its customers. Hospitals may choose to build a long-term relationship with their patients, or to focus on delivering fast and cost-effective care;
- *Channels* describe the way products and services are delivered to the customers. For eHealth services, this may include direct, face-to-face contact as well as contacts to various media, for example, computers or smartphones;
- *Revenue Streams* describe the way in which the organization is paid for its efforts. In the case of the hospital, it clarifies whether patients pay for the service delivery themselves, or if an insurance company pays the bills on their behalf. It also is about the underlying mechanisms, like, for example, does the hospital receive a standardized amount of money for a standardized treatment? The description also indicates the settlement basis, for example, effort-based, subscription-based, treatment-based, or value-based;
- *Key Activities* are the main activities carried out by the organization itself – rather than activities carried out by external partners. For a hospital, these are descriptions of the procedures and processes that are being applied within the hospital;
- *Key Resources* are the resources needed to conduct the key activities. In a hospital, these are resources, for example, the doctors and nurses with specific knowledge and skills, as well as the specific infrastructures, including instruments, housing, and equipment;
- *Key Partners* are other organizations offering intermediate products and services to the organization described by the business model. For hospitals, these are the relevant suppliers for all activities that the hospital outsources, such as housing, communication facilities, and medical equipment. If a hospital starts providing eHealth services, this almost always has major consequences for their partnerships. For example, new technology suppliers might be introduced;
- *Cost Structure* describes how the costs of the organization are distributed across the internal and external activities. If a hospital starts delivering eHealth services, this can lead to drastic changes in the cost structure. It is almost always accompanied by new activities and resources.

Non-profit Organizations

As mentioned before, the concepts and terminology of the BMC originally refer to commercial, for-profit organizations. The BMC can also be applied to non-profit organizations (NPOs) like the healthcare sector. The left-hand side of the BMC (Key Partners, Key Activities, and Key Resources) does not require adjustments when it comes to a business model for an NPO. The right-hand side of the BMC needs some further consideration. In practice, in the case of an NPO, it is useful to distinguish at least two types of Customer Segments: The 'Finance Provider' of the organization and the 'Beneficials'. Suppose the NPO is a non-commercial hospital. Here, the 'Finance Provider' could be a health insurance company, and the 'Beneficial' is the patient to be cared for. The hospital must ensure that patients are satisfied with the quality of healthcare and, at the same time, that health insurers are satisfied with the associated cost-levels. Hence, the business model in this case provides two types of value propositions, one set of value propositions for the insurance company, and one set of value propositions for the patients. The case study further on in this chapter gives an example of this.

Value Proposition Canvas

The authors of the BMC also developed an additional model to support the development of value propositions. Their Value Proposition Canvas can be used to further aid the development of *Value Propositions* and the *Customer Segments* elements of the Business Model Canvas (Osterwalder, Pigneur, Bernarda, & Smith, 2014). In literature, there are also examples in which the Value Proposition Canvas has been applied for the design and validation of concrete applications of eHealth technology (Lentferink et al., 2020; Wrede, Braakman-Jansen, & van Gemert-Pijnen, 2022), also see Chapter 7 on the CeHRes Roadmap.

The core of the BMC is the Value Proposition, which describes what benefits customers can expect from the products and services that the organization is offering (Osterwalder & Pigneur, 2010). In practice, developing Value Propositions that may be expected to be appreciated by the beneficiaries is the biggest challenge for both existing and new organizations. The Value Proposition Canvas (VPC) consists of two parts: The Customer Profile and the Value Map. The Customer Profile provides a more detailed description of a specific Customer Segment of the BMC. The Value Map gives a more detailed description of the features of a specific Value Proposition of the BMC. The authors of the VPC argue that products and services with a good fit between customer segment and value proposition have a greater chance of uptake in practice.

The Customer Profile (CP) on the right-hand side of the VPC (see Figure 10.2) is a structured way of mapping the customer's needs by looking at the jobs-to-be-done and the pains and gains of

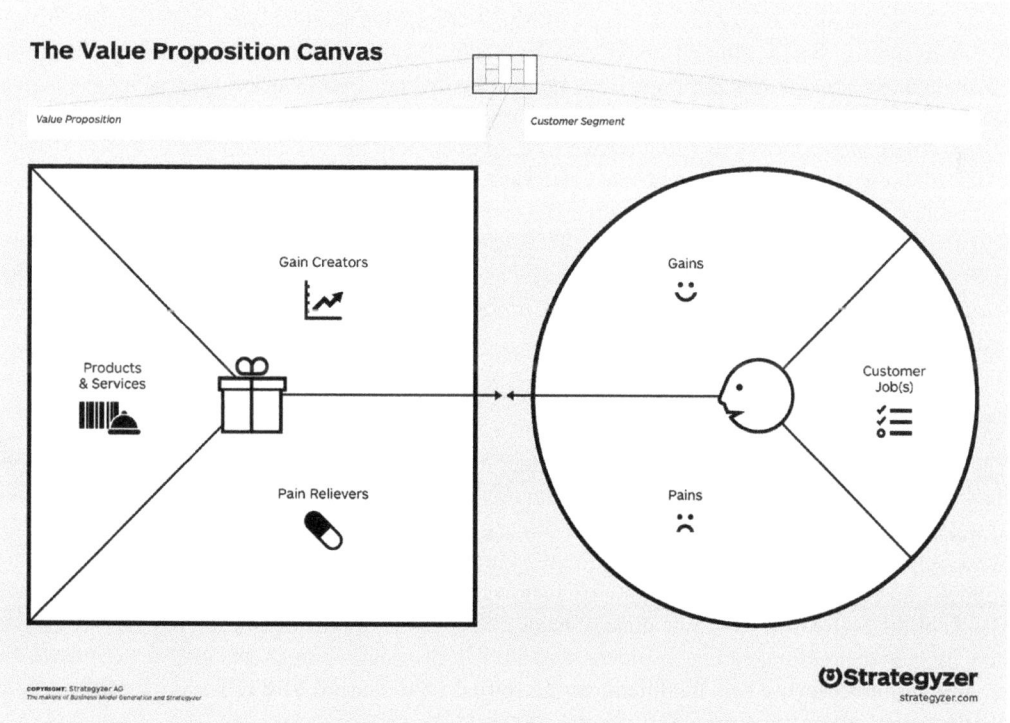

Figure 10.2 Osterwalder's Value Proposition Canvas (Alexander Osterwalder et al., 2014).

the customer. The jobs-to-be-done are about concrete targets customers may have, but also about targets with respect to social status, emotional well-being, and their context. In case of treatment from a hospital, the patient's objective is often to recover from his or her illness. The term 'pain' is used in the VPC in a metaphorical sense, but in the case of eHealth, it can also literally refer to things that the patient suffers from and would like to receive support for. Gains are about the outcomes and benefits that the customer would like to achieve. In the case of hospitals, patients benefit from, for example, shorter waiting times. Here, too, it is not just about functional utility, but also about realizing social and emotional benefits. Hence, the CP creates a concrete picture of, for example, the segment of diabetes patients, focused on what they want to achieve in their lives, what kind of problems they have with traditional treatments, and how their lives could be further improved.

The Value Map on the left-hand side of the Value Proposition Canvas (see Figure 10.2) is the counterpart of the Customer Profile. Here, we look for products and services that support their customers in achieving their goals, take away the pains and create the gains. In the case of health care, hospitals may want to use eHealth technologies to implement eHealth services that actually support diabetes patients in their daily lives, take away the difficulties they have with traditional treatments, and create additional advantages for them.

Case Study: Blended Care in Mental Healthcare

Case Description

This case study is about the use of blended care in mental healthcare, i.e., the combination of online and offline treatment. Care providers are increasingly applying blended care for, for example, depression, eating disorders, and anxiety disorders. The case study was carried out as part of a larger study on digitization in healthcare in the Netherlands (Lindenberg, van Gemert-Pijnen, & Nieuwenhuis, 2022). This case study looks at the use of a platform that consists of various components, namely online programmes, a questionnaire portal, and videoconferencing. An organization for mental healthcare wants to use the platform to meet the high demand for care, to prevent crises (emergency admissions), to improve care, to help more people, to respond to a lack of staff, a lack of budget, and long waiting times (also see Chapter 5 on eMental health).

In this case study, we wanted to build a Business Model Canvas (BMC) to systematically analyze the impact of blended care on a specific mental healthcare organization (MHO) as a whole. Different types of questions had to be answered, such as: How does it change the way of working, what investments are needed, and what is the impact on operational costs and time required from healthcare providers?

Value Proposition Canvas

The book *Value Proposition Design* (Osterwalder et al., 2014) offers specific support in filling out the VPC. Examples of suitable methods are playing cards with 'trigger and test' questions to arrive at well-formulated statements and analyses. Figure 10.3 shows a VPC for the clients of the MHO. Workshops with stakeholders were used to set up brainstorming sessions to fill out the canvas using yellow stickers with keywords. Figure 10.3 shows the Customer Profile (right-hand side) for the clients of the MHO. The job-to-be done of these clients is to remain healthy and happy. Their pains may include depression, eating disorders, and anxiety disorders. The clients may benefit from the digital platform because self-treatment can be started immediately. The self-service of the digital platform may create more flexibility for the clients.

The left-hand side of Figure 10.3 shows the Value Map for the MHO's clients. The value proposition is based on customer-oriented, online solutions with eMental health-modules that respond

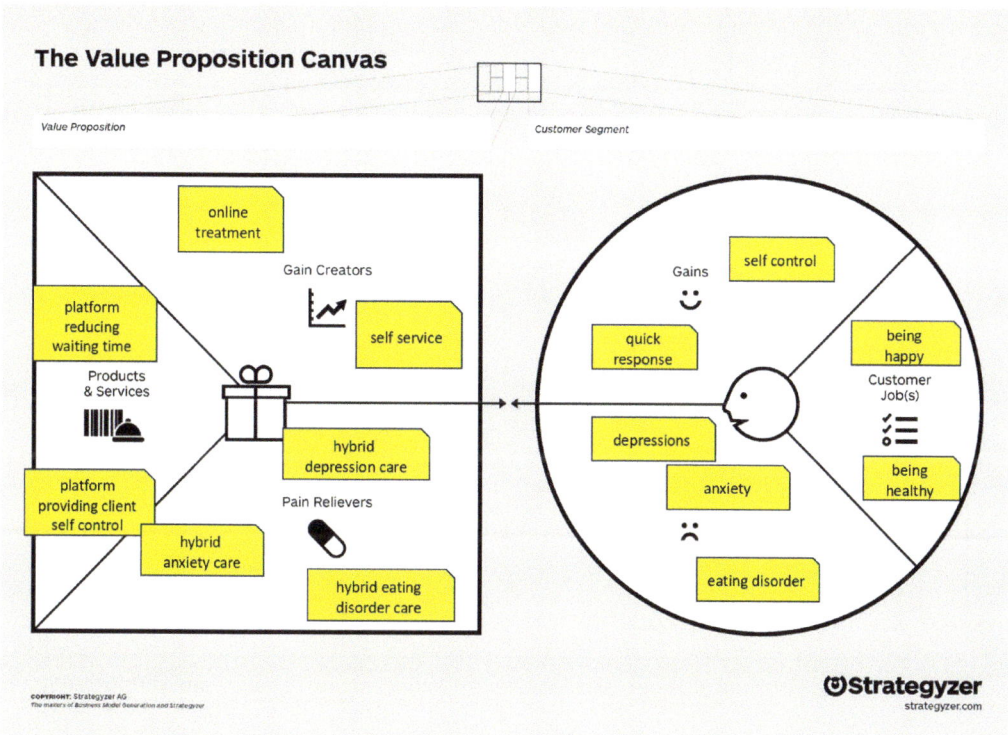

Figure 10.3 Value Proposition Canvas for mental health care clients.

to the potential problems that the clients may have. A blended way of working has been selected to respond quickly to client questions and reduce waiting time. However, the value map also showed that, if necessary, clients must be able to use the digital platform independently, without having to rely on healthcare providers. Only then can the MHO provide short-term care, due to staff shortages. Clients must be able to choose from a sufficiently broad range of solutions that meet their specific needs.

Figure 10.3 only shows the VPC for the clients of the MHO. The MHO in this case study is an NPO. The clients are the 'Beneficials' of the blended care. We did not show the VPC for the 'Finance Providers,, i.e., insurance companies and the government paying for the services. The MHO must also satisfy the needs of these 'Customer Segments'.

Business Model Canvas

Figure 10.4 shows highlights of the BMC for the MHO – providing the entire BMC is beyond the scope of this chapter. The complete BMC comprises all aspects of the entire MHO and clarifies what value the MHO creates for various client segments and finance provider and what commitment of people and resources is required to achieve this. The complete BMC indicates all customers, through which channels services are provided, and the relationships the MHO would like to maintain with them. For the implementation side, the BMC shows the activities done by partners and the activities which are carried out by the MHO itself. This also determines the staff the MHO must employ, and other resources that are required for doing so. A fully completed BMC includes the most relevant revenue streams and the largest cost items of the MHO.

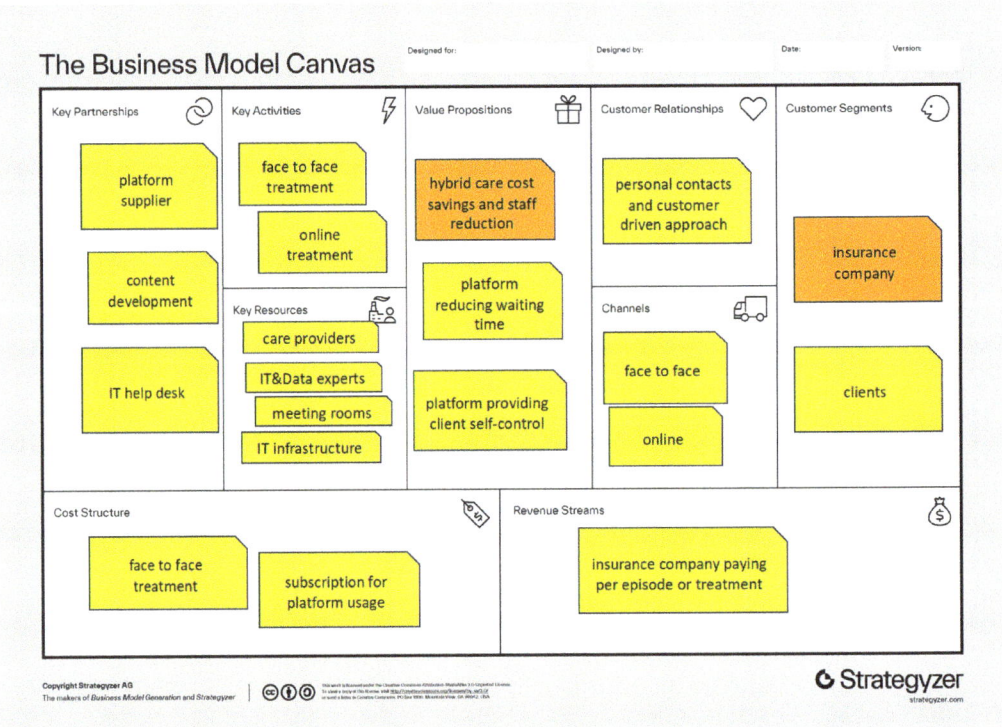

Figure 10.4 The Business Model Canvas of a mental health organization using blended care.

Figure 10.4 only shows the elements related to blended care. In addition to the value propositions from the VPC for the clients (yellow stickers) of the MHO, we also included placeholders for the value proposition for the health insurance companies reimbursing the costs for treatment (orange stickers). We assumed that blended care leads to cost savings and staff reductions. Both customer types are listed in the Customer Segments of the BMC. The MHO strives for a relationship based on a combination of a personal contacts and a customer-driven approach. This service is therefore provided via face-to-face contacts, as well as via the eHealth technology. The BMC also maps what has to be done on the part of the MHO in providing blended care. Partners are needed to supply equipment and to develop the software for the eHealth technology. Partners may also provide support in the training and education of both staff and clients. Its implementation requires additional human resources (like IT and data professionals) and employees at a permanent helpdesk. The key activities are a combination of face-to-face and online treatment.

The BMC in Figure 10.4 provides a top-level view of the MHO, with all relevant topics that need to be addressed to implement blended care. It can be considered as a sort of checklist with issues that the MHO must take care of before implementing and deploying blended care. The elaboration also requires further quantitative analyses, which are discussed in more detail in the next section.

Cost Benefit Analysis

The previous section discussed the concrete steps that an organization must take to implement an eHealth service in a sustainable manner, taking into account the context in which this organization must operate. Motives such as better care, lower costs, and fewer staff can play a role in this. Depending on the way in which healthcare is arranged in different countries in the world, there are similar motives for developing policies, for example to stimulate the development of eHealth at a national or regional level (also see Chapter 4). This section provides some guidelines for analyses of the costs and benefits of eHealth implementation. For a quantitative study on the economic impact of a nationwide implementation of eHealth, it is recommended to use an approach such as a cost-benefit analysis (Romijn & Renes, 2013). Cost-benefit analysis (CBA) is a methodology for the assessment of various future policies, the so-called project-alternatives. The project-alternatives are compared with a null-alternative, i.e., the most likely development without the new policy.

A CBA can be used to provide an overview of the effects, risks, and uncertainties of developing and deploying eHealth technologies for the welfare and well-being of society as a whole. All effects are assessed by quantifying these advantages and disadvantages and assigning values to them (in a currency such as euros or dollars). Expressing all effects in monetary terms enables us to compare all various aspects of social-welfare. A CBA provides insights expressed as the balance of the benefits minus the costs (in euros or dollars). The balance includes economic effects like direct and indirect costs and, for example, employment opportunities, but also tries to monetize the effects on our environment, safety in our community, or cultural heritage, to mention a few.

A CBA requires extensive research, which means that it often takes a long time and is quite expensive. In a full CBA, the null alternative and project alternative are fully mapped, and all impacts are then monetized. An alternative is to conduct a so-called quick-scan CBA. The main difference between a full CBA and a quick-scan CBA is that first, the main differences of the null-alternative and project-alternative are identified, and only these are being studied and monetized. The risk of a quick-scan CBA is of course that certain important effects are overlooked.

In practice, healthcare professionals and administrators of, e.g., hospitals can use even simpler approaches that are based on the principles of CBA and may give a good first impression of the financial effects of eHealth implementation. For example, in the case of the implementation of videocalls, we can compare the traditional way of working with that of using videocalls. We calculated the balance of costs and benefits. The implementation of videocalls is accompanied with costs for purchasing equipment and training and education of staff and citizens. There are also operational costs and possibly, additional costs for physicians and nurses if more time is needed compared to the traditional way of working. On the other hand, costs are saved due to reduction of travel time. The balance of these costs and benefits gives an indication of the total cost savings as a result of the implementation of this eHealth technology. Its effect on the deployment of personnel can be calculated in the same way. In this example, we may expect that the use of videocalls will reduce the overall time required from physicians and nurses.

We propose to use the simplified form of cost benefit analysis mentioned above (Kijl & Nieuwenhuis, 2011; Kijl, Nieuwenhuis, Huis in't Veld, Hermens, & Vollenbroek-Hutten, 2010) and use Activity Based Costing (ABC) (Baker, 1998; Udpa, 1996) for calculation costs of the activities within our approach. Basically, ABC identifies activities in an organization and assigns the cost to each activity. Indirect costs (like overheads) are also assigned to these costs per activity. The overall costs are calculated by counting the number of times activities are being executed (for example per treatment, or per period of time). ABC can be applied well in healthcare because it often involves recurring, well-defined medical treatment activities. It also fits well with the way in which care providers charge costs to health insurers. In practice, this concerns, for example, a nursing activity, the price per minute (based on personnel costs and the number of productive hours of a nurse) and the number of minutes required per treatment. In this approach the following five-step approach can be taken:

1. Identify the most significant actors that are affected by the eHealth implementation;
2. Identify the most significant activities that are executed for all alternatives;
3. Count the number of those activities (per unit of time, per patient treatment);
4. Determine the costs for each single activity using activity-based costing;
5. Calculate the total costs (per unit time, per patient treatment).

To summarize: For quantitative analysis we may look at the balance of benefits and costs to gain insight into the cost savings of the project-alternative (the eHealth technology) compared to the null-alternative (the traditional way of working). Because activities are linked to the amount of time a treatment requires, we also get a clear picture of the balance of hours care providers use in null-alternative and project-alternative. This allows us to analyze whether the eHealth treatment compared to the traditional treatment contributes to a reduction in healthcare personnel, and whether the eHealth alternative leads to an increase (or decrease) of labour productivity. In the next section, an eHealth case from practice is presented, in which this approach is applied.

Case Study: Telemonitoring in Heart Failure

Case Description

This case study is focused on the development of an Internet platform used for heart failure patients and centres around telemonitoring. Telemonitoring refers to the structural measurement of health-related data at home. These patient data are monitored remotely to reduce the chance of (re-)hospitalization. The case study was carried out as part of a larger study on digitization in healthcare in the Netherlands (Lindenberg et al., 2022). The patients received a tablet with software, to which the equipment for measuring blood pressure was connected via a Bluetooth connection. The measured values were sent to the hospital via an Internet connection. Daily data such as blood pressure (systolic, diastolic), heart rate, weight, and complaints were automatically transmitted to the server via the platform. An algorithm was used to determine whether data deviated from the threshold values set by cardiologists. In the event of an abnormality, the system automatically issued an alert to the patients. Nurses analyzed these alerts and contacted the patients by telephone or via a message service if the situation was viewed as threatening.

Telemonitoring was expected to shorten the duration of treatment, reduce the number of physical appointments and admissions, and improve patients' quality of life. It was expected that tasks and responsibilities would change and shift as a result of telemonitoring. Technology was seen not only as a cost-saving tool, but also as a possible solution to staff shortages and as a new treatment option. The introduction of telemonitoring had an effect on the quality and accessibility of care and on the deployment of staff. The intended effects were an improved quality of care, time and cost savings due to fewer (expensive) personnel, the creation of other types of jobs, and better accessibility.

Cost Benefit Analysis

The cost benefit analysis (CBA) of this case study was focused only on the period between when a patient with heart failure first consulted the specialist, up until the patient received adequate and stable medication. This covered a period of several months. Using the approach mentioned in the previous section, the null alternative was defined as the situation in which there is no telemonitoring. The project-alternative was the situation where patient data was monitored remotely via the eHealth technology.

Activities

The first step was to create an overview of all relevant actors and the activities they carried out. We assumed that there were no other actors than healthcare professionals and patients that would be significantly affected by the implementation of telemonitoring. For all actors, we identified all activities of the traditional treatment that would disappear, and all new activities that would be needed for telemonitoring.

Patient Contacts

The hospital and healthcare professionals measured the impact of telemonitoring for a cohort of 68 patients. In Figure 10.5, an overview of contacts patients and healthcare professionals had during the episode is provided. For both the null-alternative and project-alternative the average number of contacts and the average duration (in minutes) of the contact were calculated. An important effect was the increase from 4.96 to 6.03 outpatient visits by a healthcare provider per patient, which were mostly handled by a nurse (90%) and partly by a doctor (10%). We also observed an increase in doctor supervision activities. Telemonitoring was associated with a decrease in the average number of hospital admissions from 1.40 to 0.94 per patient. The average number of days a patient was admitted to the hospital decreased as well when telemonitoring was used: From 6.85 to 1.63 days.

Personnel and Hospitalization Costs

Many countries provide information about personnel costs for members of staff in hospitals. Once in a while, the available data is updated. We used the average hourly rate of the various actors in the year 2014 in the Netherlands (Hakkaart-van Roijen, van der Linden, Bouwmans, Kanters, & Swan Tan, 2015). We converted these data into the hourly rates for the year 2021, using price indices for the Netherlands. Similar data has been collected for health care costs in the Netherlands. Price index developments were used to convert staff and hospital costs towards 2021.

Results

The collected data originated from a cohort of 63 patients. The hospital treated 1200 patients annually using telemonitoring. The data has been scaled up to show costs and benefits for the hospital on an annual basis. With these data, a calculation model for the traditional heart failure treatment

patient contacts		0-alternative		p-alternative	
		#/patient	duration (min)	#/patient	duration (min)
outpatient clinic		4,96		6,03	
medical intake		1	60,00	1	60,00
outpatient clinic c	10%	0,50	15,00	0,60	15,00
outpatient clinic r	90%	4,46	30,00	5,43	30,00
call nurse		3,30	10,00	6,82	10,00
supervision doctor -> outpatient clinic nurse		4,46	5,00	5,43	5,00
supervision doctor -> call nurse		3,30	5,00	6,82	5,00
hospitalization doctor+patient		1,40	30,00	0,94	30,00
hospital doctor+patient		6,85	10,00	1,63	10,00
hospital discharge doctor+patient		1,40	30,00	0,94	30,00
hospitalization nurse +patient		1,40	45,00	0,94	45,00
hospital nurse+patient		6,85	45,00	1,63	45,00
hosptal discharge nurse+patient		1,40	45,00	0,94	45,00
hospital caregiver+patient		6,85	60,00	1,63	60,00

Figure 10.5 Input data for Telemonitoring Impact Model.

Actor	0-alternative	p-alternative	balance
supplier	-	420.000	-420.000
trainer	-	-	-
hospital	3.751.223	892.235	2.858.988
doctor	488.184	397.342	90.842
nurse	634.500	502.451	132.049
patient (employed)	-	-	-
patient (unemployed)	863.728	692.161	171.567
caregiver	728.981	744.371	-15.390
	6.466.616	3.648.560	2.818.057

Figure 10.6 Financial results.

and the eHealth treatment was developed. We implemented the model using commodity spread-sheet software. The annual costs were calculated for both the null-alternative and the project-alternative, using activity-based costing data. This takes into account costs for equipment, hospital costs, travel and accommodation costs, the hourly rates for the medical staff, and the time that patients and caregivers are involved in the treatment. Figure 10.6 gives an overview of the annual costs for the null-alternative, the project-alternative, and the resulting balance.

The devices used by patients were leased for €350 per patient, including training and support. The annual costs for the hospital added up to €420.000. As a consequence of using telemonitoring, the hospital costs decreased significantly from €3.7 to €0.8 million, related to additional outpatient costs but significantly less hospitalization costs. We also observed a decrease in costs for doctors and nurses due to less hospitalization. The time spent by patients and caregivers was monetized as well. There were no employed patients (almost all patients were older than 75 years). The overall CBA for telemonitoring boiled down to an annual cost saving of €2.8 million due to telemonitoring. The spreadsheet model was used to calculate the costs of personnel staff, using the number of hours they were involved in delivering treatment services to their patients. Hence, the impact of telemonitoring in heart failure on time spent by doctors, nurses, patients, and their caregivers can be extracted. Figure 10.7 gives the results in terms of working hours rather than labour costs per year. It can be seen that both doctors and nurses are saving time due to the telemonitoring. The hospital can save about 0.5 FTE doctors and 1.5 FTE nurses annually. Additionally, patients

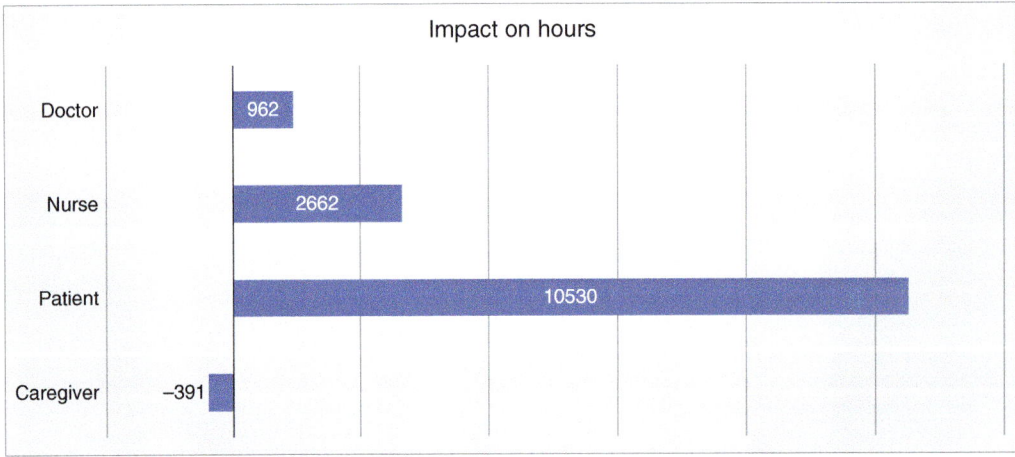

Figure 10.7 Impact on hours of medical staff, patient and caregiver.

experience a significant reduction in illness-related time due to the decrease in hospitalization. It is important to note that the time spent by caregivers slightly increases due to the additional time needed to accompany the patient to the hospital.

Conclusion of the Case Study

This case study demonstrates how activity-based costing and cost benefit analysis provide insights into the consequences of the implementation of the eHealth services in the day-to-day practice of healthcare organizations. Managers of healthcare organizations (or independent healthcare providers) use more detailed analysis to make 'business' decisions about the use of eHealth technologies. The case study demonstrates how the business impact in terms of savings of costs and human resources can be calculated in a straightforward manner.

Conclusions

After developing and using eHealth technologies, many steps still need to be taken by managers (and independent healthcare providers) before eHealth can ultimately be used in practice. To support this process, we can use commonly used business modelling tools and some simple financial methodologies. In this chapter, the importance of this approach and examples of models and methodologies were introduced. The take-home messages of this chapter are:

- A business model describes the rationale of how an organization creates, delivers, and captures value, and can be useful for the implementation of eHealth services in healthcare;
- The use of values is important for business models, but also for eHealth development, implementation, and evaluation in general;
- The Business Model Canvas and Value Proposition Canvas can be used in the context of both for-profit and non-profit healthcare organizations;
- The BMC and VPC provide insight into what needs to be done in practice to successfully introduce eHealth into practice by putting values central;
- There are different types of approaches to make rudimentary calculations which demonstrate how eHealth technology can contribute to reductions of costs and healthcare professionals.

Key References for Further Reading

Baker, J. J. (1998). *Activity-based costing and activity-based management for health care*. Jones & Bartlett Learning.

Kijl, B., & Nieuwenhuis, L. J. M. (2011). Deploying e-health service innovations; an early stage business model engineering and regulatory validation approach. *International Journal of Healthcare Technology and Management*, 12, 23–23.

Kijl, B., Nieuwenhuis, L. J. M., Huis in't Veld, R., Hermens, H. J., & Vollenbroek-Hutten, M. M. R. (2010). Deployment of e-health services—A business model engineering strategy. *Journal of Telemedicine and Telecare*, 16, 344–353.

Osterwalder, A., & Pigneur, Y. (2010). *Business model generation: A handbook for visionaries, game changers, and challengers*. John Wiley & Sons.

Osterwalder, A., Pigneur, Y., Bernarda, G., & Smith, A. (2014). *Value proposition design: How to create products and services customers want*. John Wiley & Sons.

References

Alberts, B. T., Meertens, L. O., Iacob, M.-E., & Nieuwenhuis, L. B. J. M. (2012). *A meta-model perspective on business models. International Symposium on Business Modeling and Software Design*, (pp. 64–81). Berlin, Heidelberg: Springer.

Al-Debei, M. M., & Avison, D. (2010). Developing a unified framework of the business model concept. *Eur J Inf Syst*, 19, 359–376.

Baker, J. J. (1998). *Activity-based costing and activity-based management for health care*. Jones & Bartlett Learning.

Bellman, R., Clark, C. E., Malcolm, D. G., Craft, C. J., & Ricciardi, F. M. (1957). On the construction of a multi-stage, multi-person business game. *Operations Research*, 5, 469–503.

Casadesus-Masanell, R., & Ricart, J. E. (2010). From strategy to business models and onto tactics. *Long Range Planning*, 43, 195–215.

DaSilva, C. M., & Trkman, P. (2014). Business model: What it is and what it is not. *Long Range Planning*, 47, 379–389.

Hakkaart-van Roijen, L., van der Linden, N., Bouwmans, C., Kanters, T., & Swan Tan, S. (2015). Bijlage 1: Kostenhandleiding: Methodologie van kostenonderzoek en referentieprijzen voor economische evaluaties in de gezondheidszorg.

Kijl, B., & Nieuwenhuis, L. J. M. (2011). Deploying e-health service innovations; an early stage business model engineering and regulatory validation approach. *International Journal of Healthcare Technology and Management*, 12, 23–23.

Kijl, B., Nieuwenhuis, L. J. M., Huis in 't Veld, R., Hermens, H. J., & Vollenbroek-Hutten, M. M. R. (2010). Deployment of e-health services—A business model engineering strategy. *Journal of Telemedicine and Telecare*, 16, 344–353.

Kimble, C. (2015). Business models for e-health: Evidence from ten case studies. *Global Business and Organizational Excellence*, 34, 18–30.

Lentferink, A., Polstra, L., D'Souza, A., Oldenhuis, H., Velthuijsen, H., & van Gemert-Pijnen, L. (2020). Creating value with eHealth: Identification of the value proposition with key stakeholders for the resilience navigator app. *BMC Medical Informatics and Decision Making*, 20, 76.

Lindenberg, M., van Gemert-Pijnen, L., & Nieuwenhuis, L. (2022). *A closer look at digitization in healthcare*. University of Twente, https://www.utwente.nl/en/techmed/research/research-programmes/sht/projects-and-results/meva/#.

Osterwalder, A. (2004). The Business Model Ontology – a proposition in a design science approach. Academic Dissertation, Universite de Lausanne, Ecole Des Hautes Etudes Commerciales.

Osterwalder, A, Gordijn, J., & Pigneur, Y. (2005). Comparing two business model ontologies for designing e-busines models and value constellations. 18 *The Bled eConference, eIntegration in Action*, 6–8.

Osterwalder, A., & Pigneur, Y. (2010). *Business model generation: A handbook for visionaries, game changers, and challengers.* John Wiley & Sons.

Osterwalder, A., Pigneur, Y., Bernarda, G., & Smith, A. (2014). *Value proposition design: How to create products and services customers want*. John Wiley & Sons.

Osterwalder, A., Pigneur, Y., & Tucci, C. L. (2005). Clarifying business models: Origins, present, and future of the concept. *Communications of the Association for Information Systems*, 16, 1–25.

Romijn, G., & Renes, G. (2013). *General guidance for Cost-Benefit Analysis*. In URL: https://www. Cpb. Nl/sites/default/files/publicaties/download/cba-guidance. Pdf.

Saebi, T., Lien, L., & Foss, N. J. (2016). What drives business model adaptation? The impact of opportunities, threats and strategic orientation. *Long Range Planning*, 50, 567–581.

Teece, D. J. (2010). Business models, business strategy and innovation. *Long Range Planning*, 43, 172–194.

Udpa, S. (1996). Activity-based costing for hospitals. *Health Care Management Review*, 83–96.

Wirtz, B. W., Pistoia, A., Ullrich, S., & Göttel, V. (2016). Business models: Origin, development and future research perspectives. *Long Range Planning*, 49, 36–54.

Wrede, C., Braakman-Jansen, A., & van Gemert-Pijnen, L. (2022). How to create value with unobtrusive monitoring technology in home-based dementia care: A multimethod study among key stakeholders. *BMC Geriatrics*, 22, 921.

Zott, C., Amit, R., & Massa, L. (2011). The business model: recent developments and future research. *Journal of Management*, 37, 1019–1042.

11 Human-centred Design

Tessa Dekkers & Catherine Burns

Introduction

Most people are familiar with the negative consequences of poorly designed technology: Websites with an overly complicated menu structure, smartwatches with screens that are too small to use properly, or extremely unattractive apps. These kinds of issues might cause users to stop using the technology or use it in the wrong way. In eHealth, poorly designed technology can have a negative impact on effectiveness, because the users do not optimally benefit from the content of the technology. Consequently, it is important that a design fits the needs and preferences of the users as closely as possible. Attention should be paid to this throughout the entire development process, as described in Chapter 7 on holistic eHealth development. In this chapter, specific attention is paid to how design good eHealth technologies, using methods from human-centred design.

In this chapter, the basics of a human-centred design (HCD) approach are discussed. First, HCD as a domain is introduced. After that, the rationale behind and specific methods for requirements, prototyping and formative evaluation are provided. Throughout the chapter, a case study on the design of a smartwatch for seniors is used to illustrate the application of these methods. After completing this chapter, you will be able to:

- Explain the basic principles and rationale behind human-centred design and understand their relevance for eHealth design;
- Name and explain several methods and approaches that are suitable for the different phases of HCD and connect them to eHealth design;
- Describe different types of prototypes and connect them to iterative design and the different phases of HCD;
- Explain the relevance of evaluation for HCD and compare the goals of several common evaluation techniques for different design stages;
- Name and explain different methods for remote, online HCD and understand their advantages and disadvantages.

DOI: 10.4324/9781003302049-13

Human-centred Design

What is HCD?

There is a broad range of possible end-users for eHealth technologies, for example, highly educated clinicians, busy administrators, or patients who are starting to learn to self-manage their disease. While the type of end-user differs, the same methods can be used to create an adequate and accurate design for specific user groups. Methods from human-centred design (HCD) can be used throughout the development process. HCD can include many methods but is essentially a design framework and a value system to be considered and applied by the designer. HCD begins with a deep respect for the user and a realization that the user is the most important partner in design. As partners in the development process, users co-discover their needs through assisting with requirements definition, contributing to design through iterative cycles of prototyping and providing continuous feedback. When done properly, HCD creates a partnership between designer and user, and empowers the user to engage in the improvement of their own situation.

HCD aims to develop solutions to problems by involving the human perspective in all steps of the process via observing the problem within its context and brainstorming, conceptualizing, developing, and implementing the solution. Central to HCD – sometimes also referred to as user-centred design – are the lives and desires of the people for whom the eHealth technology is designed. The design should match their needs and context. Therefore, the design process should focus on finding a solution for a real-life problem experienced by real people. The key to a human-centred design process is keeping *users* and *stakeholders* involved in the process, through requirements definition, early feedback, evaluation, and field testing (ISO, 2021).

Phases of HCD

HCD is an *iterative process* of design and redesign. Iterative means that, at each stage, the design is reconsidered and receives feedback before progressing to the next stage. This iteration is the key to continually ensuring that the design is calibrated to the needs of the users and will help them effectively. All HCD methods are based on cycles of iteration between design and testing phases (Maguire, 2001). These different phases are discussed below according to the Double Diamond Model, a prominent visualization and understanding of the design process developed by the British Design Council in 2004 and renamed as the Framework for Innovation in 2019 (Council, 2023) that has been widely applied in healthcare settings and is suitable for HCD (Melles, Albayrak, & Goossens, 2021).

The Double Diamond Model in Figure 11.1 assumes that all HCD design processes go through phases of divergence, in which issues and ideas are explored more widely, followed by phases of convergence, in which focused action and decision-making take place. This process of divergence-convergence is done both to find and define the problem the design will tackle and to develop and test a solution. The designer begins with finding out what the problem is that needs to be addressed. This includes understanding the lives and desires of the people who will eventually use the technology (the target group) – also see Chapter 8 on the contextual inquiry. After that, different ideas and prototypes are developed that could solve the problem that was analyzed. These prototypes are tested with the target group and adapted accordingly. These phases are called *Discover*, *Define*, *Design*, *Deliver* and are described in more detail below:

- **Discover**. At the beginning of the design process, designers often have very little idea of the design and target group. The designer uses this phase to learn more about the lives, attitudes, and context of users and other possibly important stakeholders through immersion, observation, and conversation (e.g., by interviewing elderly people about what motivates them to exercise). During this phase, the designer aims to understand what the actual problem is according to the people who are affected by it;

- **Define.** When the scope of the design project is better understood, and it is clear who the key users will be, the designer defines a problem statement that best describes the main challenge the design will tackle. This challenge is typically more focused than the initial brief (e.g., elderly people want an easy tool to get in more steps because they are relatively sedentary and want to avoid future health complaints). In addition, requirements (see Chapter 9) will be defined to guide the design phase;
- **Design.** Once the problem is defined and the requirements are clear, the designer, in collaboration with a range of stakeholders, prepares many different early ideas of what they think might be suitable solutions. *Low-fidelity prototypes* or *mock-ups* can be created using quick approaches (e.g., paper or simple computer-based approaches), since the intention is to modify and revise these significantly based on the input of the users;
- **Deliver.** Prototypes are tested with users. Based on the results of these user tests, promising ideas are further improved and aspects of the design that do not work are discarded.

As these four activities are iterated, the process moves closer and closer to the final design. In later iterations, the *Design* phase may involve the development of high-fidelity prototypes or mock-ups with a finished 'look and feel'. Such a high-fidelity prototype can then be used in the *Deliver* phase to do a full evaluation in which the user can perform all intended tasks, and the user experience is as realistic as can be achieved. In turn, introducing the prototype in practice may lead to an even better understanding of the issue at stake, or the *Discovery* of a potential new design problem to tackle, and so forth.

At the end of the iterative design process, a product is released. The 'final' product (e.g., the eHealth technology) is implemented in practice but is often still referred to as a prototype, because

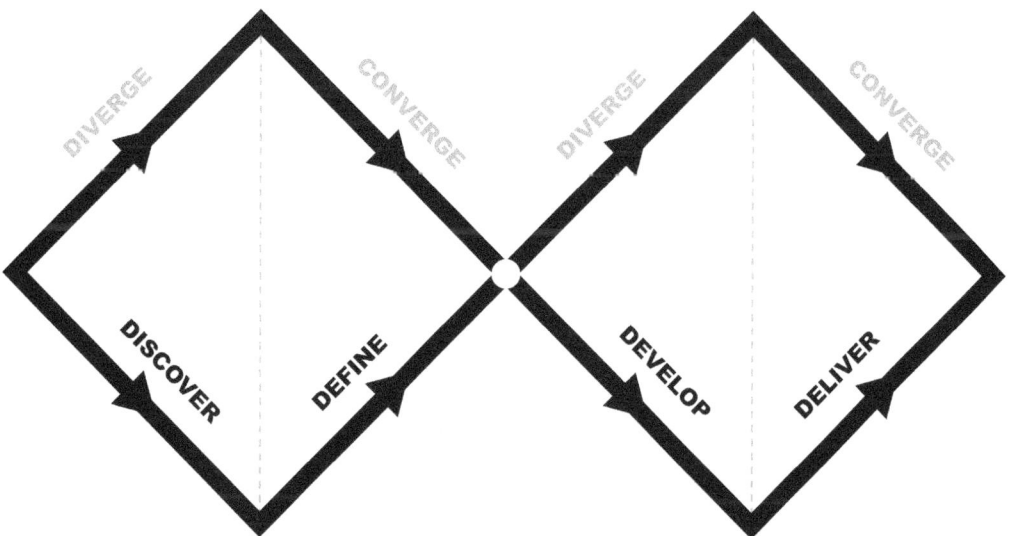

Figure 11.1 Double Diamond Model. Note: Adapted from the Double Diamond by the Design Council as licensed under a CC BY 4.0 license.

even final products should be evaluated and improved continuously. Even after the eHealth technology is released, feedback and data may be collected to begin the design cycle for the next release of the product. Constant periodic product improvement is a very good way to continually generate well-designed products.

Discovering and Defining the Problem and its Design Requirements

At the beginning of the HCD process, the designer seeks to understand the context of the user as deeply as possible, gather information, and understand the value points of the task at hand. In each case, the designer creates models of the user's work or task space, and these models are used to identify, scope, and define the design problem. In the section below, some of these methods as applied to healthcare are described. These methods partly overlap and can be combined with activities described in contextual inquiry (Chapter 8) and with methods for extracting values and requirements as described in Chapter 9.

There are several methods that are suitable for problem identification. Some methods are specifically relevant for large, complex design problems with many stakeholders, while others are more suitable for relatively straightforward, simple design problems without too many components. There also is a relationship between the method and the gathered information: Some methods result in information that is mainly centred on work processes, while others contain information about the user perspective. The choice for a method also depends on the availability of the user to participate in the design process, because some methods are a lot more time-consuming than others. Therefore, the use of a method is often based on not just substantive considerations, but also on practical constraints.

In Table 11.1 an overview is provided of possible methods and accompanying design problems, types of information that can be gathered, the required access to users, an example of a relevant eHealth technology, and a key source for further reading. More information on these methods is provided in the section below the table.

Contextual Inquiry and Design

As was described in Chapter 8, a *contextual inquiry* entails the activities that are undertaken to get a good grasp of the context in which the design problem is present. Contextual design aims to aggregate data from stakeholders in the context where they are living and working and apply these findings to a final product (Beyer & Holtzblatt, 1997). Consequently, the goal is to get a thorough understanding of the prospective users, other important stakeholders, and their environment, which can be achieved by both qualitative and quantitative methods such as interviews and questionnaires.

Patient Journey Mapping

Patient journey mapping is an adaptation of customer journey mapping, specifically tailored to healthcare settings (Simonse et al., 2019). It is used to create a graphic representation of a health service and its procedures from the patient perspective, including feelings and interactions with healthcare staff. The central activity in patient journey mapping is to 'walk the journey') in which the designer follows a patient in real time while noting emotions, interactions, and actors throughout (Trebble et al., 2010). A critical advantage of patient journey mapping is that it allows designers to look at the entire picture instead of a singular touchpoint. This provides more insight into possible problems to tackle in the design. Furthermore, the graphical output is easily shared and discussed with a multi-disciplinary team.

Table 11.1 Methods to discover and define the design problem.

Method	Design problem involves	Information gathered	Access to users	eHealth example	Key source
Contextual Inquiry and design	Complex team or environment interactions	Rich descriptions of the problem	Deep access with hours shadowing the user	Work engagement of nurses after introduction of a chat function for patient-provider communication (Cajander, Larusdottir, & Hedström, 2020).	(Beyer and Holtzblatt, 1997; Cooper, Reimann, Cronin, and Noessel, 2014)
Patient Journey Mapping		Representation of the health service and its procedures, including relationships and feelings from a patient perspective	Whole-day access to clinical staff and patients	Experience of hand and wrist surgical patients in public and private hospitals (Ridder, Dekkers, Porsius, Kraan, & Melles, 2018).	(Trebble, Hansi, Hydes, Smith, & Baker, 2010; Simonse, Albayrak, & Starre, 2019).
Cognitive work analysis	Hard-to-understand equipment or complex processes	Understanding of physical relationships and strategies of experts	Access to experts, trainers and manuals	Key pathways to successful blood pressure control (Burns, Rezai, & Maurice, 2018; Dikmen & Burns, 2022).	(Vicente, 1999)
Cognitive task analysis	Lack of efficiency and workflow	Task maps and ways to make common tasks more efficient	Access to users for observations and interviews	Mobile app for delivering crucial information about antipsychotic drugs (Roosan et al., 2019).	(Ramos, Utne, & Mosleh, 2019)
Persona-based design	Specific user group, lack of user engagement and satisfaction	Characteristics of specific user groups	Brief access to users through observation, surveys, interviews, and/or existing marketing research.	Biopsychosocial personas of older patients with heart failure (Holden, Kulanthaivel, Purkayastha, Goggins, & Kripalani, 2017).	(Adlin & Pruitt, 2010)
Participatory design and co-design		User perception of what the design should be like, what they need	Access to users, typically in groups	Asthma self-management app informed by young people's lived experience (Peters et al., 2017).	(Clemensen, Rothmann, Smith, Caffery, & Danbjorg, 2017; Sanders & Stappers, 2008)
Generative design		Tacit and latent knowledge of user needs	Access to users for a longer period of sensitization followed by (group) interviews.	Communication and information services for people receiving hip or knee surgery (Groeneveld et al., 2020).	(Stappers, 2014)

Cognitive Work Analysis

Cognitive work analysis (Vicente, 1999) is a work-centred conceptual framework that aims to analyze cognitive work and is widely applied in healthcare (Jiancaro, Jamieson, & Mihailidis, 2014). It first evaluates the system already in place, and then develops recommendations for design. Within Cognitive Work Analysis, people who interact with information are considered as actors in work-related actions rather than users of a system. Human-information interaction is viewed in the context of human work activities. A basic presumption is that in order to design good systems that work with humans, one has to understand the work that people (actors) do (e.g., enter values in a personal health record), their information behaviour (e.g., reading the information off the screen of a blood-glucose meter), the context in which they work (e.g., at home, on the couch) and the reason for their actions (e.g., to gain an overview of their blood-glucose levels during the day) (Fidel & Pejtersen, 2004).

Cognitive Task Analysis

The primary goal of *cognitive task analysis* is to dissect 'mental work' into more manageable constructs that shed light on a particular problem. It is seen as an extension of traditional task analysis techniques by collecting information about the knowledge, thought processes and goal structures that underlie observable task behaviour (Schraagen et al., 2000). Often, observable behaviour and the covert cognitive functions are seen as an integrated whole, so it is advisable to not separate them and focus on the cognitive functions alone (Gordon & Gill, 1997). This knowledge can be used in the design of technology that supports human work.

Persona-based Design

Personas are specific, concrete representations of fictitious persons that represent the target group and are used to put a face on the user. This enables the designers to get a thorough understanding of the people that will use their technology. Personas are a useful way to communicate this understanding to all members of the team (Adlin & Pruitt, 2010). There are many different kinds of personas used for various purposes (Floyd, Jones, & Twidale, 2008). Personas can be created in a systematic way, for example, by using tables or templates (LeRouge, Ma, Sneha, & Tolle, 2013; Acuña, Castro, & Juristo, 2012) or by statistically stratifying relevant data collected from electronic patient records, interviews, questionnaires or log data to user subgroups (Ten Klooster et al., 2022). In this way, personas can be used to easily disseminate demographic characteristics, daily roles and tasks, skills, and knowledge, and personal as well as psychological or medical details about the target group. Since a persona synthesizes data about the users, it can assist in identifying what the product should do to satisfy users' needs during the requirement elicitation (Acuña et al., 2012).

Participatory Design and Co-design

Participatory design and co-design have multiple definitions, but all approaches stress the importance of actively involving relevant persons during the development of technologies (Simonsen & Robertson, 2013). These important people can be users, but other stakeholders can also be involved during the mapping of the context and accompanying requirements (van Gemert-Pijnen, Peters, & Ossebaard, 2013). There are multiple ways in which users can be involved in the participatory development process. In 'informant' design, users are asked for input and feedback on some, but not all, design choices. They provide suggestions but don't actually make the decisions and designs themselves (Scaife, Rogers, Aldrich, & Davies, 1997). In 'co-design', users are closely involved in the creation of the design and are seen as equal design partners (DeSmet et al., 2016).

Generative Design

Generative design is closely related to participatory design. It is focused on the making (*generating*) of artefacts by users to help reflect on their lived experience and preferences of the design. These artefacts may include mind maps, collages, sketches, scale models, or prototypes. This allows access to tacit and latent knowledge. Tacit knowledge refers to things users know, but are unable to articulate through words, and latent knowledge is subconscious and dormant knowledge about the future, based on past experiences (Sanders & Stappers, 2008). Through the act of creating, users are confronted with a concrete representation of what they do (not) like, which allows them to better articulate their needs. This concrete approach to codesign may be specifically helpful when working with vulnerable populations of different cognitive capabilities and literacy levels, including people with severe mental illness (Schouten et al., 2022), people with dementia (Wang, Marradi, Albayrak, & van der Cammen, 2019), or children (Van Mechelen, 2016).

Generative design and participatory design are often combined. Both actively involve users and stakeholders directly in the design process and share underlying principles of democracy, mutual learning, multiple layers of knowledge, and collective creativity (Vandekerckhove, de Mul, Bramer, & de Bont, 2020).

Case Study Physical Activity of Seniors – Part 1: Problem Finding

Throughout this chapter, a fictional case study on physical activity of seniors is provided to illustrate some of the important HCD methods. Most older adults have a sedentary lifestyle and do not engage often enough in physical activity, despite the evidence that regular exercise can increase life expectancy and delay the onset and progression of chronic diseases (Chodzko-Zajko et al., 2009). The first part of this case study provides an example of a (simplified) problem finding process by which the designers discover what the exact problem is they are trying to solve, which technology could be applicable, what the technology should do and what kind of experience it should provide.

Selection of methods

The technology that will be developed has to reflect the needs of the user group consisting of seniors, since they may have very specific requirements. Because the target group is so specific, the project would benefit most from methods as Contextual Inquiry and Generative Design. Methods such as Cognitive Work or Task Analysis would be less suitable because they include an analysis of already existing complex tasks which is not the case.

Contextual inquiry

To perform a contextual inquiry for this design problem, the designer would need to visit some older adults and spend time with them. They can be asked to talk about their day, when they walk and when they use technology. Important information would be:

- Who do they talk to, email to, phone and visit, and what are their communications about?
- What daily tasks do they perform and what do they find difficult?
- What environments are they in? Do they have electronic access? Are their environments crowded, noisy, indoors or outdoors?
- How do they structure their homes? Is there an area for computing?
- How do they relate to technology and people around them? What cultural aspects might influence them?

184 Tessa Dekkers & Catherine Burns

These *observations* can be used to develop flow models (e.g., how people communicate and coordinate to accomplish work), sequence models (e.g., detailed steps performed to accomplish each task), cultural models (e.g., culture and policy that constrains how work is done), artefact models (e.g., what is created and used in doing the work) and models of their physical environment (e.g., what supports or gets in the way of doing the work) (Beyer & Holtzblatt, 1997). From a contextual inquiry, one might learn information like the following:

- They mostly talk to their family and some neighbours;
- They find things like remembering to take medication or where they parked their car difficult;
- They enjoy walks outdoors in sunshine, but prefer to walk with someone else, both for company and in case they fall;
- Most of their environments are quiet. But with hearing changes, they might still miss auditory notifications;
- Most do not have a computer workspace but can use their mobile phone and tablet with help of their (grand)children;
- They feel intimidated calling technical support and are more likely to ask a friend or relative for help, so the technology needs to be suitable for them too.

Generative design

Now that the designer has some understanding of the physical and social context in which older adults (do not) engage in exercise, they can further clarify how a technology could promote physical activity in older adults by inviting them to a generative design workshop. There are various creative activities they could do to help the design team better understand their attitude towards physical activity. Some tools focus on making artefacts, others on telling stories and others on enacting possible futures (see also (Sanders & Brandt, 2010)). Design activities could include for example:

- Make photographs of items and people that help them lead more active lives;
- Make a timeline of a typical day in their lives, focusing on moments in which they are physical active and when they are not;
- Make a collage of what being active means to them, using a toolkit of pre-selected photographs, quotes, stickers, and/or other materials;
- Tell or write a story about a time when they were more physically active;
- Act out their ideal walk in the park using a hypothetical technology that can do anything they want.

This may uncover the following findings in addition to the contextual inquiry:

- Some older adults use mobility aids. They enjoy the freedom they provide, but dislike feeling dependent;
- They consider gardening and cleaning physical activities;
- Some older adults experience pain when walking. They are on a waiting list for hip surgery, but this could take another six months;
- They would like to learn something about the history of the environment when going on a stroll.

Likely, the designer will get a lot of rich information from both the contextual inquiry as well as the generative design workshops, some of which might not be directly applicable to the design. That is okay, since the goal of problem finding is to first diverge and consider many different areas and problems that the eHealth technology may address before converging on a definite problem to solve. Based on the findings described above, design directions one may formulate to increasing physical activity of older adults through eHealth are:

- A smart mobility aid that automatically recognizes and corrects instable gait;
- A smartwatch that invites the user to log steps and partake in walks;
- An app to help elderly stay active in physical hobbies like gardening while coping with pain; and
- Augmented reality glasses that provide information and history of neighbourhood parks.

Any of the directions could be feasible. The choice of which design direction to follow should be made by the multidisciplinary team in relation to their budget, interest, and/or existing techno-logical focus. In this chapter, we will continue our example with a smartwatch.

Designing a Solution

Once the design problem is specified and requirements are set, it is time to develop the actual eHealth technology that will tackle the problem. This will also involve requirement specification, as discussed in Chapter 9. But requirements are not just magically integrated into a finished, ready-to-use design. During the design process, numerous prototypes that incorporate the requirements have to be developed, tested with users and adapted accordingly.

What are Prototypes?

The word prototype comes from the Greek 'prototypos': Protos meaning 'first' and typos meaning 'mould', 'pattern', or 'impression'. This original meaning still defines low-fidelity (lo-fi) proto-typing, which is an initial, raw representation of an idea. While there are also high-fidelity (hi-fi) prototypes, the design process usually starts with lo-fi prototypes. These kinds of prototypes do not have to look like the final technology at all. A lo-fi prototype is suitable for communicating the general goal and ideas behind the technology to users and, if necessary, other stakeholders. The most important features of the idea should be present in the lo-fi prototype so that users, experts or stakeholders can evaluate these features. Hi-fi prototypes, however, have a higher resemblance to the final version of the eHealth technology. People can interact with hi-fi prototypes and they are suitable for testing specific details of the technology that is being developed. Throughout all adaptations and improvements, it is important to constantly check whether the requirements are still present in the prototypes (Newman & Landay, 2000).

Prototyping Methods

As was described before, a HCD process entails multiple phases in which the designer gains clarity of the problem and develops and tests multiple solutions before settling on the definitive design. For each phase in the design process, specific ways and goals of prototyping are most suitable, also see Table 11.2.

At the beginning of the design process, designers still have very little idea of the design, so the prototypes that are recommended for this stage – moodboards, sketches, storyboards and quick prototypes – are intended to facilitate exploratory conversation. During this stage, the designer may prepare some early ideas of what they think might be suitable. These prototypes should be created using quick, cheap approaches (paper or simple computer-based approaches) since the intention is still to modify and revise these prototypes significantly. As previously discussed, in a participatory design process not only the designer engages in early prototyping. Other stakeholders may also develop sketches and paper prototypes to express their vision of what may be suitable or necessary to solve the design problem.

Later in the design process, the designer can work out more specific features of the eHealth technology, such as what the navigation of the system might look like, the layout of the screens or some early screen designs. Early on, keeping a 'rough' look-and-feel to these prototypes can encourage a broader discussion, as users will sometimes be more willing to critique a 'rough' looking sketch than product that looks more finished. This also prevents a focus on details that are not relevant for this specific stage in the process. After this, the focus lies on the finer details of the design. The prototypes at this stage should likely be built on a computer to ensure that the look appears quite finished. However, the prototype itself is still usually developed in some software that enables quick changes. Some simple simulation of how the design would interact is also possible. Usually, the interaction may simulate the navigation and presentation of new screens, or simple interactions. The prototype would not be connected to working software such as databases. Prototypes at this stage can be tested with simple user tasks such as finding information, understanding a clinical situation or entering data.

For testing, a high-fidelity prototype or mock-up may be developed. The intention of the high-fidelity prototype is to do a full evaluation during which the user, other stakeholders or experts on design or content can perform all intended tasks, and the user experience is as closely comparable to the actual experience as can be achieved. The high-fidelity prototype can be recognized, as it may look indistinguishable from the final product. Differences from the final product in scope or functionality are hidden from the user to make the interaction experience seem realistic.

Finally, once the product is released, it is often still referred to as a prototype, since even final products should be evaluated continuously through their life cycle. Products should constantly be improved to ensure that a product stays well designed.

In Table 11.2, different types of prototypes and accompanying design questions that can be answered with that kind of prototype are described.

As can be observed in Table 11.2, multiple types of prototypes can be used, and most of them have a different place in the design process. These different prototypes and their main goals are described below.

- **Sketch**. A sketch (see Figure 11.2 for an example) is a freehand drawing on paper that gives a really low-fidelity representation. It is a really fast way to get an idea ready for brainstorming and can describe it better than words;
- **Storyboard**. A storyboard is often a series of roughly drawn comic-book style frames that visualize key moments in (the use of) a design and can be used to build a short narrative. This method can assist in fine-tuning an idea and provide insight in who will use it, where and how;

Table 11.2 Prototypes and design questions.

Prototype type	Design questions that can be answered
Sketch, or storyboard, paper prototype (Buxton, 2007; Snyder, 2003)	What is the scope of functionality that should be covered? Who are the key stakeholders? What is the compelling use story for this product? How do the stakeholders see this product?
Sketches, wireframes, rough mock-ups, paper prototype	Can the functionality be further understood? What is the information architecture underlying this system? How will people navigate? What are the basic design needs?
Low-fidelity paper and digital prototypes	Is the content and scope, ok? Does it have the right look and feel? Do the screens have the right information and the right interaction opportunities?
High-fidelity digital prototypes with interaction developed	Can users perform the tasks as intended? Do they make errors? Are they efficient? How do they find the user experience?
Full product	How are people actually using the design? Do they have feedback? How is it changing their behaviour or their work processes?

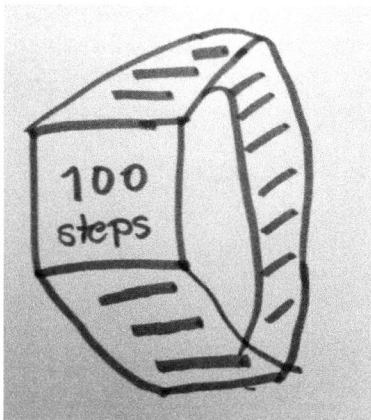

Figure 11.2 An example of a basic starting sketch for initiating design discussions.

- **Wireframe**. A wireframe (see Figure 11.3 for an example) represents the skeleton or simple structure of a design. It can describe the functionality of a product and what happens, for example, when you click a certain button. Decisions on what content to put where in the design are often made via wireframes;
- **Mock-ups.** Mock-ups provide medium-fidelity representations of a design. Elements such as colours, fonts, texts, images, and logos are used for the mock-up. These elements are integrated in the structure as was determined via the wireframes;
- **Paper prototype**. Paper prototypes of an interface can be created with materials such as paper, pencils, paint, sticky notes, cards, and coloured paper. In paper prototyping, users can perform realistic tasks by interacting with a paper representation of the interface. This interaction can be manipulated by a person (researcher) who 'acts as the computer' (Snyder, 2003);
- **Digital prototype**. Digital prototyping (see Figure 11.4 for an example) mainly has the same principle of paper prototyping. The interface is represented in a simple way in order to give the user an idea about the final technology. Digital 2D prototyping is mainly different in its form. Instead of paper, programmes can be used, which enables the designer to make the prototype clickable. Digital prototypes can be low-fidelity or high-fidelity, depending on whether and how many interactions are developed.

Case Study Physical Activity of Seniors – Part 2: Prototyping, Iteration and Evaluation

This case study further elaborates on the findings presented in the case study on the development of a smartwatch specifically for seniors. This second part focuses on several methods of prototyping that might be relevant to design the smartwatch. Some evaluation techniques are also already presented, as prototyping and evaluating are two intertwined processes, because you always have to check whether the requirements were successfully implemented in the design and whether the design truly matches the needs of the intended users. It is important to note that when evaluating prototypes, more requirements may be discovered. In reality, the phases of HCD are always overlapping.

Participatory design

In a participatory design exercise, the users may look at sketches and early ideas, and offer direct suggestions on the design. One way in this example might be to have a focus group of four or five seniors and present some early ideas.

Paper and pens can be brought to encourage them to join the design process. An example of a participatory design in this example might present the front face of the watch via a sketch of a digital display and a number reflecting the steps taken that day (Figure 11.2). The focus group can start with confirming the group's understanding of the design, and then asking them what they like and how it should be different. From this process it would be possible to learn things like:

• Whether they want a digital or analogue clock display;
• Where and how large should the font for the step count be?
• What colours might be good, and how large should the typeface be?
• If they pressed a button on the side, what would they expect to happen?

Participatory design can be a great way to understand ergonomic, user experience and content requirements (see Chapter 9).

Sketches and storyboards

Sketches (such as in Figure 11.2) and storyboards are prototyping methods that are used in the earlier phases of design and are often useful to explore requirements, for example, in individual interviews or focus groups. The sketch and/or storyboard is shown, the context of use is explained, including an explanation of how the technology would work. Based on that, new sketches or storyboards can be presented. At each point, the designer asks for feedback on the design and tries to figure out what the users would expect to see next and what could be improved. Other stakeholders may also be involved in this process. For the smartwatch design, this may include family members of older adults who may be asked to fix, calibrate, or help maintain the watch. All of these people can give valuable feedback on early design ideas. Again, because storyboards provide a concrete representation of how the design will be used in context, this may be a particular accessible method to use with vulnerable populations. For example, (Faber et al., 2023) used storyboards to codesign asthma digital medication adherence interventions for and with asthma patients with low health literacy.

Wireframes

Wireframes allow the exploration of the method of navigating the product and basic layout and structure of the screens. The wireframes do not focus on specific design details yet. In a wireframe for this smartwatch, the designer may need to decide on things like:

• Is the time always visible?
• How much of the screen space goes to the time and how much to other information like notifications or step counts?
• Is there navigation information on the watch? Is it a touchscreen?

Wireframes can also be evaluated to gather feedback. The wireframe in Figure 11.3 indicates that the watch will have navigation at the top and bottom of the screen and will reserve the middle of the screen for content. With this wireframe, the designer could assess whether the up/down arrows are understandable for navigation and whether users were satisfied with the time, battery and connectivity not being shown.

Early digital prototype

A first digital prototype often shows how the various screens can look like, with anticipated colours, typeface, and graphics. This prototype is often just a set of linked screens and does not have a 'back-end' behind it. In the case of the smartwatch, this means that the prototype is not yet capable

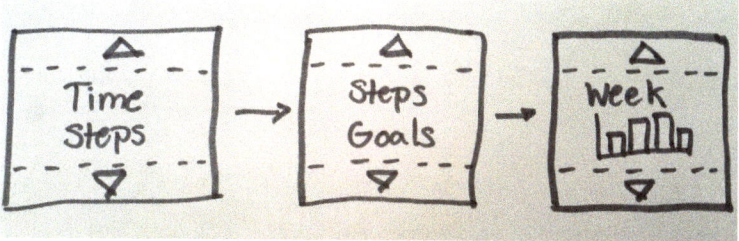

Figure 11.3 An example of a possible wireframe for the smartwatch.

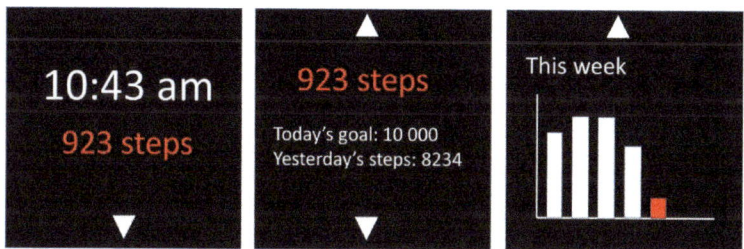

Figure 11.4 An example of a possible early digital prototype for the smartwatch.

of tracking the number of steps and does not collect any data. However, it is often not too hard to at least link up the navigation so users can press a button and move to the next appropriate screen so that users can experience what it would look like when their activity is tracked. Figure 11.4 shows an example of three possible smartwatch screens that would be seen in series. In this design, the designer has chosen a certain typeface to indicate low activity with red and has retained the navigation and layout from the wireframe in Figure 11.3.

Evaluation of early paper or digital prototypes with users can provide valuable information. They can be given small tasks that require them to find information on different screens and navigate through the product. For example, despite being just an early prototype, users can be asked about where they would click to perform a certain action. In the example in Figure 11.4, the designer might want to make sure people understand the navigation from screen one to screen three and back. The designer can also determine if they understand and like the colour scheme, particularly the red coding. The users that participate in the testing should reflect the user groups, as identified earlier. Personas can provide very good guidance on who to include in testing phase.

While user evaluations are of course valuable, this is also a good stage to consult some experts or colleagues in user experience design. Do they see any problems with the design? Has anything been missed? Is everything clear and consistent?

High-fidelity prototype

A high-fidelity prototype should look, feel and operate as close to the eventual product as possible. In the case of the smartwatch, the high-fidelity prototype will respond to notifications and button presses and can also generate sounds or vibrations. This kind of prototype can be tested in quite realistic tasks. At this stage, the designer can understand with depth and detail how users will interact with the product and make adaptations accordingly. In the smartwatch example, a high-fidelity prototype must have the same size and scale as the final watch (see Figure 11.5).

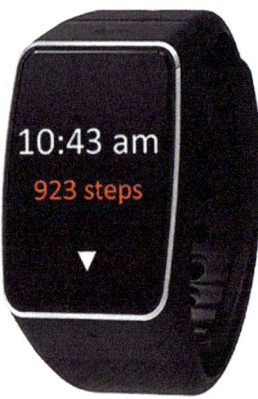

Figure 11.5 The smartwatch design progressed to a high-fidelity prototype.

Delivering and Evaluating the Design

What is Evaluation in HCD?

As mentioned before, a prototype needs to be continuously tested and evaluated with prospective users (also see the section on formative evaluation in Chapter 7). Some exemplary questions that can be answered are: To what extent do the users find the design is useful? What elements of the design do and do not appeal to them? Do they find it engaging? What about its functionalities? Designers can use evaluation methods to observe how end user interacts with the system, to test the ease of use and user-friendliness of the technology, and to assess whether user requirements are correctly translated into the design. Information on these kinds of topics can be used to improve the design. There are various methods of evaluation that can be considered to evaluate prototypes. The evaluation methods vary in terms of the design stage at which they can be applied, and the individuals involved in the evaluation process. Broadly speaking, there are two ways of evaluating prototypes: Expert-based and user-based.

- **Expert-based**. In this kind of evaluation, *experts* on design or the subject the technology is aimed for are conducting the *usability* evaluation. They use their own knowledge about good design, the target group and/or the subject;
- **User-based**. Here, the evaluation is performed with *potential end-users*.

In *expert-based testing*, the experts use their own knowledge about design and/or the target group. Of course, it is important to have the right experts: ideally you want people who are experts in both usability and in the subject that you are designing an eHealth technology for. Likewise, in *user-based testing* it is also important to have the right users: They must be members of the target group.

From research, we know that the best results occur when both expert-based and user-based methods are used (Jaspers, 2009). Usually, the flaws and issues that experts and users find do overlap, but both groups also find issues that the other group did not identify. Experts tend to find more flaws related to the general working of the prototype and point out things that can make the experience smoother. Users tend to find more flaws in how the technology can help them achieve their goals (Jaspers, 2009).

Table 11.3 Methods of evaluation for HCD.

Method of evaluation	Participants needed	Minimum prototype level	Types of results to expect
Heuristic evaluation	User experience and human-computer interaction experts	Paper prototype, low-fidelity prototype, wireframes	Quick identification of where usability guidelines are not being followed (e.g., places of inconsistency, incomplete navigation opportunity, poor interaction choices)
Cognitive walkthrough	User experience and human-computer interaction experts	Sketch, paper prototype, low-fidelity prototype, wireframe	Confirmation of the scope of the design, first reactions, learnability, understandability, navigation expectations
Usability test	End-users from the intended target group(s)	High-fidelity mock-ups with interaction developed	User ability to perform and complete tasks, accuracy, errors, path efficiency, qualitative user reactions to the experience, learnability, discoverability (Tullis & Albert, 2008)
Performance test	End-users from the intended target group(s), balanced and recruited to be able to test for significant effects	High-fidelity mock-ups with interaction developed	Accuracy, errors, fault detection or diagnosis, workflow or performance measures, confidence of measurable performance difference compared with a different design
Field test	Actual end-users who use the product in context	Final product	Insights in how people actually use the design in practice and the design's long-term impact on people's behaviour and work processes. Feedback for future iterations of the design

Methods for Formative Evaluation

Several commonly used methods for *formative eHealth evaluation* during design are presented in Table 11.3. Information on the types of participants and the minimum prototype level that are required to conduct the evaluation is provided.

Heuristic Evaluation

In *heuristic evaluations*, experts review a design. This can be done at any point in the design cycle but may be most valuable at an early prototype stage (i.e., mock-up, paper prototype), when it is easier to make changes to the design following the outcomes of the heuristic evaluation. A heuristic evaluation is considered an 'inspection' method since the evaluator does not actually interact with the design. Experts look through the design in a systematic way, looking for common usability problems. They usually try to access and use all features of the system and sometimes intentionally do the 'wrong' thing to see how the system handles error input. Usability experts are almost twice as good in finding system flaws as novice evaluators. Double experts (experts both in usability and the subject area) are almost three times as good as novices. When using double experts for usability testing, three to five experts can find approximately 75% of all prototype flaws (Jaspers, 2009). The evaluator is often aided by a worksheet or checklist that reminds them of the key problems to look for. Nielsen's *heuristics* (Nielsen, 1994) are one of the most commonly used lists of usability heuristics:

1. Visibility of system status;
2. Match between system and the real world;
3. User control and freedom;
4. Consistency and standards;
5. Error prevention;
6. Recognition rather than recall;
7. Flexibility and efficiency of use;
8. Aesthetic and minimalist design;
9. Help users recognize, diagnose, and recover from errors;
10. Help and documentation.

Cognitive Walk-through

Another common approach used in evaluation is a *cognitive walk-through* (Wharton, Rieman, Lewis, & Polson, 1994). Similar to the heuristic evaluation, the cognitive walk-through (CW) is also performed with experts, but in a very structured, task-oriented way. Before giving instructions to the expert, the researcher specifies the tasks that a user would want to perform with the system. In the CW, the expert will perform these tasks by analyzing which steps are needed. For each step, the expert will answer questions, for example:

- Will the user try to achieve the correct action?
- Will the user notice that the correct action is available?
- Will the user associate the correct action with the desired effect?
- Will the user notice that progress is made in accomplishing his or her goals?

In the CW, fewer problems are often identified than in a heuristic evaluation, but the problems that are found are often severe and essential to address. This is why a CW is often preferred when there are time or financial constraints on a project (Jaspers, 2009).

Usability Test – Think-aloud Method

The think-aloud method is a user-based usability method. Simply put, members of the target group use the prototype to complete scenarios that are provided by the designer. While completing these scenarios, the user is asked to '*think aloud*' – in other words to verbalize their thoughts and why they are performing certain actions within the system. Both the user's actions and their verbalized thoughts provide input for improving the system. In the think-aloud method, the more severe and recurring problems that are important to the target group are often identified. Therefore, it's very important that these participants are part of the target group of the technology that is being developed. When the right participants are found and realistic scenarios are used, a think-aloud usability test with five to eight end users will yield valuable insights for improving the technology (Jaspers, 2009), although in many cases using around 15 end users will provide more stable results (Van den Haak, 2008).

Performance Test

The performance test requires a product or a prototype that looks and feels as much as possible to the eventual product. For a full *performance evaluation*, significant numbers of users may be recruited to have adequate statistical power. A performance evaluation needs to occur with reference to some level of benchmark performance. Benchmark performance may be established by recording performance with an existing system or by comparing two designs in the evaluation. Design comparisons are usually between the new design and an older existing design, or between two new designs that have different design characteristics. The evaluation will require recruitment of participants who reflect the range of possible users. Both test groups are given the same tasks to perform with the design. Good evaluations will capture quantitative 'end result' performances such as total task time or accuracy but will also capture 'process' performance (navigation pathways, mid process errors, missed information) in order to understand how the end results occurred. A performance evaluation should ideally also include qualitative data collection. This may entail experiences with communication, feelings of comfort or trust in the design, impressions of usability or satisfaction with the design.

Field Test

Field testing is focused on the use of a technology once it is close to being finished and is used by the end users. In eHealth research, this may also be referred to as a pilot test to indicate that it is the first situated evaluation of the final prototype. Multiple qualitative and quantitative evaluation methods such as *log data* analysis, interviews and questionnaires can be used to determine how people are actually using the final product, what their experiences are and what influence it has on their work processes.

Case Study Physical Activity of Seniors – Part 3: Field Testing

Some user and expert evaluation methods for the case study on the smartwatch for seniors were already presented in the second part of the case study. However, it would be possible to also conduct a field test once the design is finished. Such a field test would involve giving functioning smartwatches to a test group for a period of time, for example, three months. The watches might be programmed to collect log data. The field test is also an opportunity to explore issues that cannot be discovered in the earlier tests, such as:

- Are they still wearing it after a few weeks?
- Do they find the watch easy to charge?
- Is the strap comfortable after repeated use?
- What aspects of the watch are often used, and which ones not?
- Do they feel more comfortable using technology and want to move to more advanced features?
- How do their families feel about it? Do they feel their older family member is more active, or more in contact with them?

Remote and Online Human-centred Design

Up until now, this chapter discussed methods for HCD under the assumption that these will take place face-to-face, for example a journey mapping session in the hospital ward, or an interview in the living room of someone with a chronic illness. However, HCD activities may also take place remotely online, for example if this better suits the participants, to save costs, to include participants at hard-to-reach locations, or if the wider context demands it, e.g., the COVID-pandemic. For example, online whiteboard platforms (like Miro.com (Miro, 2023)) offer the possibility to collaborate on a digital canvas in real-time. Users can use a wide range of drawing and annotation tools including sticky notes to share ideas. These platforms also often come with a variety of pre-designed templates to help jumpstart a participatory design workshop or brainstorm. Other options for remote and online HCD include remote interviews, virtual prototyping, and remote usability testing.

Remote Interviews

Remote interviews have traditionally been seen as a sub-optimal compromise to consider only if face-to-face interviews were not possible. However, as videoconferencing services advanced and are now more widely used, they enable designers to conduct high-quality online interviews remotely (Keen, Lomeli-Rodriguez, & Joffe, 2022). Many researchers have turned to online video interviews during the COVID-19 pandemic and advantages and disadvantages are now being reflected on within qualitative research, including HCD. A common advantage mentioned is better inclusion of sensitive, stigmatized, and marginalized populations through the convenience of online video interviews. Remote interviews may also be specifically relevant when prospective users of the technology live in remote or rural areas. For example, (Lathen & Laestadius, 2021) use of online video focus groups facilitated geographically dispersed African American adults with low socio-economic status to participate regardless of physical location. (Walker, 2023) noted that through online recruitment and online interviews, it was easier to reach people with dementia who were reluctant to self-identify as living with dementia in-person. As there is no need to physically travel to participate in a remote interview, these may also be more accessible to people with chronic conditions or informal care responsibilities, making online interviews a particularly interesting option for eHealth designers to obtain a more diverse sample of people who would otherwise not be able to participate. Another benefit is that online interviews may improve ecological validity of HCD research. Videoconferencing captures the participant at a time and location of their choice, without physical presence of the designer. This allows designers to unobtrusively observe how a participant uses a system.

Still, disadvantages of video interviews are also present. Researchers have warned for digital exclusion, in which vulnerable populations who do not have access to videoconferencing software- and hardware, or may lack familiarity with these tools, are less likely to be included in research (Lathen & Laestadius, 2021). And while videoconferencing has great convenience in capturing more data (e.g., person in context, audio and video), this exchange of (potentially sensitive) health information does require special attention to consent, confidentiality, and data security (Keen et al., 2022; Valkonen, Karisalmi, Kaipio, & Kujala, 2021). A broader review focussed on remote and online participatory research approach in general settings (i.e., not health specific) discussed that in addition to these points, costs of Internet data, limited IT literacy, lack of accessibility for visual or hearing-impaired participants, limited confidentiality & privacy, and problems with initiating & maintaining an interpersonal relationship with remote participants can form additional barriers to remote HCD (Hall, Gaved, & Sargent, 2021).

Virtual Prototyping and Remote Usability Testing

Tools like Figma (Figma, 2023) and Miro.com (Miro, 2023) can be used to create digital mappings, sketches, wireframes, mock-ups, and prototypes, that users can interact with over a remote video interview. Virtual prototyping can allow participants to be directly involved in the participatory design process. For example, in their project on embedding the stories of people with multiple chronic health conditions in electronic health records, (Cummings, Bradley, & Teal, 2022; Cummings & Teal, 2023) shared mood boards, maps, and other interactive online prototypes with participants over a series of remote video interviews. Participants could directly comment and collaborate on the designs in real-time. Another using remote HCD in the development of a shared decision-making tool for chronic pain study (Smaradottir, Bellika, Fredeng, & Fagerlund, 2020) has noted that participants could be more frequently involved in the iterative design process due to the convenience and accessibility of virtual prototyping tools. However, designers should also be aware that these complex, digital tools may also not be accessible and overwhelming to people unaccustomed to working with them.

When interactive, digital prototypes are paired with options such as screensharing, remote control, eye-tracking through webcams, and mouse-tracking software to record the user's cursor clicks, this can enable a highly efficient remote usability test to comprehensively understand users' interaction with the prototype and possible areas for improvement. Many types of asynchronous and synchronous remote usability testing methods have been proposed, including synchronous remote testing, web-based surveys, remote post use interviews, diaries, feedback, and log analysis, each with their own benefits when used in a health setting (Hill, Brown, Campbell, & Holden, 2021).

In general, remote usability testing methods share the same benefits as remote interviews. They also allow for more diverse sampling and hold high ecological validity, as they allow the participants' interaction with the prototype to be observed directly in the envisioned context of use (i.e., in their own home, on their own device). However, remote usability methods may also result in the identification of fewer, or less useful, usability problems (Hill et al., 2021). Finally, many of the factors (e.g., user characteristics, quality of the Internet connection, digital instructions) that could affect validity, reliability or efficiency of remote usability tests of eHealth technologies have not been studied yet (McLaughlin et al., 2020).

Summary

Human-centred design is an iterative process of divergence and convergence and of design and redesign. At each stage the design is reconsidered and taken for feedback before progressing to the next stage. The key to a human-centred design process is keeping users and stakeholders in the process through involving them in identifying the actual problem, early feedback, codesign, and evaluation. The take-home messages for this chapter are:

- Developing a meaningful eHealth technology requires (re)discovery and definition of the actual problem according to the people who are affected by it;
- Using and combining results of different methods is important to understanding an eHealth design problem thoroughly;
- Designs develop in stages, so it is important to involve users at each stage and continually evaluate your design;
- Prototyping and evaluating are intertwined, iterative activities;
- Remote and online HCD methodology may support diverse sampling and continuous involvement of users with high ecological validity but may also hold disadvantages that are not yet fully explored.

Key References for Further Reading

Beyer, H., & Holtzblatt, K. (1997). *Contextual design: Defining customer-centered systems*. San Francisco, CA: Morgan Kaufmann.

Maguire, M. (2001). Methods to support human-centred design. *International Journal of Human-Computer Studies*, *55*(*4*), 587–634.

Nielsen, J. (1994). *Usability engineering*. San Francisco, CA: Morgan Kaufmann.

Sanders, E. B. N., & Stappers, P. J. (2008). Co-creation and the new landscapes of design. *Co-design*, *4*(1), 5–18.

Snyder, C. (2003). *Paper prototyping: The fast and easy way to design and refine user interfaces*. San Francisco, CA: Morgan Kaufmann.

References

Acuña, S. T., Castro, J. W., & Juristo, N. (2012). A HCI technique for improving requirements elicitation. *Information and Software Technology*, *54*(*12*), 1357–1375.

Adlin, T., & Pruitt, J. (2010). *The essential persona lifecycle: Your guide to building and using personas*. San Francisco, CA: Morgan Kaufmann.

Beyer, H., & Holtzblatt, K. (1997). *Contextual design: Defining customer-centered systems*. San Francisco, CA: Morgan Kaufmann.

Buxton, B. (2007). *Sketching user experiences: Getting the design right and the right design*. San Francisco, CA: Morgan Kaufmann.

Cajander, Å., Larusdottir, M., & Hedström, G. (2020). The effects of automation of a patient-centric service in primary care on the work engagement and exhaustion of nurses. *Quality and User Experience*, 5. doi:10.1007/s41233-020-00038-x

Chodzko-Zajko, W. J., Proctor, D. N., Fiatarone Singh, M. A., Minson, C. T., Nigg, C. R., Salem, G. J., & Skinner, J. S. (2009). American College of Sports Medicine position stand. Exercise and physical activity for older adults. *Med Sci Sports Exerc*, 41(7), 1510–1530. doi:10.1249/MSS.0b013e3181a0c95c

Clemensen, J., Rothmann, M. J., Smith, A. C., Caffery, L. J., & Danbjorg, D. B. (2017). Participatory design methods in telemedicine research. *J Telemed Telecare*, 23(9), 780—785. doi:10.1177/1357633x16686747

Cooper, A., Reimann, R., Cronin, D., & Noessel, C. (2014). *About face: The essentials of interaction design*. Indianapolis, IN: John Wiley & Sons.

Cummings, M., Bradley, J., & Teal, G. (2022). Patient co-design of digital health storytelling tools for multimorbidity: A phenomenological study. *Health Expectations*, 25(6), 3073–3084. doi:https://doi.org/10.1111/hex.13614

Cummings, M., & Teal, G. (2023). Healing fabulations: A dialogic methodology for digital codesign in health research. *CoDesign*, 19(1), 74–90. doi:10.1080/15710882.2022.2157837

DeSmet, A., Thompson, D., Baranowski, T., Palmeira, A., Verloigne, M., & De Bourdeaudhuij, I. (2016). Is participatory design associated with the effectiveness of serious digital games for healthy lifestyle promotion? A meta-analysis. *J Med Internet Res*, 18(4), e94. doi:10.2196/jmir.4444

Dikmen, M., & Burns, C. (2022). The effects of domain knowledge on trust in explainable AI and task performance: A case of peer-to-peer lending. *International Journal of Human-Computer Studies*, 162, 102792. doi:https://doi.org/10.1016/j.ijhcs.2022.102792

Faber, J. S., Poot, C. C., Dekkers, T., Romero Herrera, N., Chavannes, N. H., Meijer, E., & Visch, V. T. (2023). Developing a digital medication adherence intervention for and with patients with asthma and low health literacy: Protocol for a participatory design approach. *JMIR Form Res*, 7, e35112. doi:10.2196/35112

Fidel, R., & Pejtersen, A. M. (2004). From information behaviour research to the design of information systems: The cognitive work analysis framework. *Information Research: An International Electronic Journal*, 10(1), n1.

Figma. (2023). How you design, align and build matters. Do it together with Figma. Retrieved from https://www.figma.com/

Floyd, I., Jones, M., & Twidale, M. (2008). Resolving incommensurable debates: A preliminary identification of persona kinds, attributes, and characteristics. *Artifact*, 2. doi:10.1080/17493460802276836

Gordon, S. E., & Gill, R. T. (1997). Cognitive task analysis. *Naturalistic Decision Making*, 131–140.

Groeneveld, B. S., Dekkers, T., Mathijssen, N. M. C., Vehmeijer, S. B. W., Melles, M., & Goossens, R. H. M. (2020). Communication preferences in total joint arthroplasty: Exploring the patient experience through generative research. *Orthop Nurs*, 39(5), 292–302. doi:10.1097/nor.0000000000000694

Hall, J., Gaved, M., & Sargent, J. (2021). Participatory research approaches in times of Covid-19: A narrative literature review. *International Journal of Qualitative Methods*, 20, 16094069211010087. doi:10.1177/16094069211010087

Hill, J. R., Brown, J. C., Campbell, N. L., & Holden, R. J. (2021). Usability-in-place—Remote usability testing methods for homebound older adults: Rapid literature review. *JMIR Form Res*, 5(11), e26181. doi:10.2196/26181

Holden, R. J., Kulanthaivel, A., Purkayastha, S., Goggins, K. M., & Kripalani, S. (2017). Know thy eHealth user: Development of biopsychosocial personas from a study of older adults with heart failure. *Int J Med Inform*, 108, 158–167. doi:10.1016/j.ijmedinf.2017.10.006

ISO. (2021). IEC 62366-1:2015. Medical devices — Part 1: Application of usability engineering to medical devices. Retrieved from https://www.iso.org/standard/63179.html

Jaspers, M. W. (2009). A comparison of usability methods for testing interactive health technologies: Methodological aspects and empirical evidence. *International Journal of Medical Informatics*, 78(5), 340–353.

Jiancaro, T., Jamieson, G. A., & Mihailidis, A. (2014). Twenty Years of Cognitive Work Analysis in Health Care. *Journal of Cognitive Engineering and Decision Making*, 8, 22–23.

Keen, S., Lomeli-Rodriguez, M., & Joffe, H. (2022). From challenge to opportunity: Virtual qualitative research during COVID-19 and beyond. *International Journal of Qualitative Methods*, 21, 16094069221105075. doi:10.1177/16094069221105075

Knapp, J., Zeratsky, J., & Kowitz, B. (2016). Sprint: How to solve big problems and test new ideas in just five days. New York, NY: Simon & Schuster.

Lathen, L., & Laestadius, L. (2021). Reflections on online focus group research with low socio-economic status African American adults during COVID-19. *International Journal of Qualitative Methods*, 20, 16094069211021713. doi:10.1177/16094069211021713

LeRouge, C., Ma, J., Sneha, S., & Tolle, K. (2013). User profiles and personas in the design and development of consumer health technologies. *International Journal of Medical Informatics*, 82(11), e251–e268.

Maguire, M. (2001). Methods to support human-centred design. *International Journal of Human-Computer Studies*, 55(4), 587–634.

McLaughlin, A. C., DeLucia, P. R., Drews, F. A., Vaughn-Cooke, M., Kumar, A., Nesbitt, R. R., & Cluff, K. (2020). Evaluating medical devices remotely: Current methods and potential innovations. *Human Factors*, 62(7), 1041–1060. doi:10.1177/0018720820953644

Melles, M., Albayrak, A., & Goossens, R. (2021). Innovating health care: Key characteristics of human-centered design. *International Journal for Quality in Health Care*, 33(Supplement_1), 37–44. doi:10.1093/intqhc/mzaa127

Miro. (2023). Retrieved from https://miro.com/nl/

Newman, M. W., & Landay, J. A. (2000). Sitemaps, storyboards, and specifications: A sketch of Web site design practice. In *Proceedings of the 3rd conference on designing interactive systems: Processes, practices, methods, and techniques* (pp. 263–274). New York, NY: ACM.

Nielsen, J. (1994). *Usability engineering*. San Francisco, CA: Morgan Kaufmann.

Peters, D., Davis, S., Calvo, R. A., Sawyer, S. M., Smith, L., & Foster, J. M. (2017). Young people's preferences for an asthma self-management app highlight psychological needs: A participatory study. *J Med Internet Res*, 19(4), e113. doi:10.2196/jmir.6994

Ramos, M., Utne, I., & Mosleh, A. (2019). Collision avoidance on maritime autonomous surface ships: Operators' tasks and human failure events. *Safety Science*, 116, 33–44. doi:10.1016/j.ssci.2019.02.038

Ridder, E., Dekkers, T., Porsius, J., Kraan, G., & Melles, M. (2018). The perioperative patient experience of hand and wrist surgical patients: An exploratory study using patient journey mapping. *Patient Experience Journal*, 5, 97–107. doi:10.35680/2372-0247.1273

Roosan, D., Li, Y., Law, A., Truong, H., Karim, M., Chok, J., & Roosan, M. (2019). Improving medication information presentation through interactive visualization in mobile apps: Human factors design. *JMIR mHealth and uHealth*, 7(11), e15940.

Saiedian, H., & Dale, R. (2000). Requirements engineering: Making the connection between the software developer and customer. *Information and Software Technology*, 42(6), 419–428.

Sanders, E. B. N., Brandt, E., & Binder, T. (2010, November). A framework for organizing the tools and techniques of participatory design. In: *Proceedings of the 11th biennial participatory design conference* (pp. 195–198).

Sanders, E., & Stappers, P. J. (2008). Co-creation and the new landscapes of design. *CoDesign*, 4, 5–18. doi:10.1080/15710880701875068

Scaife, M., Rogers, Y., Aldrich, F., & Davies, M. (1997). Designing for or designing with? Informant design for interactive learning environments. In *Proceedings of the CHI 97 SIGCHI conference on human factors in computing systems* (pp. 343–350). New York, NY: ACM Press.

Schouten, S. E., Kip, H., Dekkers, T., Deenik, J., Beerlage-de Jong, N., Ludden, G. D. S., & Kelders, S. M. (2022). Best-practices for co-design processes involving people with severe mental illness for eMental health interventions: A qualitative multi-method approach. *Design for Health*, 6(3), 316–344. doi:10.1080/24735132.2022.2145814

Schraagen, J. M, Chipman, S. F., & Shalin, V. L. (Eds.). (2000). *Cognitive task analysis*. Mahwah, NJ: Lawrence Erlbaum Associates.

Simonse, L., Albayrak, A., & Starre, S. (2019). Patient journey method for integrated service design. *Design for Health*, 3(1), 82–97. doi:10.1080/24735132.2019.1582741

Simonsen, J., & Robertson, T. (Eds.). (2013). *Routledge international handbook of participatory design*. New York, NY: Routledge.

Smaradottir, B. F., Bellika, J. G., Fredeng, A., & Fagerlund, A. J. (2020). User-centred design with a remote approach: Experiences from the chronic pain project. *Stud Health Technol Inform*, 275, 197–201. doi:10.3233/shti200722

Snyder, C. (2003). *Paper prototyping: The fast and easy way to design and refine user interfaces*. San Francisco, CA: Morgan Kaufmann.

Stappers, S. (2014). *Convival toolbox: Generative research for the front end of design*. Amsterdam: BIS.

Ten Klooster, I., Wentzel, J., Sieverink, F., Linssen, G., Wesselink, R., & van Gemert-Pijnen, L. (2022). Personas for better targeted eHealth technologies: User-centered design approach. *JMIR Hum Factors*, 9(1), e24172. doi:10.2196/24172

The Design Council. (2023). Framework for innovation. Retrieved from https://www.designcouncil.org.uk/our-resources/framework-for-innovation/

Trebble, T. M., Hansi, N., Hydes, T., Smith, M. A., & Baker, M. (2010). Process mapping the patient journey: An introduction. *BMJ*, 341, c4078. doi:10.1136/bmj.c4078

Tullis, T., & Albert, W. (2008). *Measuring the user experience: Collective analyzing, and presenting usability metrics*. San Francisco, CA: Morgan Kaufmann.

Valkonen, P., Karisalmi, N., Kaipio, J., & Kujala, S. (2021). Remote interviews and visual timelines with patients: Lessons learned. *Stud Health Technol Inform*, 281, 845–849. doi:10.3233/shti210298

Vandekerckhove, P., de Mul, M., Bramer, W. M., & de Bont, A. A. (2020). Generative participatory design methodology to develop electronic health interventions: Systematic literature review. *J Med Internet Res*, 22(4), e13780. doi:10.2196/13780

Van Den Haak, M. J. Van den (2008). A penny for your thoughts: Investigating the validity and reliability of think-aloud protocols for usability testing. Doctoral dissertation, University of Twente, Enschede, The Netherlands.

Van Gemert-Pijnen, J. E. W. C., Peters, O., & Ossebaard, H. C. (Eds.). (2013). *Improving eHealth*. The Netherlands: Eleven International Publishing.

Van Mechelen, M. (2016). Designing technologies for and with children: A toolkit to prepare and conduct co-design activities and analyse the outcomes. Ph.D. Thesis, University of Hasselt, Hasselt, Belgium.

Vicente, K. J. (1999). *Cognitive work analysis: Toward safe, productive and health computer-based work*. Mahwah, NJ: Lawrence Erlbaum Associates.

Walker, M. (2023). Developing and sustaining a doctoral study in design research involving participants living with dementia during COVID-19. *Design for Health*, 7(1), 108–119. doi:10.1080/24735132.2023.2187151

Wang, G., Marradi, C., Albayrak, A., & van der Cammen, T. J. M. (2019). Co-designing with people with dementia: A scoping review of involving people with dementia in design research. *Maturitas*, 127, 55–63. doi:https://doi.org/10.1016/j.maturitas.2019.06.003

Wharton, C., Rieman, J., Lewis, C., & Polson, P. (1994). The cognitive walkthrough method: A practitioner's guide. In J. Nielsen & R. L. Mack (Eds.), *Usability inspection methods* (pp. 105–140). New York, NY: John Wiley & Sons, Inc.

12 Persuasive Health Technology

Nienke Beerlage-de Jong, Lisette (J.E.W.C.) van Gemert-Pijnen, Harri Oinas-Kukkonen, & Saskia M. Kelders

Introduction

As explained in Chapter 2, behaviour change is important to improve health and well-being. Behaviour change techniques can be applied in the design of eHealth technology to support users in reaching their goals. Persuasive technology can partly be considered the technological instantiation of these behaviour change techniques. Indeed, when technology is persuasive, it can increase the chances of people using the technology and reaching its health and well-being goals. Chapter 10 has shown that methods from human-centred design can be employed to make a technology that is appealing and fits the users' needs. In this chapter, it is shown that technology can be more than just appealing. It can also be persuasive and in this way be an excellent support for users to reach their own goals.

In this chapter, the added value of persuasive health technology is explained. The chapter starts with an introduction to persuasive technology and how such technology has been applied in the context of improving health and well-being. In addition, the Persuasive Systems Design (PSD) model (Oinas-Kukkonen & Harjumaa, 2009) and how it can be used to develop and evaluate eHealth technologies are introduced. After completing this chapter, you will be able to:

- Explain what persuasive technology is, and in what way domains such as persuasive communication, health promotion, social marketing, technology acceptance, and human-media interaction are its underlying foundations;
- Analyze the added value of persuasive technology in the context of improving health and explain its relation to behaviour change (techniques);
- Explain the PSD model, name the four categories, and provide examples of accompanying persuasive features;
- Explain in what way persuasive technology can be used to develop and evaluate eHealth technologies;
- Provide examples of how persuasive features can be integrated into an eHealth technology.

What is Persuasive Technology?

Increased interactivity and engagement of users through modern information and communication technologies (ICTs) have opened up many opportunities to influence users' behaviours. For instance, digital interventions have been developed to educate, inform, or increase their health and well-being. However, despite the potential of ICT to influence users' behaviours, achieving actual

DOI: 10.4324/9781003302049-14

(and sustained) behaviour change remains challenging. Behaviour is complex and influenced by a multitude of intra-, inter-personal, and environmental factors. Therefore, interventions to change behaviour are also usually complex and multi-faceted. The smallest identifiable components of such – online or offline – interventions are referred to as 'Behaviour Change Techniques' (see also Chapter 2; Michie et al., 2013). They for example entail 'self-monitoring', 'goal-setting', or 'feedback'. This means that an intervention that aims to increase physical activity could, for example, ask its user to formulate and commit to a specific goal, i.e., goal-setting ('at least twice a week I will go for a half-hour brisk walk'), and to reflect on the progress towards reaching that goal, i.e.' self-monitoring (showing a diary of daily activities). It is known that basing an intervention on (theory driven) techniques like these will increase its likelihood of success (Webb, Joseph, Yardley, & Michie, 2010). Yet, there is more that can be done.

As stated in the introduction, technology itself can also try to persuade the user to change their behaviour. In the late 1990s, Fogg suggested that this could be called persuasive technology: A field that studies any interactive information technology intentionally designed to change users' attitudes or behaviour. Since then, this field has received growing interest among both researchers and practitioners. Based on Fogg's work, Oinas-Kukkonen and Harjumaa more recently defined persuasive systems as 'computerized software or information systems designed to reinforce, change or shape attitudes or behaviours or both without using coercion or deception' (Oinas-Kukkonen & Harjumaa, 2009). It is important to note in this definition that persuasive systems are by definition voluntary. Therefore, while other forms of persuasion, including deception, coercion, and monetary inducements may sometimes be effective, they are not what we call persuasive technology.

Important to note is that persuasive technology is not limited to the health domain. In many other domains, technology has been designed to change behaviour as well. For example, in marketing, persuasive technology has been used to increase online sales, and in the ecological domain, it has been used to decrease individuals' energy consumption. However, the promotion of health and well-being is one of the most prominent areas for application of persuasive technology, and the focus of this chapter. In the remainder of the chapter, when referring to persuasive technology, we refer to persuasive technology in the field of health and well-being, or: Persuasive eHealth technology.

Why do we Need Persuasive Technology?

When looking at what persuasive technology (PT) can offer, there are two broad reasons for using it in the domain of health and well-being. The first one is to increase the effectiveness of eHealth interventions. As stated, PT can be seen as the technological instantiation of BCTs, and BCTs are key ingredients of interventions. We have already established that research shows that interventions that are based on (theory driven) techniques such as the BCTs are more likely to succeed (Webb et al., 2010). Now, for example, if an intervention aimed at increasing physical activity uses the BCT 'goal setting' to get its user to commit to concrete exercise goals ('at least twice a week I will go for a half-hour brisk walk'), it could use PT in the form of sending 'reminders' to help people actually attain the set goals. So, in this way, PT can help people to improve their health-related behaviour. The second reason is that PT can persuade people to keep using the eHealth interventions that help them improve their health-related behaviour. This is needed because, despite this promise, many existing eHealth interventions in practice do not show the great (health) benefits that were expected (Elbert et al., 2014; Hadjiconstantinou et al., 2016; Kooij, Groen, & van Harten, 2017). There is strong evidence that this may have a lot to do with the technologies not being used as intended. This is analogous to literature on medication use, indicating that medication adherence has a big impact on its health outcomes (Burkhart & Sabaté, 2003). The dose-response curve describes this effect in pharmaceutical research: It shows the normalized amount of effect (i.e., response) that is to be expected after exposure to different doses of the medication. For eHealth technologies, such a curve could describe the 'usage' of the technology, often measured as the number of times it has been used or the number of elements of the technology that were used (Sieverink, Kelders, & van Gemert-Pijnen, 2017). However, with an increased focus on tailoring interventions to the individual user combined with different goals of users, it might not be necessary that every user uses as many elements as possible, or that every user uses a technology as often as possible. That is where the concept of 'adherence' comes to play. Adherence refers to 'the degree to which the user followed the program as it was designed' (Donkin et al., 2011). Achieving such adherence to eHealth interventions is notoriously challenging, but making use of persuasive design has been shown to contribute to it (Kelders, Kok, Ossebaard, & van Gemert-Pijnen, 2012). Therefore, the second reason to use persuasive technology for health and well-being is to increase the use of and adherence to a (technology driven) intervention.

The Foundations of Persuasive Technology

Although the field of persuasive technology is only a few decades old, it is grounded in various well-researched theories stemming from different areas. These include theories that focus on the 'persuasive' qualities of persuasive technologies, and theories that focus on the technological qualities of persuasive technologies. The theoretical foundations from some of these fields are described below.

Focus on Persuasion

Persuasive communication

Persuasive technology involves communication; people interact with technology or with other people through technology. Persuasive communication intends to describe, explain, and predict the factors that contribute to changing attitudes and behaviours (Ajzen, 1992; Dillard & Pfau, 2002; Perloff, 1993). For example, persuasive communication describes and explains the four layers of communication that influence the understanding of information (Schulz von Thun, 1981). These are (1) the factual layers, which refers to facts, data; (2) the expressive layer, referring to the relationship between sender and receiver; (3) the self-revealing layer, expressing something about the sender's emotions, values and so on; and (4) the appellation layer, referring to the desire, advice, instructions, and effects. The four layers of the communication model are part of the process of persuasion, since these four aspects influence the coding (sending) and decoding (receiving) of information. The way this coding and decoding is done grounds theoretical models about health communication to promote public health (e.g., infectious diseases campaigns) or to promote a healthier lifestyle in chronic care (Kreps, Bonaguro, & Query Jr, 2003; Kreps & Maibach, 2008; Rimal & Lapinski, 2009). In the field of social psychology, the communication model has, for example, been used to further describe and explain the mediating processes of information exchange by searching for characteristics that play a role in communication and understanding how these characteristics influence each other. Some of these influential characteristics are the sender, receiver, messages, channels, and the settings. In particular, the processes of getting attention, comprehension of information, and acceptance of information have been studied in the area of persuasive communication to change attitudes and behaviours (McGuire, 1985).

Health promotion

In health promotion the theory of planned behaviour (TPB) (Ajzen, 1991; Fishbein, 1979) and the elaboration likelihood model (ELM) (Petty & Cacioppo, 1986) have been dominant in researching the persuasiveness of technologies. The concepts of the TPB and ELM (see Chapter 2 for a more elaborate explanation) are used in persuasive technology to understand and influence how people act.

For persuasive technology, the TPB (Ajzen, 1991) implies that an intervention should ideally influence an individual's behavioural attention by changing negative (or reinforcing positive) attitudes with regard to behaviour, it should offer support to build confidence in one's own abilities, and it should demonstrate that significant others (e.g., peers) are also positive about the behaviour.

The ELM (Petty & Cacioppo, 1986) is of specific interest to persuasive technology researchers, as it states that there are two routes for persuading people. The central route underscores reason and argument. The peripheral route builds upon social cues (e.g., source credibility, aesthetics, popularity) (Chang, Lu, & Lin, 2020) and often on the way arguments are provided, instead of the quality and content of arguments.

Social marketing

In social marketing the focus is on principles, or general rules, to influence a target audience to voluntarily accept, reject, modify, or abandon a behaviour for the benefit of individuals, groups, or society as a whole (Kotler, Roberto, & Lee, 2002). These principles are often used as techniques to persuade. The basic principles from social marketing are social norms, conformity, and compliance to realize goal-directed behaviours. Social norms refer to rules and standards that are understood by members of a group that guide and/or constrain social behaviour without the force of laws. Conformity refers to the willingness of people to conform to others because of the social benefits of being accepted by them. Principles of compliance, which increase the chance of people complying with a suggestion or request, are (Cialdini, 2001):

- Reciprocity: People feel obligated to return a favour;
- Scarcity: When something is scarce, people value it more;
- Authority: People are more inclined to comply with authorities;
- Commitment and constancy: People do as they said they would;
- Consensus: People do what others do;
- Liking: People say yes to people they like.

Focus on Technology

The theories above focus on the persuasion aspect of persuasive technology. The technological aspect remains underexposed in these theories. Two additional approaches provide theories specifically focused on the technological aspects: Acceptance of technology and human-media interaction.

Acceptance of technology

Theories of acceptance of technology are mainly based on cognitive psychology. They are used to investigate and influence predictors for acceptance of technologies, especially web-based interventions for health promotion. The Technology Acceptance Model (TAM and TAM 2) (Davis, 1985; Venkatesh & Davis, 2000) and Unified Theory of Use and Acceptance (UTAUT) (Venkatesh, Morris, Davis, & Davis, 2003) have their roots in these theories. Important aspects that influence the intentions to use a certain technology from these models are perceptions about ease of use, performance and effort expectancies, and social influence. These perceptions are assumptions people have about whether they are able to use a technology and can benefit from that use. Although perceptions are important to fine-tune a technology to people's reported expectations, in practice this might not predict the actual use of a technology. Perceptions and expectations might be a good predictor for the intention to use a technology, but when there are barriers that hinder actual use, these intentions may remain intentions only (see Chapter 13 and (Abd-Alrazaq, Bewick, Farragher, & Gardner, 2019)).

Human-media interaction

Theories on human-media interaction and computer-mediated communication are used to investigate how people interact with and are influenced by information technology. These fields cover, for example, the design of interfaces to interact with technology and how technology can support people to perform tasks, to do exercises, or to communicate with others. A frequently adopted paradigm to study said interaction, is the Computers Are Social Actors (CASA) paradigm. This paradigm is used to explain that users can engage in all kinds of social behaviours towards a technology. To some extent, this is related to anthropomorphism, in which human traits are attributed to non-human artefacts (de Graaf & Ben Allouch, 2013; Nass, Steuer, & Tauber, 1994). More recently, it was shown that mindless anthropomorphism explained a relatively large part of the social presence between user and technology (Xu, Chen, & Huang, 2022). This refers to a kind of anthropomorphism that occurs unintentionally, without extensive thought, thus relying on an automatic psychological process. In other words: People tend to unconsciously attribute human traits to a technology, and therefore are more likely to engage in a social interaction with it. Chapter 10 on human-centred design provides some examples of methods used in human-media interaction and computer-mediated communication domains to study aspects like the CASA paradigm.

The Challenges of Persuasive Technology

Many things make developing a good persuasive technology challenging, ranging from its development to its actual design. To develop technologies that facilitate the achievement of people's goals, a deep understanding is needed of how people interact with and are influenced by technology. As we have seen, this requires an interdisciplinary approach, using insights from fields like persuasive communication, social psychology, engineering, and human-centred design.

This interdisciplinary approach is not a 'one-way street' in that, for instance, theories on persuasive communication and social psychology can only be used to inform the design and understand the influence of persuasive technology. Rather, the use of technologies as persuaders can also shed a new light on the interaction process and refine existing theories. Within persuasive technology, the interaction takes place between a system and different users (known or unknown), where the system can be seen as the 'representative' of the designers of a certain technology. Therefore, computer-human persuasion is more complex than a traditional sender-receiver interaction via face-to-face or text, because of an additional influential medium: The technology. Although human-computer interactions are social in nature and people see computers as social actors (i.e., the CASA paradigm as introduced earlier), it is largely unknown how these interactions reshape attitudes, beliefs, and emotions, or how they actually change behaviour. Moreover, as humans interact with technologies, the role and importance of a certain technology can change over time. This suggests that how a technology is used can differ between and (over time) within users, requiring technology to be dynamic and continuously adapt.

This means that persuasion is also not a static ad hoc event but an ongoing and dynamic process. This implies that behaviour models and techniques should also be dynamic and context- and process-driven, while more static models such as the theory of planned behaviour or the Technology Acceptance Model could be of lesser value. Yet, these more dynamic theoretical frameworks and conceptual models that may provide a bridge between behaviour change and technology are still scarce (Hagger & Weed, 2019; Hekler et al., 2016; Patrick et al., 2016; Riley et al., 2011). As many eHealth interventions struggle with adherence, sustained engagement, and effectiveness, challenges of designing persuasive technology have become a critical area of focus within eHealth intervention development. The employment of persuasive strategies into the design can increase the adherence to interventions, and the likelihood of its desired effects being achieved (Kelders, Kok, Ossebaard, & van Gemert-Pijnen, 2012; Wildeboer, Kelders, & van Gemert-Pijnen, 2016).

Approaches to Persuasive Technology

As we saw in Chapter 7, persuasive technology is integrated in the CeHRes Roadmap to design technologies that are user-friendly and that motivate and engage users to change their attitudes and behaviours. There are several approaches that can be used to actually design a persuasive technology. Two examples of those are described below: Design with intent and Fogg's behavioural model. However, most attention is paid to the Persuasive Systems Design (PSD) model (Oinas-Kukkonen & Harjumaa, 2009), which plays an important role in the application of persuasive features to increase engagement and adherence to technologies – with the intent to change behaviours.

Design with intent

The first approach is 'Design with intent' (DwI), which draws from insights from a multitude of disciplines (ranging from urban planning to medical and persuasive website design) to offer cross-domain guidance for designers who intend to change a target audience's behaviour. DwI is defined as 'design intended to influence or result in certain user behaviour' (Lockton et al., 2010). In essence, there are two 'modes' that designers can use the model in, depending on their aims: The inspirational mode and the prescriptive mode. For both modes goes that the DwI offers input as food for discussion or even thought provocation during design meetings. The inspirational mode is mostly useful for designers who prefer to work from a more creative stance. In this mode, many pre-existing design patterns (or design examples), grouped in six 'lenses' (e.g., visual, security) are used to inspire the design of a persuasive technology. An example of such design patterns are 'prominence and visibility' (see Figure 12.1) or 'surveillance', but there are many more.

Each pattern consists of a few examples of existing designs where a certain persuasive element was used. The prescriptive mode is more useful for designers who are more procedure driven. In this mode, a target behaviour is used as the starting point of the process. For each target behaviour, the most applicable design patterns are suggested which can then be tested.

Fogg's behavioural model

According to Fogg, three factors together determine if a behaviour occurs: Motivation, ability, and a prompt (i.e., B=MAP). The motivation and the ability are dependent on the person: Are

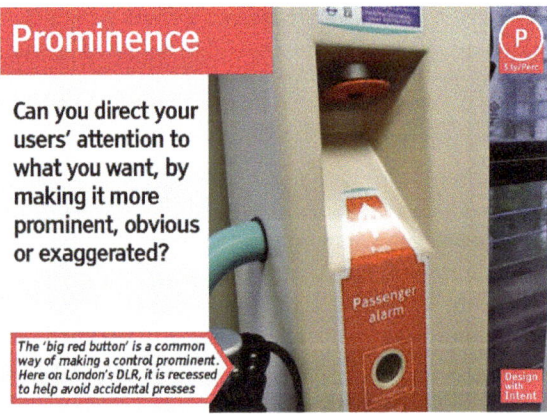

Figure 12.1 The design pattern 'prominence' as an example of the Design with intent approach (Lockton, Harrison, & Stanton, 2010).

they highly or hardly motivated to change, is the behaviour hard or easy to do? These two factors can, to some extent, also compensate for one another. If motivation is low, a higher ability can somewhat make up for that. And that is understandable because think about it, if one is not really motivated to learn a new task, one is more likely to succeed if the new task is easy than when it is really tough and requires a lot of effort. The latter factor, the prompt, is where external factors can play a role: Users should be prompted at the right time to perform the behaviour. Fogg argues that prompts have the biggest chance of provoking change, if its dosage and timing fits the amount of ability and motivation a user has. Technology can play a role in supporting each of these factors. For example, motivation can be increased through gamification (e.g., completing levels to visualize progress), ability can be increased through tunnelling to make the task easier (e.g., remove detours from the behaviour), prompts can be sent at the right time (e.g., based on information from wearables). To be successful in doing so, persuasive technology can be of added value. Fogg's seminal book *Persuasive Technology* (2002) presented the first conceptualization for helping software designers to create technology that can influence its users. Fogg states that, for its users, information technology can be persuasive in the role of a tool (e.g., making a task easier), a medium (e.g., providing an experience), or a social actor (e.g., levering principles from social influence).

The Persuasive Systems Design model

The Persuasive Systems Design (PSD) model, as described by Oinas-Kukkonen & Harjumaa (2009) provides a framework to decide and test what kind of features could be applied within a persuasive eHealth technology, depending on, for example, the target group and desired goals to be achieved. It is a well-known and often applied model and as such, it is connected to the design stage of the CeHRes Roadmap. The PSD model consists of premises that form the foundation of any PT, as well as concrete techniques that can be used in the design, content, and functionality of the PT.

The seven premises describe the assumptions that should be accounted for when designing the PT. They are preconditions for the successful design of a technology that is actually used and trusted, and truly has an impact without using deception or coercion. The premises are (Oinas-Kukkonen & Harjumaa, 2009):

1. Information technology, at least philosophically, is **never neutral**, but rather always influences its user(s) in one way or another. In other words, even technology that was not intended to be 'persuasive', to some degree still will be;
2. Being able to build persuasive systems requires **insight from both software design and psychology**. On the one hand designers must have knowledge on BCTs that could be used, on the other hand they need insight into what (kind of) technology is most suitable to communicate those BCTs;
3. Persuasion is often **incremental**, a gradual process of smaller steps. It is quite uncommon for a person to go from not exercising at all to running a marathon overnight. Change takes time, and practice;
4. The **direct and indirect routes** (ELM) are key persuasion strategies. This means that designers should not just think about the information they convey, but also about the optimal way to reach their target audience (e.g., gamification or providing background information);
5. Software design requirements call for persuasive systems to be both **useful and easy to use**. If one of these does not hold true, it is unlikely that the technology will succeed in achieving long-term engagement;
6. Persuasion through these systems must **fit the life, work or thought processes** that are involved in performing a user's primary tasks;
7. Persuasion should always be **transparent**. Without it, technologies would be unethical (e.g., misleading or deceptive towards its users) since it does not disclose its intentions and background.

Taking these premises into account, designing a PT starts with a careful analysis of the context of persuasion. This includes the targeted users and the intended use of the system as well as the users' intentions to change behaviours. Also included are the environment (locations, etc.) and strategies for persuasion that are suitable to be applied in the given context. Analyzing the context for persuasion is needed for all stages of design and evaluation of persuasive systems, ranging from evaluating software specifications in the early stages of systems development to studying fully-fledged commercial applications. This is needed because it is pivotal to check the fit between persuasion and context, at every stage of development and evaluation.

Last, the PSD model defines four categories of software features for persuasive systems, namely, primary task support, computer-human dialogue support, system credibility support, and social support, which are explained in a bit more detail in Box 12.1. Thus, different types of persuasive software features can be implemented to support the user's primary activities, the computer-human dialogue, the credibility of information being presented, and to leverage social influence. Tables 12.1 through 12.4 show the design features of each category, and Figure 12.2 illustrates the operationalization of some of these persuasive features. It is important to note that the seven features in each category are not exhaustive: There are other possible features imaginable that can support each of the four categories. Moreover, the model does not put forward a claim that all imaginable software features should be implemented into a persuasive system or that more is always better.

Box 12.1 Description of PSD model categories.

Primary task support

Primary task support facilitates the performance of the user in carrying out the primary activities to reach the goal of the intervention (e.g., decrease depressive symptoms, improve self-management of diabetes). The purpose of these features is to increase the understandability of the information by presenting it in personalized and small steps. These strategies are also aimed at breaking up the target behaviour into tiny steps to make it easier to achieve goals, as well as to provide monitoring strategies of users' performance and progress towards such goals.

Dialogue support

Dialogue support facilitates the interaction between a system and the user by providing persuasive features that aim to motivate and engage the user to achieve desired goals with the system. For example, the technology can take on a social role, through an avatar that guides you through the process.

System credibility support

Credibility support refers to the trustworthiness and reliability of the system. With the use of the persuasive features, the foundations of the systems can be made clear, e.g., who were involved in its creation, what was their expertise, what was their aim? Users need that information, particularly to decide whether or not they want to be persuaded by it.

Social support

Social support features motivate users by leveraging social influence of other people. The system can help users to compare themselves with others, such as relatives or unknown people, or share information with those who have the same goal to achieve desired behaviours.

Table 12.1 PSD model features for primary Task Support (adapted from: Oinas-Kukkonen & Harjumaa, 2009).

Design feature	Explanation	Example operationalization
Reduction	The system reduces complex behaviour into simple tasks	A complex and long question is divided into multiple short and simple yes/no questions (Beerlage-de Jong, Eikelenboom-Boskamp, Voss, Sanderman, & van Gemert-Pijnen, 2014a).
Tunnelling	The system guides the user through a process or experience	Users are guided through educational content in a predefined, sequential order, (Dekkers, Melles, Vehmeijer, & de Ridder, 2021) and at times some of the information or navigational options are not available.
Tailoring	The system provides information and services that are tailored to its user group	Platform provides advice tailored to 'people like you' based on log-data and questionnaire responses (Bente et al., 2023).
Personalization	The system provides information and services that are personalized to the individual user	An eCoaching system adapts its coaching strategy based on self-tracking data, and the user's inputs on personal health goals and coaching needs (Lentferink et al., 2017).
Self-monitoring	The system allows the user to track their behaviour (change)	Progress is shown in a progress bar and domes around completed areas (tasks) (Ludden, Kelders, & Snippert, 2014).
Simulation	The system provides a way to observe the link between behaviour and effect	The relation between target behaviour (e.g., exercise, sleep) and outcome (e.g., weight loss) is visualized (Asbjørnsen et al., 2022).
Rehearsal	The system enables the user to rehearse the target behaviour	A VR environment resembling the real world allows the user to practice behaviour in a safe environment (Klein Tuente et al., 2020).

Table 12.2 PSD model features for Dialogue Support (adapted from: Oinas-Kukkonen & Harjumaa, 2009).

Design feature	Explanation	Example operationalization
Praise	The system uses praise as positive reinforcement of the target behaviour	Positive feedback messages close to target behaviour when reaching individual goals (Asbjørnsen et al., 2022).
Rewards	The system offers virtual rewards for performing the target behaviour	Animated rewards (e.g., confetti) are shown when a (self-selected) target is reached (Dekkers et al., 2023).
Reminders	The system reminds the user to perform the target behaviour	A pop-up reminds users to retrospectively add relevant information when it becomes available (Beerlage-de Jong et al., 2014a).
Suggestion	The system suggests appropriate behaviours to the user	The app suggests sharing an anonymous code with the user's network to alert them to potential exposure to an infectious disease (Bente et al., 2021).
Similarity	The system is similar to its user in some meaningful way	A VR environment allows you to speak with an avatar that looks like the user (Kip, 2021).
Liking	The system's look and feel is appealing to the user	The use of images is considered attractive and helpful in explaining risks about COVID-19 (Bente et al., 2021).
Social role	The system adopts a social role towards the user	An avatar of a professor coaches the user (Ludden et al., 2014).

Table 12.3 PSD model features for Credibility Support (adapted from: Oinas-Kukkonen & Harjumaa, 2009).

Design feature	Explanation	Example operationalization
Trustworthiness	The system provides truthful, fair, and unbiased information	A supporting website describes how the system works and what it was based on (Beerlage-de Jong et al., 2014a).
Expertise	The system displays its knowledge, experience, and competence	A website lists and describes the experts who were involved in development of the system (Beerlage-de Jong et al., 2014a).
Surface credibility	The system looks and feels competent at first glance	Integrate the system in an established website and include project logo on every screen (Beerlage-de Jong et al., 2014a).
Real-world feel	The system provides insight into the organization or people behind its content and services	An 'about us' page highlights contributions of all stakeholders (e.g., researchers, healthcare organization, designers) (Dekkers et al., 2023).
Authority	The system refers to authoritative people	An app refers to authoritative institutes that support its messages (Bente et al., 2021).
Third-party endorsements	The system is visibly endorsed by respected third parties	When downloading an app, the national government's logo (who endorses its use) is displayed (Bente et al., 2021).
Verifiability	The system's information is verifiable via outside sources	A website provides links to scientific papers that are used for the system's algorithms (Beerlage-de Jong et al., 2014a).

Table 12.4 PSD model features for Social Support (adapted from: Oinas-Kukkonen & Harjumaa, 2009).

Design feature	Explanation	Example operationalization
Social learning	The system shows activities and outcomes of others who are performing the target behaviour	A system shows the physical activity (cycling) and performance of other users (Barratt, 2017).
Social comparison	The system allows the user to compare how they are doing with the published performance of others	A system compares a user's 'personal best' scores to those on a leaderboard (Barratt, 2017).
Normative influence	The system allows the user to gather likeminded people and communicates social norms	A public health campaign deploys social media influencers to increase flu vaccination willingness (Bonnevie et al., 2020).
Social facilitation	The system shows information about other users that perform the target behaviour	An app shows how many and which other users partake in an activity (Kanstrup, Bertelsen, & Knudsen, 2020).
Cooperation	The system supports and enables cooperation between users	An app allows users to connect and start 'healthy cooperations' with peers who want to engage in physical activity (Kanstrup et al., 2020).
Competition	The system supports and enables competition between users	A website and mobile app allows cyclists to compete with other (virtual) users of the system (Barratt, 2017).
Recognition	The system provides a means for public recognition for users who perform the target behaviour	A system publicly displays the top 10 best performing users on a leaderboard (Barratt, 2017).

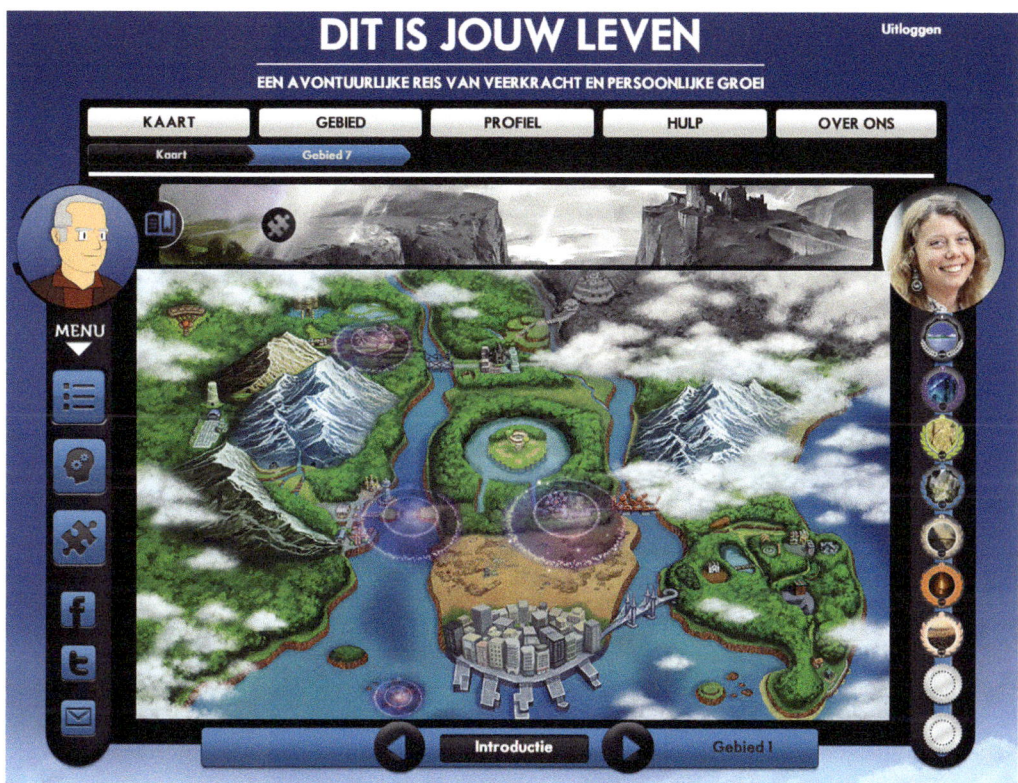

Figure 12.2 Screenshot from This is Your Life, a gamified intervention to promote well-being (Kelders, Sommers-Spijkerman, & Goldberg, 2018).

To illustrate some of the strategies in more detail, and to show how these are used in actual interventions, Figure 12.2 contains a screenshot of the eMental Health intervention 'This is Your Life' (introduced in Chapter 5) with several persuasive features.

Tunnelling can be seen as the guided route participants take throughout the map, therewith omitting irrelevant content or navigational options. These are the lessons that guide the users through the intervention. One could argue that the intervention is also somewhat *personalized* by providing a picture of the user on the screen. *Self-monitoring* is present as the user can see the progress she made, visualized by the progress bar/picture on the top of the screen and the 'domes' around some of the areas indicating that after completing these areas the user improved on the outcome measures of that area. *Rewards* are visible as the badges the user has earned, shown on the right of the screen. Arguably, *liking* is present due to the whole design of the intervention being attractive to the users, which was ensured by actively engaging them in a participatory design process. Last, *social role* is present as the avatar of the professor. With this avatar, the system itself adopts a social role, in this case a coaching professor, which makes the system more persuasive.

Evaluating Persuasive Technology

In recent years, considerable research has been conducted using the PSD model as an evaluation framework to understand the impact of persuasive eHealth technology and to improve this impact. The focus has mostly been on the relationship between specific persuasive features (and combinations of features) and perceived persuasiveness, adherence, and effectiveness of eHealth interventions. This will be elaborated upon in the section below.

Perceived Persuasiveness

To measure what features matter in supporting adherence and (health) outcomes, research has been conducted into the perceived persuasiveness of technologies. Up until recently, it was merely assessed whether a persuasive feature is present or not, and the quality or extent of the feature, or whether end-users actually perceive the presence of the feature were not taken into account. This may entail that even the slightest use of tailoring is interpreted by one researcher as 'present', while others would interpret this as not enough to merit the feature as being present, or while end-users do not notice the feature being present.

A different way of studying the influence of persuasive features is to investigate whether a system with these features is perceived as more persuasive by its users, and whether a system that is perceived as more persuasive is actually more effective in changing behaviour. In this way, the assumptions that employing persuasive features increases the persuasiveness of the system, and that this increased persuasiveness makes a system more effective, can be tested.

To attain more insight into if and how (potential) end-users of a persuasive technology perceive its persuasive features, the Perceived Persuasiveness Questionnaire (PPQ) was developed (Drozd, Lehto, & Oinas-Kukkonen, 2012; Lehto, Oinas-Kukkonen, & Drozd, 2012). The PPQ consists of a 31-item scale that covers all four categories of the PSD model, but also four additional but related constructs (unobtrusiveness, effort, effectiveness, and perceived persuasiveness). Although it holds promise for studies that aim to gain more insight into the working mechanisms of persuasive technologies, it has not been (psychometrically) validated yet and shows room for improvement when it comes to its construct validity (Beerlage-de Jong, Kip, & Kelders, 2020). For example, on the one hand the questionnaire includes constructs that are *part of* persuasion, such as perceived unobtrusiveness. The technology's fit with daily life (routines) is known to be an important factor for the success of an eHealth technology (Beerlage-de Jong et al., 2014b; Laurie & Blandford, 2016). At the same time, the PPQ also includes constructs that *predict* persuasion, such as perceived effort. In literature, (perceived) effort is considered a part of usability, which in turn is a necessary precondition (but not part of) persuasion (Lehto et al., 2012).

However, despite the challenges that remain with the PPQ in its current form it most certainly holds promise for the field of research on persuasive technologies. Early research on the concept of perceived persuasiveness indicates that it is related to the intention and actual use of persuasive eHealth technology (Drozd, Lehto, & Oinas-Kukkonen, 2012; Oinas-Kukkonen, 2013). Having a valid and reliable measure of *perceived* persuasiveness available will make a strong contribution to the much-needed research into what elements of a technology actually contribute to its success.

Influence on adherence

Few studies have investigated the relationship between persuasive features and adherence (e.g., using an intervention as intended by the developers, for instance, in terms of duration and features, see Chapter 15). As persuasive technology has the ability to motivate users and change their behaviour, it seems logical to assume that it can consequently influence the way and frequency by which eHealth interventions are used. Persuasive features could be important to increase adherence when the appropriate principles are deployed in those critical moments when non-adherence starts (Kelders & van Gemert-Pijnen, 2013). A reminder at the right time, or a smart reward, may give the user just a little bit of extra motivation to stick with the programme.

This hypothesis is supported by a large systematic review including 83 web-based interventions to improve health and well-being (Kelders et al., 2012). The review showed that increased employment of dialogue support features increased the adherence to web-based interventions. Although social support features were hardly used, it seemed that interventions that did employ these features more elaborately achieved higher adherence rates. Primary Task Support did not show a significant contribution to adherence. The study showed the importance of a persuasive design of the interaction between the system and its users for the sustained use of technology, while also showing that the possibilities to do this are still hardly employed in web-based interventions in the health area.

Influence on effectiveness

Studies have shown that persuasive systems as a whole tend to be effective in improving health and well-being (Hamari, Koivisto, & Pakkanen, 2014). However, these kinds of studies often compare a persuasive system to no intervention or 'care as usual'. Therefore, no claims can be made about the influence of the persuasiveness of the technology (rather than the technology as a whole), or which features are most effective. To shed more light on these questions, some studies have investigated the relationship between the number of persuasive features and effectiveness, or between specific features and effectiveness.

It seems that there is a positive relationship between the number of persuasive features and effectiveness (Wildeboer et al., 2016; Xu, Chomutare, & Iyengar, 2014), suggesting that persuasive technology indeed adds to the effectiveness of eHealth technology. However, it cannot be concluded that the more such features are used, the more effective a technology is. It may be more important to focus on what combinations of features yield the best possible outcomes. Studies have shown that some PSD features work well together while others don't. Using features that supplement each other can strengthen the persuasive effects. For example, rewards can supplement *suggestion*, making this an effective combination (Räisänen, Lehto, & Oinas-Kukkonen, 2010). Also, the combination of tunnelling, tailoring, reminders, social learning, social comparison, with or without similarity, seems to contribute to higher effect sizes (Wildeboer et al., 2016). However, weakening persuasiveness by implementing features that have low synergy must be avoided. For example, abundant use of reduction makes tunnelling redundant (Räisänen et al., 2010).

It appears that it is important to employ features from different categories to be most effective, but more research is needed to verify this hypothesis. Moreover, research is needed to ground the use of (combinations of) features in behaviour change techniques, persuasive communication, and social psychology. In most studies, the rationale behind the choice of features and the users' evaluation of the persuasiveness of the eHealth technology is lacking. In most cases, the underlying theories or principles for persuasion are not reported (Langrial et al., 2012; Lehto et al., 2012; Oinas-Kukkonen, 2013). Often, no information is given on how these interventions were developed (Kelders et al., 2012), and the persuasive context (intent, event, strategy) for developing the interventions were not specified (Langrial et al., 2012). This makes it difficult to draw generalizable conclusions about which features to employ in which contexts.

Evaluations of Persuasiveness as Input for Design

Both the PSD model itself and insights from evaluation research have been used as guidelines for the design of persuasive eHealth technologies in formative research. For instance, the PSD model itself is intended as a guideline for the design, where developers need to address the premises and the context, as well as employ primary task, dialogue, credibility, and/or social support features to create a persuasive eHealth technology. Also, recommendations on how to design eHealth technologies have come from studies on specific persuasive technology strategies, from both theories and theory-based studies. This has led to general design guidelines and guidelines on ways to use a specific feature such as 'suggestion' (Andrew, Borriello, & Fogarty, 2007; Consolvo, McDonald, & Landay, 2009; Ploderer, Reitberger, Oinas-Kukkonen, & van Gemert-Pijnen, 2014). Although these studies provide valuable insights, more in-depth work needs to be done on validating and studying the effects of using these design guidelines. Specifically, attention needs to be paid to the ways in which the persuasive design of eHealth technology can improve the usability and fit with its users.

Improving usability

From evaluation research we know that users of eHealth technologies face usability issues: They get lost in interventions (Sieverink, Kelders, Braakman-Jansen, & van Gemert-Pijnen, 2014), have issues finding exercises that should be done daily (van Gemert-Pijnen, Kelders, & Bohlmeijer, 2014), or they do not know what features they should use to reach their goals (Akkersdijk, Kelders, & van Gemert-Pijnen, 2016). Persuasive technology can provide support to help users overcome these usability issues.

These features can be designed in the system in advance when usability issues are expected. However, sometimes these issues only surface after a system is implemented. Log data can provide insight into where and when persuasive features are needed to improve usability (see Chapters 8 and 14). For example, within an eMental health intervention for people with depressive symptoms, log data revealed that many users occasionally log in to the system without accessing any of the features (Kelders, Bohlmeijer, & van Gemert-Pijnen, 2013). This points towards a non-effective usage of the system. Additional investigation found that users use these logins only to see whether they can start the next session. To improve the usability, a persuasive feature such as reminders ('Your new session is ready!') can be used to avoid these unnecessary logins, or a feature as suggestion or rehearsal can be used to make these short sessions more useful (e.g., a message when logging in to the system saying 'Your next session is not yet ready, but it would be very beneficial to do this exercise again').

Improving fit with users

A last question within the design of persuasive eHealth technology is how to create a technology that fits with the users. As discussed in Chapter 13, this fit can lead to high user engagement, and a good fit can be beneficial to effectiveness, adherence, and implementation in practice. However, to date, not much is known on how to personalize interventions to achieve this fit.

Studies have investigated whether user characteristics such as personality, gender, and gamer type can be used to match users to persuasive features (Beerlage-de Jong, Wrede, van Gemert-Pijnen, & Sieverink, 2017; Drozd et al., 2012; Oinas-Kukkonen, 2013; Halko & Kientz, 2010; Orji, Vassileva, & Mandryk, 2014). All of these studies have shown that these characteristics impact the effectiveness of different features. They indicate that persuasion might be more effective when tailored to the user rather than implementing a 'one size fits all' version of a technology. However, as there may be many user characteristics that impact the effectiveness of persuasive features, and it may be that the influence of these characteristics varies in different contexts, it seems to be unfeasible to explore all characteristics that influence persuasiveness in all contexts.

Other approaches have tried to overcome this issue by, for example, using the concepts of persuadability and engagement. Kaptein et al. have used questionnaires to create a persuadability score of each individual (Kaptein, Lacroix, & Saini, 2010). This persuadability score is a measure of the tendency of a person to comply with the different persuasive strategies. The study showed that people with a high persuadability score are more persuaded by health-related messages that employ these persuasive strategies than people with a low persuadability score. Although there are limitations of this study (e.g., it investigated short-term effects on a single behaviour), it is important because it shows that differences in the persuadability of people (and therefore in the potential effectiveness of persuasive technology) can be assessed and utilized, at least from a theoretical starting point. In the same way, it has been posited that selecting the persuasive features that invoke the most engagement in each individual may be a way to personalize interventions. Such knowledge can be used to design more effective eHealth interventions and to increase adherence to these interventions.

The Dark Side of Persuasion

Ethics are an important part of persuasive technology. An ideal system literally persuades its users to adopt the target behaviour. Computer-mediated persuasion means that people are persuading others through computers, for example, via instant messages or social networking systems. In the case of persuasive systems, there are always stakeholders who have the intention of influencing someone's attitudes or behaviour, because computers do not have intentions of their own, at least at this point in time.

The 'dark sides' of persuasion can include strategies like manipulation or coercion, forcing people to do something on a non-voluntary basis. For all of these goes that the underlying premise is that a technology is *not* transparent in what it aims to do. This is out of the scope of the 'positive' oriented approach of supporting people to behave healthier, as is the case with persuasive (eHealth) technology. However, it is imaginable that a certain form of manipulation can be (and is) used to push people in the right direction to control their behaviours. For example, nudging people to support decision making on a healthier lifestyle can be considered as manipulation by providing a limited spectrum of choices (just providing 'good' products or services), especially when a system is not transparent in which goals it's striving to achieve. Another, relatively new, phenomenon that is an example of the dark side of persuasion, is the massive spread of misinformation about health-related topics such as SARS-CoV-2 vaccines through social media. The aim of such information is to instil fear and (mis)lead people to take a certain health-related decision that is considered desirable by its sender. In this case, people are persuaded to accept false information since the technology is not being transparent about the credibility of that information. Then, people are persuaded by that false information to act in a certain way.

Some of the ethical issues one should think of when developing a persuasive eHealth technology are (National Advisory Committee on Bioethics, 2015):

- **Responsibility**. Whose responsibility is it that people lead healthy lives? When developing a persuasive eHealth technology to stimulate people to lead more healthy lives, the assumption may be that the developers of the technology have a responsibility in the self-management of people. However, using a persuasive technology and not, for instance, more firm techniques such as rules or legislation, also emphasizes the free choice aspect of behaviour. This in turn might push people towards being wholly responsible for their own well-being (or the lack of), while not everyone may be able to deal with this responsibility;
- **Autonomy**. This is the right of individuals to make their own choices, based on their own values. Persuasive technology may limit autonomy by first deciding on what the desired behaviour is, for example, based on social norms, thus limiting the person's autonomy to choose their own desired behaviour. Second, the technology will also nudge people towards behaving in that specific way, limiting the choice of people behaving in different ways. A way to overcome this potential threat is to always be transparent about how and why the technology influences people's autonomy;

- **Impact on self-control**. It may be that being persuaded to behave a certain way actually limits an individual's self-control in the long term: It may make it even harder to behave in a desired way when not having a specific persuasive eHealth technology to assist him or her. Thus, there is a chance people might become too dependent on technology;
- **Equity**. Although technology may make healthcare more accessible to many different people, persuasive eHealth technology may also hinder equity in different ways. First, as these technologies make decisions about certain desired behaviours, they may only reach people that already share these ideas and norms. Second, some of the persuasive techniques might be more effective for different people, therefore influencing them in different ways. For example, people with lower literacy skills may lack the ability to carefully weigh arguments but may defer to authority more readily, making them more influenced by the use of authority figures.

All the aspects mentioned above are potential threats to the integrity of the technology. However, it does not mean that it is impossible to create 'integer technology', as long as the mentioned threats are properly accounted for during development and critically appraised during evaluation.

The Future of Persuasive Health Technology

Persuasive technology, when aimed at changing behaviours in the domain of health and well-being, is a promising field. However, we need to have more theoretical insights in what works best for whom and keep an eye on the 'dark sides' of using persuasive features to nudge people to do what we think is best for them. To design health technologies that are usable and that motivate users to improve behaviours, we need more insight in persuasive features to understand and predict factors that improve adherence to and effectiveness of eHealth technologies. More research is needed on, for example:

- Understanding how behaviour change techniques can be implemented as persuasive features (see Chapter 2). For example, behaviour change techniques are used to set goals in health promotion interventions, and although these techniques provide a feasible framework to change behaviour, it is rather unknown how these techniques can be translated to design persuasive eHealth technologies;
- Understanding and predicting factors that improve adherence, for example, understanding what features matter most for whom by using log data to observe real-time use of an eHealth technology. In future research, artificial intelligence (e.g., machine learning) may well be used to optimize adherence via personalization of the technology because of using knowledge on the patterns of usage, predicting non-usages, and creating user profiles;
- Identifying what features are most effective and in what combinations. Experimental research designs (see Chapter 14) can be used to investigate which (persuasive) features and which combinations within eHealth technology have most impact;
- Creating persuasive eHealth technologies that have a fit with the users. A promising approach is to design technologies that increase engagement (see Chapter 13). Engagement may also provide an opportunity to personalize interventions: Different people can be engaged by different persuasive features. An optimal intervention for everyone can be composed by selecting only those features that invoke high engagement.

Summary

This chapter has shown that persuasive design is pivotal in using technology to change behaviour and improve health. It can persuade people to continue using the eHealth intervention and can increase its effectiveness. There are several approaches to design persuasive technology, of which the Persuasive Systems Design model is discussed in more detail. Careful consideration of the aims, user, and use context is necessary when deciding what persuasive features to apply in an intervention. The take-home messages of this chapter are:

- The field of persuasive technology is grounded in various theories, e.g., persuasive communication, health promotion, social marketing, acceptance of technology, and human-media interaction;
- Persuasive technology can contribute to the sustained use and the effectiveness of eHealth interventions;
- The Persuasive Systems Design model consists of four categories of software features that can be applied to support the user's primary activities, the computer-human dialogue, the credibility of presented information, and to leverage social influence;
- Decisions about which software features to apply should carefully consider the aims, user, and use-context of the intervention.

Key References for Further Reading

Beerlage-de Jong, N., Kip, H., & Kelders, S. M. (2020). Evaluation of the Perceived Persuasiveness Questionnaire: User-centered card-sort study. *Journal of Medical Internet Research*, 22(10), e20404.

Fogg, B. J. (2002). Persuasive technology: Using computers to change what we think and do. *Ubiquity*, 2002 (December), 5.

Kelders, S. M., Kok, R. N., Ossebaard, H. C., & van Gemert-Pijnen, J. E. (2012). Persuasive system design does matter: A systematic review of adherence to web-based interventions. *Journal of Medical Internet Research*, 14(6).

Oinas-Kukkonen, H. (2013). A foundation for the study of behaviour change support systems. *Personal and Ubiquitous Computing*, 17(6), 1223–1235.

Oinas-Kukkonen, H., & Harjumaa, M. (2009). Persuasive systems design: Key issues, process model, and system features. *Communications of the Association for Information Systems*, 24(1), 28.

References

Abd-Alrazaq, A. A., Bewick, B. M., Farragher, T., & Gardner, P. (2019). Factors that affect the use of electronic personal health records among patients: A systematic review. *Int J Med Inform*, 126, 164–175. doi:10.1016/j.ijmedinf.2019.03.014

Ajzen, I. (1991). The Theory of Planned Behavior. *Organizational Behavior and Human Decision Processes*, 50, 179–211. doi:10.1016/0749-5978(91)90020-T

Ajzen, I. (1992). Persuasive communication theory in social psychology: A historical perspective. *Influencing Human Behaviour*, 1–27.

Akkersdijk, S., Kelders, S., & van Gemert-Pijnen, J. (2016). The grid, classification of eHealth applications towards a better (re)design and evaluation. Paper presented at the eTELEMED 2016: The eighth international conference on eHealth, telemedicine, and social medicine.

Andrew, A., Borriello, G., & Fogarty, J. (2007). Toward a systematic understanding of suggestion tactics in persuasive technologies. *Persuasive Technology*, 259–270.

Asbjørnsen, R. A., Hjelmesæth, J., Smedsrød, M. L., Wentzel, J., Ollivier, M., Clark, M. M., . . . Solberg Nes, L. (2022). Combining persuasive system design principles and behavior change techniques in digital interventions supporting long-term weight loss maintenance: Design and development of eCHANGE. *JMIR Hum Factors*, 9(2), e37372. doi:10.2196/37372

Barratt, P. (2017). Healthy competition: A qualitative study investigating persuasive technologies and the gamification of cycling. *Health Place*, 46, 328–336. doi:10.1016/j.healthplace.2016.09.009

Beerlage-de Jong, N., Eikelenboom-Boskamp, A., Voss, A., Sanderman, R., & van Gemert-Pijnen, J. (2014a). Combining user-centered design with the persuasive systems design model: The development process of a web-based registration and monitoring system for healthcare-associated infections in nursing homes. *International Journal on Advances in Life Sciences*, 6, 262–271.

Beerlage-de Jong, N., Kip, H., & Kelders, S. M. (2020). Evaluation of the Perceived Persuasiveness Questionnaire: User-centered card-sort study. *J Med Internet Res*, 22(10), e20404. doi:10.2196/20404

Beerlage-de Jong, N., Wentzel, M. J., Kelders, S. M., Oinas-Kukkonen, H., & van Gemert-Pijnen, J. E. W. C. (2014b). Evaluation of perceived persuasiveness constructs by combining user tests and expert assessments. In A. Öörni, S. M. Kelders, J. E. W. C. van Gemert-Pijnen, & H. Oinas-Kukkonen (Eds.), *BCSS 2014: Behaviour Change Support Systems* (pp. 7–15). (CEUR workshop proceedings; Vol. 1153). CEUR-WS.org.

Beerlage-de Jong, N., Wrede, C., van Gemert-Pijnen, J., & Sieverink, F. (2017). Storyboarding persuasion to match personality traits. Paper presented at the 12th international conference on persuasive technology, Amsterdam, The Netherlands.

Bente, B. E., van 't Klooster, J. W. J. R., Schreijer, M. A., Berkemeier, L., van Gend, J. E., Slijkhuis, P. J. H., ... van Gemert-Pijnen, J. E. W. C. (2021). The Dutch COVID-19 contact tracing app (the CoronaMelder): Usability study. *JMIR Form Res*, 5(3), e27882. doi:10.2196/27882

Bente, B. E., Wentzel, J., Schepers, C., Breeman, L. D., Janssen, V. R., Pieterse, M. E., . . . van Gemert-Pijnen, L. (2023). Implementation and user evaluation of an eHealth technology platform supporting patients with cardiovascular disease in managing their health after a cardiac event: Mixed methods study. *JMIR Cardio*, 7, e43781. doi:10.2196/43781

Bonnevie, E., Rosenberg, S. D., Kummeth, C., Goldbarg, J., Wartella, E., & Smyser, J. (2020). Using social media influencers to increase knowledge and positive attitudes toward the flu vaccine. *PLoS One*, 15(10), e0240828. doi:10.1371/journal.pone.0240828

Burkhart, P. V., & Sabaté, E. (2003). Adherence to long-term therapies: Evidence for action. *J Nurs Scholarsh*, 35(3), 207.

Chang, H. H., Lu, Y.-Y., & Lin, S. C. (2020). An elaboration likelihood model of consumer respond action to Facebook second-hand marketplace: Impulsiveness as a moderator. *Information & Management*, 57(2), 103171. doi:https://doi.org/10.1016/j.im.2019.103171

Cialdini, R. B. (2001). *Influence: Science and practice* (4th ed.). Boston: Allyn & Bacon.

Consolvo, S., McDonald, D. W., & Landay, J. A. (2009). Theory-driven design strategies for technologies that support behaviour change in everyday life. In *Proceedings of the SIGCHI conference on human factors in computing systems*.

Davis, F. D. (1985). *A technology acceptance model for empirically testing new end-user information systems: Theory and results*. Cambridge, MA: Massachusetts Institute of Technology.

Dekkers, T., Heirbaut, T., Schouten, S. E., Kelders, S. M., Beerlage-de Jong, N., Ludden, G. D. S., . . . Kip, H. (2023). A mobile self-control training app to improve self-control and physical activity in people with severe mental illness: Protocol for 2 single-case experimental designs. *JMIR Res Protoc*, 12, e37727. doi:10.2196/37727

Dekkers, T., Melles, M., Vehmeijer, S. B. W., & de Ridder, H. (2021). Effects of information architecture on the effectiveness and user experience of web-based patient education in middle-aged and older adults: Online randomized experiment. *J Med Internet Res*, 23(3), e15846. doi:10.2196/15846

Dillard, J. P., & Pfau, M. (2002). *The persuasion handbook: Developments in theory and practice*. London: *Sage Publications*.

Donkin, L., Christensen, H., Naismith, S. L., Neal, B., Hickie, I. B., & Glozier, N. (2011). A systematic review of the impact of adherence on the effectiveness of e-therapies. *J Med Internet Res*, 13(3), e52. doi:10.2196/jmir.1772

Drozd, F., Lehto, T., & Oinas-Kukkonen, H. (2012). Exploring perceived persuasiveness of a behavior change support system: A structural model (Vol. 7284).

Elbert, N. J., van Os-Medendorp, H., van Renselaar, W., Ekeland, A. G., Hakkaart-van Roijen, L., Raat, H., . . . Pasmans, S. G. (2014). Effectiveness and cost-effectiveness of ehealth interventions in somatic diseases: A systematic review of systematic reviews and meta-analyses. *J Med Internet Res*, 16(4), e110. doi:10.2196/jmir.2790

Fishbein, M. (1979). A theory of reasoned action: Some applications and implications. *Nebraska Symposium on Motivation*, 27, 65–116.

Fogg, B. J. (2002). Persuasive technology: Using computers to change what we think and do. *Ubiquity*, 2002(December), 5.

Fogg, B. J. (2019). Fogg Behaviour Model. Retrieved from https://behaviormodel.org/

Graaf, de M. M. A., & Ben Allouch, S. (2013). Exploring influencing variables for the acceptance of social robots. *Robotics and Autonomous Systems*, 61(12), 1476–1486.

Hadjiconstantinou, M., Byrne, J., Bodicoat, D. H., Robertson, N., Eborall, H., Khunti, K., & Davies, M. J. (2016). Do web-based interventions improve well-being in type 2 diabetes? A systematic review and meta-analysis. *J Med Internet Res*, 18(10), e270. doi:10.2196/jmir.5991

Hagger, M. S., & Weed, M. (2019). DEBATE: Do interventions based on behavioral theory work in the real world? *Int J Behav Nutr Phys Act*, 16(1), 36. doi:10.1186/s12966-019-0795-4

Halko, S., & Kientz, J. (2010). Personality and persuasive technology: An exploratory study on health-promoting mobile applications. *Persuasive Technology*, 150–161.

Hamari, J., Koivisto, J., & Pakkanen, T. (2014). Do persuasive technologies persuade? A review of empirical studies. Paper presented at the International Conference on Persuasive Technology.

Hekler, E. B., Michie, S., Pavel, M., Rivera, D. E., Collins, L. M., Jimison, H. B., . . . Spruijt-Metz, D. (2016). Advancing models and theories for digital behavior change interventions. *Am J Prev Med*, 51(5), 825–832. doi:10.1016/j.amepre.2016.06.013

Kanstrup, A. M., Bertelsen, P. S., & Knudsen, C. (2020). Changing health behavior with social technology? A pilot test of a mobile app designed for social support of physical activity. *Int J Environ Res Public Health*, 17(22). doi:10.3390/ijerph17228383

Kaptein, M., Lacroix, J., & Saini, P. (2010). Individual differences in persuadability in the health promotion domain. *Persuasive*, 6137, 94–105.

Kelders, S. M., Bohlmeijer, E. T., & van Gemert-Pijnen, J. E. (2013). Participants, usage, and use patterns of a web-based intervention for the prevention of depression within a randomized controlled trial. *Journal of Medical Internet Research*, 15(8).

Kelders, S. M., Kok, R. N., Ossebaard, H. C., & van Gemert-Pijnen, J. E. W. C. (2012). Persuasive system design does matter: A systematic review of adherence to web-based interventions. *J Med Internet Res*, 14(6), e152. doi:10.2196/jmir.2104

Kelders, S. M., & van Gemert-Pijnen, J. E. L. (2013). Using log-data as a starting point to make eHealth more persuasive. Paper presented at the International Conference on Persuasive Technology.

Kelders, S. M., Sommers-Spijkerman, M., & Goldberg, J. (2018). Investigating the direct impact of a gamified versus nongamified well-being intervention: An exploratory experiment. *J Med Internet Res*, 20(7), e247. doi:10.2196/jmir.9923

Kip, H. (2021). The added value of eHealth in treatment of offenders. Improving the development, implementation and evaluation of technology in forensic mental healthcare. PhD Thesis, University of Twente, Enschede, the Netherlands.

Klein Tuente, S., Bogaerts, S., Bulten, E., Keulen-de Vos, M., Vos, M., Bokern, H., . . . Veling, W. (2020). Virtual Reality Aggression Prevention Therapy (VRAPT) versus waiting list control for forensic psychiatric inpatients: A multicenter randomized controlled trial. *J Clin Med*, 9(7). doi:10.3390/jcm9072258

Kooij, L., Groen, W. G., & van Harten, W. H. (2017). The effectiveness of information technology-supported shared care for patients with chronic Disease: A systematic rview. *J Med Internet Res*, 19(6), e221.

Kotler, P., Roberto, N., & Lee, N. (2002). *Social marketing: Improving the quality of life*. London: *Sage Publications*.

Kreps, G. L., Bonaguro, E. W., & Query Jr, J. L. (2003). The history and development of the field of health communication. *Russian Journal of Communication*, 10, 12–20.

Kreps, G. L., & Maibach, E. W. (2008). Transdisciplinary science: The nexus between communication and public health. *Journal of Communication*, 58(4), 732–748.

Langrial, S., Lehto, T., Oinas-Kukkonen, H., Harjumaa, M., & Karppinen, P. (2012). Native mobile applications for personal well-being: A persuasive systems design evaluation. Paper presented at the PACIS.

Laurie, J., & Blandford, A. (2016). Making time for mindfulness. *Int J Med Inform*, 96, 38–50. doi:10.1016/j.ijmedinf.2016.02.010

Lehto, T., Oinas-Kukkonen, H., & Drozd, F. (2012). Factors affecting perceived persuasiveness of a behavior change support system. Paper presented at Thirty-Third International Conference on Information Systems, Orlando, Florida.

Lentferink, A. J., Oldenhuis, H. K., de Groot, M., Polstra, L., Velthuijsen, H., & van Gemert-Pijnen, J. E. (2017). Key components in eHealth interventions combining self-tracking and persuasive eCoaching to promote a healthier lifestyle: A scoping review. *J Med Internet Res*, 19(8), e277. doi:10.2196/jmir.7288

Lockton, D., Harrison, D., & Stanton, N. (2010). The Design with Intent Method: A design tool for influencing user behaviour. *Applied Ergonomics*, 41(3), 382–392.

Ludden, G. D. S., Kelders, S. M., & Snippert, B. H. J. (2014). 'This Is Your Life!'. Paper presented at the International Conference on Persuasive Technology, Cham.

McGuire, W. (1985). Attitudes and attitude change. In L. Gardner & A. Elliot (Eds.), *Handbook of social psychology* (volume 2). New York: Random House.

Michie, S., Richardson, M., Johnston, M., Abraham, C., Francis, J., Hardeman, W., . . . Wood, C. E. (2013). The behavior change technique taxonomy (v1) of 93 hierarchically clustered techniques: Building an international consensus for the reporting of behavior change interventions. *Ann Behav Med*, 46(1), 81–95. doi:10.1007/s12160-013-9486-6

Nass, C., Steuer, J., & Tauber, E. R. (1994). Computers are social actors. Paper presented at the Proceedings of the SIGCHI Conference on Human Factors in Computing Systems, Boston, Massachusetts, USA.

National Advisory Committee on Bioethics (2015). *Nudging in public health – An ethical framework. A report by the national advisory committee on bioethics*. Ireland: Department of Health.

Oinas-Kukkonen, H. (2013). A foundation for the study of behaviour change support systems. *Personal and Ubiquitous Computing*, 17(6), 1223–1235.

Oinas-Kukkonen, H., & Harjumaa, M. (2009). Persuasive Systems Design: Key issues, process model, and system features. *Communications of the Association for Information Systems*, 24. doi:10.17705/1CAIS.02428

Orji, R., Vassileva, J., & Mandryk, R. L. (2014). Modeling the efficacy of persuasive strategies for different gamer types in serious games for health. *User Modeling and User-Adapted Interaction*, 24(5), 453–498.

Patrick, K., Hekler, E. B., Estrin, D., Mohr, D. C., Riper, H., Crane, D., . . . Riley, W. T. (2016). The pace of technologic change: Implications for digital health behavior intervention research. *Am J Prev Med*, 51(5), 816–824. doi:10.1016/j.amepre.2016.05.001

Perloff, R. M. (1993). Third-person effect research 1983–1992: A review and synthesis. *International Journal of Public Opinion Research*, 5(2), 167–184.

Petty, R. E., & Cacioppo, J. T. (1986). The elaboration likelihood model of persuasion. *Advances in Experimental Social Psychology*, 19, 123–205.

Ploderer, B., Reitberger, W., Oinas-Kukkonen, H., & van Gemert-Pijnen, J. (2014). *Social interaction and reflection for behaviour change*. Dordrecht: Springer.

Räisänen, T., Lehto, T., & Oinas-Kukkonen, H. (2010). Practical findings from applying the PSD model for evaluating software design specifications. *Persuasive Technology*, 185–192.

Riley, W. T., Rivera, D. E., Atienza, A. A., Nilsen, W., Allison, S. M., & Mermelstein, R. (2011). Health behavior models in the age of mobile interventions: Are our theories up to the task? *Transl Behav Med*, 1(1), 53–71. doi:10.1007/s13142-011-0021-7

Rimal, R. N., & Lapinski, M. K. (2009). Why health communication is important in public health. *Bulletin of the World Health Organization*, 87(4), 247–247a.

Scholten, M., Kelders, S., & van Gemert-Pijnen, J. (2017). Self-guided web-based interventions: A scoping review on user needs and on the potential of embodied conversational agents to address them. *Journal of Medical Internet Research*.

Schulz von Thun, F. (1981). *Miteinander reden 1. Störungen und Klärungen. Allgemeine Psychologie der Kommunikation*. Rowohlt Taschenbuch Verlag: Reinbek bei Hamburg.

Sieverink, F., Kelders, S. M., Braakman-Jansen, L. M., & van Gemert-Pijnen, J. E. (2014). The added value of log file analyses of the use of a personal health record for patients with type 2 diabetes mellitus: Preliminary results. *Journal of Diabetes Science and Technology*, 8(2), 247–255.

Sieverink, F., Kelders, S. M., & van Gemert-Pijnen, J. E. W. C. (2017). Clarifying the concept of adherence to eHealth technology: Systematic review on when usage becomes adherence. *J Med Internet Res*, 19(12), e402. doi:10.2196/jmir.8578

Van Gemert-Pijnen, J. E., Kelders, S. M., & Bohlmeijer, E. T. (2014). Understanding the usage of content in a mental health intervention for depression: An analysis of log data. *Journal of Medical Internet Research*, 16(1).

Venkatesh, V., & Davis, F. D. (2000). A theoretical extension of the technology acceptance model: Four longitudinal field studies. *Management Science*, 46(2), 186–204.

Venkatesh, V., Morris, M. G., Davis, G. B., & Davis, F. D. (2003). User acceptance of information technology: Toward a unified view. *MIS Quarterly*, 425–478.

Webb, T. L., Joseph, J., Yardley, L., & Michie, S. (2010). Using the Internet to promote health behavior change: A systematic review and meta-analysis of the impact of theoretical basis, use of behavior change techniques, and mode of delivery on efficacy. *J Med Internet Res*, 12(1), e4. doi:10.2196/jmir.1376

Wildeboer, G., Kelders, S. M., & van Gemert-Pijnen, J. E. (2016). The relationship between persuasive technology principles, adherence and effect of web-based interventions for mental health: A meta-analysis. *International Journal of Medical Informatics*, 96, 71–85.

Xu, K., Chen, X., & Huang, L. (2022). Deep mind in social responses to technologies: A new approach to explaining the Computers are Social Actors phenomena. *Computers in Human Behavior*, 134, 107321.

Xu, A., Chomutare, T., & Iyengar, S. (2014). Systematic review of behavioural obesity interventions and their persuasive qualities. Paper presented at the International Conference on Persuasive Technology.

13 Innovation, Improvement, and Implementation – Conceptual Frameworks for Thinking Through Complex Change

Chrysanthi Papoutsi & Trish Greenhalgh

Introduction

Contemporary healthcare is characterised by rapid change as new treatments and (eHealth) technologies are introduced. Translating an innovation (such as a research finding, a medical device, or a piece of software) into business as usual in a healthcare organisation is difficult and complex. This chapter begins by distinguishing between three related processes: Innovation, improvement, and implementation, and introducing other key concepts such as complexity, spread, scale up, and sustainability. We then describe three frameworks which were all developed to support and evaluate efforts in innovation, improvement and implementation and are thus relevant for eHealth implementation: The diffusion of innovations (DOI) framework, the consolidated framework for implementation research (CFIR), and the nonadoption, abandonment, scale up, spread and sustainability (NASSS) framework. The first two frameworks cover innovation and implementation respectively but were not designed with digital technologies in mind. NASSS was developed more recently to consider the many different domains of complexity in digital technology implementation, making it especially suitable for eHealth. We also include some brief worked examples to illustrate the concepts and frameworks in this chapter.

After reading this chapter you will be able to:

- Explain in broad terms why, eHealth technologies, research findings, and other innovations often fail to get taken up to their full potential;
- Distinguish between innovation, improvement, and implementation;
- Define complexity and explain why complex phenomena are different from complicated ones;
- Explain different framework (such as DOI, CFIR, or NASSS) to a real initiative to implement an eHealth innovation or achieve an improvement in services;
- Provide examples of how the NASSS framework can be applied to implementation of technology in healthcare.

Introduction and Terminology

Change is a defining feature of modern medicine and healthcare. New drugs, medical devices and eHealth technologies are constantly being developed. Healthcare relies heavily on information and communication technologies (ICTs), which develop rapidly and may thus also quickly become

DOI: 10.4324/9781003302049-15

obsolete. New ways of working (in teams rather than individually, for example) may be shown to be more efficient and effective. New research may show that drugs we had thought were effective are actually ineffective and perhaps harmful: Patients taking those drugs should discontinue them. Or a new eHealth technology (e.g., virtual reality in mental healthcare) may be developed that has to be used by practitioners as soon as possible. In short, evidence is constantly emerging that should prompt us to make changes to tests, treatments, and the way services are organised. We need to be able to implement these changes as quickly and widely as possible.

Here is an example. Fifty years ago, hip fracture in older people carried a high mortality. An apparently well 80-year-old would fall, break their hip, be admitted to hospital and then – despite a successful operation to fit a replacement hip – deteriorate and die within a few days or weeks. Research studies identified several areas for improvement in the *care pathway* (the various assessments, tests, and interventions that occur when someone breaks their hip). For example, patients were spending hours in the accident and emergency department before being examined and sent for X-ray. Pain relief was often inadequate, causing needless suffering and stress to the nervous system. Operations were sometimes delayed, and patients lay in bed afterwards for many days before being helped to mobilise, causing many to develop thrombosis. A high proportion became confused and delirious during their hospital stay. Care on orthopaedic wards focused mainly on bones, but attention to patients' other illnesses (such as high blood pressure or urine infections) was suboptimal. By the time patients were discharged – typically after a month or more in hospital, most had become deconditioned, despondent, and osteoporotic (thinning of the bones from disuse). Many died, and many more were unable to return to independent living.

The management of hip fracture was one of the first topics addressed in a comprehensive quality improvement effort (Leigheb et al., 2012). 'Evidence-based' changes – that is, ones that were strongly backed up by research findings – included prompt assessment on admission (including of coexisting illnesses), adequate pain relief, fast-track to X-ray, urgent operation, early mobilisation (patients were to be up and walking within 24 hours), active physiotherapy and rehabilitation, anticoagulants, and compression stockings to prevent thrombosis, and holistic care planning for return home. You do want this package for your own grandparent. But even though all these proposed changes were evidence-based, implementing them was not straightforward. How do you get hold of a geriatrician to assess a patient promptly in the accident and emergency department when the clinician in charge is an orthopaedic surgeon? How do you fast-track someone to X-ray if the junior doctor is not around to sign the request form? Even when everyone is willing in principle, the logistics may be prohibitive. The remainder of this chapter offers ways of unpacking those logistics and the contexts in which they play out.

Let's start by clarifying terminology. Innovation, improvement, and implementation are closely related concepts, but they are not synonymous.

Innovation, Improvement, and Implementation

Innovation

Innovation in healthcare delivery and organisation has been defined as 'a novel set of behaviours, routines, and ways of working that are directed at improving health outcomes, administrative efficiency, cost effectiveness, or users' experience and that are implemented by planned and coordinated actions' (Greenhalgh et al., 2004, p. 582). The defining feature of innovation is *discontinuous* change: It involves something new and different from what has happened up to now. As in the hip fracture care pathway example above, everyone must do something different (or do what they were previously doing more quickly or in a different order), and it all has to be carefully coordinated. The innovation *may* involve a new eHealth technology such as a structured care pathway embedded in the patient's electronic medical record (EMR), which would allow different members of the multidisciplinary team to enter data on their own contribution and see what other professionals are doing for the patient. Such a technology would also – in theory at least – allow key data on performance (such as 'time to first assessment', 'time to operation' and 'length of stay') to be extracted at a later date, aggregated electronically, and presented on digital dashboards for clinical directors and managers to scrutinise.

Improvement

Improvement in healthcare is generally seen as a more organic and continuous process of identifying something to improve, making a change and evaluating its success (Grol et al., 2007), though strictly speaking, innovation is a kind of improvement. In the hip fracture care pathway example, the introduction of a formal care pathway is an *innovation*, but the ongoing work to monitor and further improve how well the pathway is followed (for example by auditing how long the average patient with hip fracture spends in the accident and emergency department before being assessed, how quickly their operation happens, and how long they stay in hospital) will be a year-on-year *improvement effort*. In other words, after the introduction of an innovation, there may need to be a more over-arching, longer improvement process. Hopefully, the quality improvement team will see steady reduction in the metrics chosen to monitor performance.

Implementation

Implementation is the effort put in by individuals, teams and organisations to help the uptake of an innovation or a quality improvement initiative. It consists of things like following through on strategic decisions (e.g., making a purchase of a new eHealth technology or ICT system), introducing the idea of the change to staff (and perhaps patients) and dealing with their concerns, training people to use any new equipment, adjusting work practices and routines, and identifying and applying measures and metrics to evaluate and monitor the change. As a research field, implementation science focuses on "the scientific study of methods to promote the systematic uptake of research findings and other evidence-based practices into routine practice" (Nilsen, 2015, p. 2). For example, it examines how the finding that the length of time in hospital increases mortality from hip fracture can be best 'translated' into faster assessment, throughput, and discharge (while ensuring that patients remain supported) (Graham et al., 2006; Kitson & Straus, 2010).

Complexity

Innovation, improvement and implementation are challenging because of complexity – an inherent feature of modern healthcare. Complexity refers to the extent that phenomena are dynamic, unpredictable, and interdependent with other phenomena (Greenhalgh & Papoutsi, 2018). A *simple* task (one that is entirely predictable and has few interactive components – such as making a sandwich) and a *complicated* task (one that has multiple components but is still largely predictable and can be protocolised – such as building a rocket) are the same kind of problem. But a *complex* task (such as raising a child) is fundamentally different because it cannot be fully captured in a step-by-step protocol. However many guidelines and evidence-based textbooks on child-rearing you have, raising your own particular child will involve unique and unpredictable events and interactions. What worked for your first child may not work for the next.

So, it is with much of healthcare. Some aspects of hip fracture management are identical for every patient, but many aspects have to be tailored to take account of the patient's other illnesses, sociocultural factors (perhaps the patient is a Jehovah's witness who will not accept a blood transfusion), and local contingencies (perhaps the hospital has only one operating theatre; perhaps the surgeon is stuck in traffic; perhaps the hospital formulary does not list the drug of choice). In short, the patient in the guideline never fully corresponds to the patient in the bed. However, advanced the innovation, it has to be implemented in an imperfect world.

Complexity means that well-intentioned changes sometimes seem to worsen the very problems they were introduced to solve. For example, adding in a 'triage' step when a patient wants to book an appointment to see their family physician is *intended* to reduce workload by filtering out people who can safely be given advice to self-manage. But in reality, triage frees up few appointments and may lead to 'triple-handling' (patients receive one phone call to triage their request, another phone call to assess the problem, and then a face-to-face appointment to examine them in person). Another example would be the introduction of internet-based interventions in mental healthcare. While they are designed to save time by allowing the patient to work on parts of their treatment individually, in practice, they often take up more time from the therapist; they must be trained for and get acquainted with the intervention, and they must introduce it to their patients, and help patients who have technical or content-related difficulties with working on these interventions.

Complex healthcare journeys these days involve multiple kinds of digital technologies: to access (or provide a gateway to) care; to assess the patient; to code and bill particular diseases or procedures; to collate and present performance data; to present research findings and support evidence-based decision making; to hasten communication; to coordinate work routines; to bring together different professionals for multidisciplinary team meetings. And technologies bring their own complexities – such as material features (more or less 'clunky' to use), bugs (a piece of software may conflict with something else on the system), access controls (try using a digital device when you've forgotten your password), and the limitations of pull-down menus and algorithms that don't cover the situation you're trying to address.

As we have seen, healthcare is complex, amongst other things because patients are unique; illness plays out in unpredictable ways; both patient and professional behaviour is shaped by social, cultural, and other influences; drugs, devices, and procedures need regulating; organisations have practical and material constraints; resources are not infinite; technologies work in particular ways and sometimes do not work as intended; and so on. Because of this complexity, it's hard enough to get innovations taken up in one setting, such as supporting an outpatient clinic to introduce video consultations. It's even harder to get that same innovation taken up in other settings (such as other clinics in the same hospital or other hospitals in the same or a different country). There are two key processes here. *Spread* refers to the process of implementing innovations in settings beyond those from where they originally emerged or were first adopted, for example, extending video consulting from a single outpatient clinic to different clinical areas or different hospitals (Papoutsi et al., 2023). *Scale-up* focuses on the processes by which the necessary infrastructure is put in place to enable spread in different settings, for example, increasing network bandwidth to enable widespread adoption of video consulting (Papoutsi et al., 2023). Innovations, especially complex ones, require modifications to be implemented successfully elsewhere – such as allocating a larger budget and hiring more staff as part of the spread and scale-up effort (Côté-Boileau et al., 2019).

Sustainability

Sustainability presents another key challenge. An innovation deployed successfully during an initial adoption period may not continue to be used routinely over time and its implementers may revert to their previous ways of working (Lennox et al., 2018). In the hip fracture example, there may be an initial flurry of activity as staff pull together to improve the patient experience and reduce mortality rates, but after months or years, the energy and enthusiasm for this initiative fades and the performance metrics start to slide. This means the improvement effort may not achieve sustainability, which has been defined as '*the continuation of programme or programme components, or the continuation of outcomes, after initial implementation efforts, staff training or funding has ended*' (Braithwaite et al., 2020).

In some cases it is important to sustain an innovation as it was originally conceptualised (in which case the original performance metrics would remain valid), while in other cases it becomes critical to further develop it as new research evidence emerges (in which case, you may need new metrics to define and measure success) (Greenhalgh et al., 2012). In hip fracture management, for example, the original care pathway innovation centred mainly on reducing the time patients spent in the different steps of the care pathway; more recent improvements to the pathway have included novel anticoagulant drugs; advances in anaesthetics for the elderly; and new ways of preventing, detecting and treating delirium (Sermon et al., 2021). Whereas the focus 25 years ago was on promptly treating the fracture itself, new developments have focused on managing common comorbidities – an issue of increasing importance as the population ages.

De-implementation may also be important to discontinue practices that are obsolete, detrimental or do not provide added value (Norton & Chambers, 2020). A recent study examined the impact of de-implementing scoring tools used to assess inpatient falls risk in hospital settings, reverting instead to clinical decision making and judgement. Clinicians had complained that the scoring tool was administratively burdensome and risked overshadowing what they felt was their expert clinical judgement. By comparing fall rates between hospitals sustaining routine use of scoring tools and those that discontinued them, the authors found de-implementation did not lead to inferior outcomes (Morris et al., 2021).

There is no process, formula or checklist that will enable a person or team to ensure that an innovation such as an eHealth technology gets implemented and sustained. But there are several conceptual frameworks that can guide our thinking. The remainder of this chapter looks at three such frameworks. All were designed to address the challenges of complexity when attempting to achieve or evaluate change in a healthcare setting, and all are relevant to planning or evaluating eHealth implementation. All propose thinking through the complexity of the change project in a series of domains. As with child-rearing manuals, these frameworks provide a useful guide on what to think about, but they do not (and cannot) tell you precisely how to handle every eventuality in a complex system.

The Diffusion of Innovations Framework

The original diffusion of innovations *theory* was developed in the 1950s by Everett Rogers, a social psychologist, to explain adoption of innovations by individuals (Rogers, 1995). Rogers studied mainly farmers, who can make their adoption decisions more or less independently. Healthcare staff, on the other hand, work in organisations, which means they have to obey rules and procedures laid down by others. For this reason, Greenhalgh et al (2004) extended Rogers' original model to incorporate organisational and system elements of healthcare innovation. This healthcare-adapted diffusion of innovations *framework* is shown in Figure 13.1. In this section we first introduce Rogers' version of diffusion of innovations and then explain why and how it has been extended for healthcare settings.

The Innovation

The first domain of Figure 13.1 comes from the work of Rogers. In his original diffusion of innovations theory, Rogers proposed six attributes of an innovation – that is, characteristics which, in the perception of potential adopters, explain whether and to what extent adoption will actually happen. These are shown in the first domain ('The Innovation') in Figure 13.1. The first and by far the most important attribute of an innovation is relative advantage: Unless the person believes that

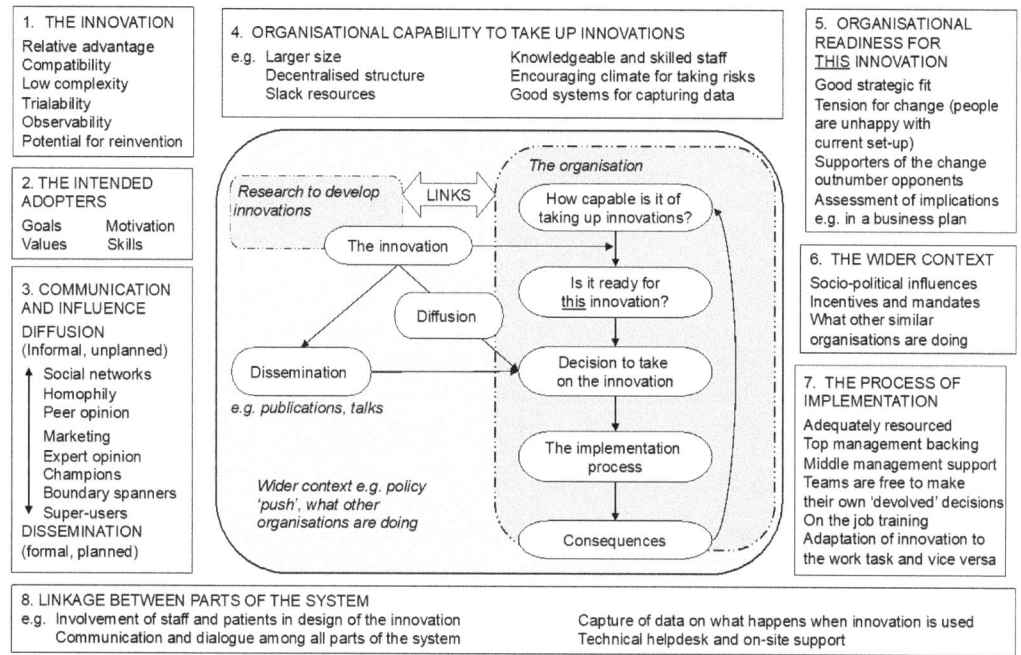

Figure 13.1 Greenhalgh et. al.'s (2004) diffusion of innovations framework for healthcare organisations. The first three domains are from Rogers (1995).

the innovation is *better than what is currently being used*, they will have no incentive to adopt it. Other attributes are also important: Low complexity (is the innovation simple to use?), compatibility (does it align with the person's values and ways of working?), trialability (can it be tried out before committing?), observability (can results be seen?), and potential for reinvention (can it be adapted to better embed it locally?). An example of how Rogers' framework can be used is shown in Box 13.1.

Box 13.1 Example of Rogers' attributes of innovation in practice.

The electronic stethoscope has certain *advantages* over a conventional stethoscope. For example, it reveals murmurs even when the person wearing the stethoscope is unable to hear them, and it allows them to share these data with others. There are some *disadvantages*, however: It's more expensive, more easily damaged, and requires batteries. Different potential users will weigh these pros and cons differently. The electronic stethoscope is also more *complex* (you may have to spend an hour or so learning to use it); it may not be *compatible* with all aspects of your role (for example, if you used it in an exam you might be accused of cheating); you could *try one out* before you buy and *directly observe* the visual representation of the murmur; and it doesn't offer much scope for you to improve its functionality (*reinvention*), so you may find it becomes obsolete as better versions are developed.

The Intended Adopters

The second domain in the diffusion of innovations framework comes also from Rogers' work and refers to the intended adopters. Different people have different propensity to adopt innovations. Rogers' original theory, which he developed during his PhD studies in the 1950s, divided people into 'innovators' (people who are usually the first to adopt something new), 'early adopters' (people who follow soon after), 'early majority' and 'late majority' (most of the rest, who come on board with the trend in their own time) and 'laggards' (who continue to refuse to take up the innovation). Later in his career, Rogers realised that these categories are not fixed personality traits, but dependent on how the person values a particular innovation and any concerns they have about it. A person may be an 'innovator' for one innovation - for example, they may be quick to install WhatsApp on their smartphone and form closed social networking groups, but a 'laggard' for another – for example, they may resist using a novel smartphone app designed to share patient data because they believe it is vulnerable to security breaches. Here is a quote from Rogers' book on this (Rogers, 1995, p. 425):

> *Back in 1954, one of the Iowa farmers that I personally interviewed for my PhD dissertation research rejected all of the chemical innovations that I was then studying: weed sprays, cattle and hog feeds, chemical fertilisers, and a rodenticide. He insisted that his neighbours, who had adopted these chemicals, were killing their songbirds and the earthworms in the soil. I had selected the new farm ideas in my innovativeness scale on the advice of agricultural experts at Iowa State University; I was measuring the best recommended farming practice of that day. The organic farmer in my sample earned the lowest score on my innovativeness scale and was categorised as a laggard.*

With the wisdom of 40 years' hindsight, Rogers reflects that the man he has categorised as a 'laggard' for refusing to adopt intensive farming methods in the 1950s was actually ahead of the pack and an 'innovator' of organic farming methods! The later Rogers rejected pejorative terms such as 'laggard' and became more interested in other characteristics of intended adopters (shown in domain 2 in Figure 13.1) – such as their goals (what do they want to *do* – and will the innovation help them do it?), motivation (what would incentivise them?), values (what do they see as good practice?), and existing skills (are they able to use digital devices for example?).

Communication and Influence

Domain 3 in the diffusion of innovations framework – communication and influence – also comes from Rogers. This domain refers to how the innovation is communicated to its intended audience. He proposed that whilst awareness of innovations is often significantly raised by mass media interventions (hence, the importance of things like branding and public awareness campaigns), actual uptake of innovations among individuals occurs primarily through social influence, where individuals persuade others to adopt the innovation in one of several ways, including acting as peer and expert opinion leaders (respected people whom others seek to copy), champions (people who extol the benefits of an innovation to others, including at board level where decisions are made), boundary-spanners (people who work in two different roles or settings, who can spread ideas between them), and technology 'super-users' who help others develop skills and confidence and act as local troubleshooters.

Domains 4 to 8 in the diffusion of innovations framework were added to Rogers' original model to make this framework more useful for looking at healthcare innovations, which occur in an organisational context (Greenhalgh et al., 2004).

Organisational Capacity to take up Innovations

Domain 4 addresses the organisation's capability of taking up any innovation in general. Features of an organisation that make it more likely to be able to identify and assimilate innovations include its size (large organisations are generally better able to do this than small ones), a decentralised, non-hierarchical structure, slack resources (spare staff and money that can be channelled into the innovation effort), a high proportion of knowledgeable and skilled staff, a climate in which it's OK to take risks (failed initiatives are seen as opportunities to learn rather than reasons to blame and punish), and good systems for capturing data (for example, on the process which the innovation is intended to help with).

Organisational Readiness for this Innovation

Domain 5 addresses organisational readiness for a particular innovation, e.g., a specific eHealth intervention. This domain covers the strategic fit between the innovation and the organisation's mission; tension for change (people are unhappy with the current set-up), perhaps even a sense of urgency (a 'burning platform'), the fact that supporters of the change outnumber opponents and are more strategically placed, and an assessment or business plan that generates confidence that the innovation will be feasible to implement and bring benefits.

The Wider Context

Domain 6 is the wider context, which relates to prevailing socio-political context (for example, whether there is a policy push or indeed policy opposition for the innovation) and also to what other organisations are doing (if they have already adopted the innovation, this serves as a powerful prompt for others to follow).

The Process of Implementation

The 7th domain of the diffusion of innovations framework for healthcare organisations is the process of implementation. Factors shown to be important in this aspect include adequate resourcing (if enough financial and human resources are available for the implementation process), top and middle management support (whether key leaders meaningfully and actively support implementation), devolvement of decision making to local teams (whether implementers have the opportunity to take initiative and make decisions to fit their local circumstances), a hands-on approach to training and implementation (rather than passive adoption), and what has been termed 'tinkering' – adapting the innovation to the work task and vice versa.

Linkage between Parts of the System

Diffusion of innovations is greatly aided by the eighth domain in the framework – linkage: That is, effective and ongoing links between all elements of the innovation process, including user involvement in the design and development of the innovation, good communication and dialogue between different parts of the system, and high-quality data capture to monitor progress.

Box 13.2 shows an example of how the diffusion of innovations framework for healthcare organisations can be used to look at an eHealth innovation.

Box 13.2 Example diffusion of Computed Tomography (CT) scanners.

First used in a London hospital in 1972, CT scanners creating detailed internal images of the body illustrate how the same innovation may be implemented differently in different settings (Robert et al., 2009).

When they were originally introduced, CT scanners had high relative advantage compared to other technologies (they produced much more detailed images, for example). Their results were easily demonstrated and they were compatible with accepted procedures and values of healthcare provision. Yet, they were extremely complex to use and required a specialist skill set. Furthermore, it was not possible to pilot them locally before committing a substantial budget and there was little scope for local adaptation.

Given this complexity, diffusion could not be explained entirely in terms of the attributes of the innovation. Organisational factors and wider context played a significant role. Initially, CT scanners were adopted by large organisations (such as regional referral centres and large hospitals) with an appetite for innovation, available human and financial resources and top management support. Clinicians who championed the technology in these organisations also had external links with industry and the university sector. The wider socio-political environment favoured evidence-based, technological solutions to improve patient care and made financial incentives available, eventually leading to CT scanners becoming the norm across organisations and relevant training becoming part of standard courses.

For a more detailed analysis of the way CT scanners resulted in different interaction patterns and relationships see Barley (1986).

The Consolidated Framework for Implementation Research (CFIR)

Greenhalgh et al.'s diffusion of innovations framework for healthcare was developed in a wide-ranging systematic review which drew heavily on empirical findings from organisational science, at a time before implementation science had emerged as an interdisciplinary field. Five years later, Damschroder et al. (2009) adapted the diffusion of innovations framework by incorporating ideas from the new discipline of implementation science, to form the consolidated framework for implementation research (CFIR). The CFIR synthesises existing theories on effective implementation to present an overarching typology. It has many parallels with the diffusion of innovations framework and incorporates most of its concepts and domains, but as its name implies, it places less emphasis on the process of innovation, for example, developing an interactive portal for patients to record and monitor their blood pressure levels which interfaces with the patient's electronic clinic record). The CFIR focuses more on the process and evaluation of implementation. In other words: The steps needed to inform and engage staff members and mobilise their efforts to get the innovation up and running in the organisation. For example, how will this technology be made 'live' and used in real time, how will staff be trained to navigate and understand the data it generates, and what kind of problems does the IT support helpdesk get asked to resolve. The CFIR framework was recently (in 2022) updated, with version 2.0 including a revised set of constructs explaining implementation successes and failures (Damschroder et al., 2022).

The updated CFIR 2.0 comprises five interacting domains, each underpinned by a number of contextual implementation determinants:

- **Domain 1** covers innovation-related influences on implementation effectiveness, including stakeholder perceptions about the credibility of the innovation, quality of supporting evidence, relative advantage versus alternative solutions, potential for adaptation to local settings, potential for small scale piloting, innovation complexity, design quality and overall cost;
- **Domain 2** covers the outer setting (wider context), including disruptive external events that influence the implementation process, broader sociocultural values, and attitudes (e.g., about

the value of supporting the intended user group), economic or political conditions, partnerships with relevant organisations or entities, external pressures (e.g., societal, market- or performance-related), and relevant policies, regulations, or financial incentives;

- **Domain 3** focuses on the inner (organisational) setting and emphasises such things as structural aspects (e.g., space, infrastructure, division of labour), formal and informal communication channels, shared norms and values, and constructs related to appetite for change, compatibility with existing workflows, innovation importance and relative priority, organisational incentives, evaluation and targets, alignment with wider organisational goals, availability of resources required, and access to relevant information and knowledge to deliver change;
- **Domain 4** places emphasis on organisational actors, including the involvement of individuals with defined roles such as formal and informal leaders at different levels (e.g., high-level leaders, opinion leaders, and implementation leaders), and the extent to which individuals have the need, capability, opportunity, and motivation required to fulfil these roles in the implementation context;
- **Domain 5** covers a series of activities deemed essential as part of the implementation process: Joint working and collaboration including bringing a team together; needs and context assessment to understand the priorities of those involved and the particularities of the setting; planning in terms of devising a course of action; adopting context-sensitive strategies tailored to local circumstances; engaging relevant stakeholders (e.g., implementers and intended innovation users); executing the plan by starting with small steps; reflecting and evaluating (i.e., collecting feedback on whether outcomes have been achieved); and modifying the innovation.

The CFIR can be used to guide planning and evaluation of a change, with a focus on optimising the implementation process and enabling adoption, spread, scale-up and sustainability. As noted by Birken et al. (2017) and Damschroder et al. (2022), the CFIR can also be combined with more specific theories of psychology such as Michie et al.'s theoretical domains framework (2005) (see Chapter 2).

Box 13.3 shows an example of using the CFIR to evaluate a large-scale weight management programme.

Box 13.3 Example evaluation of a large-scale weight management program.

Below we provide an example of a study drawing on the original CFIR framework to demonstrate its logic. The CFIR framework was recently (in 2022) updated, with version 2.0 including a revised set of constructs explaining implementation successes and failures. However, the key domains are unchanged from version 1. At the time of writing, there are no published examples of the application of CFIR 2.0.

In their evaluation of a large-scale weight management programme in Veteran Affairs (VA) medical centres in the US, Damschroder and Lowery (2013) used CFIR to explain variability between sites and identify contextual influences on implementation. They interviewed people in each site, synthesised their narratives into case reports and assigned ratings to different CFIR elements emerging as important in each setting. By comparing and contrasting between settings, they identified patterns that explained different levels of implementation effectiveness.

Of all CFIR elements, those identified as important to successful programme implementation included: Staff perceptions about relative advantage of the innovation compared to alternatives, organisational factors (appetite for change, perceived priority of the innovation compared to other needs, established communication channels, goals and feedback, learning environment, and leadership support) and aspects related to the approach executing the plan and evaluating implementation.

Only some of the CFIR elements played a significant role in this context; others appeared to have a neutral effect, were not applicable (e.g., competitive market forces) or existed equally across sites (e.g., access to materials), therefore could not be used to explain differences in implementation success.

The Nonadoption, Abandonment and Challenges to Scale-up, Spread and Sustainability (NASSS) Framework

The nonadoption, abandonment and challenges to scale-up, spread and sustainability (NASSS) framework (Figure 13.2) was developed as an extension of the diffusion of innovations framework – in this case specifically to address *digital* innovations in a healthcare context (Greenhalgh et al., 2017). eHealth technologies are often viewed as the route to better, safer and more efficient care, but attempts to improve care by introducing an eHealth component to a service rarely deliver all the anticipated benefits. This is usually because the technologies or their associated workflows are too complex – and because the complexity is sub-optimally handled.

NASSS was developed during a large programme of empirical work in which various digital health and social care projects were studied, as a way to guide our narrativizing of the multiple interacting influences that can potentially derail such projects. Both 'heavy' technologies such as major new organisational hardware, such as the servers and terminals for a networked IT system, and 'light' technologies such as smartphone apps were studied, and covered a very wide range of service models and settings (Greenhalgh et al., 2018).

In these case studies and our previous research, it was found that planners and policy makers were usually overly focused on technologies and distracted by simplistic models and metaphors of

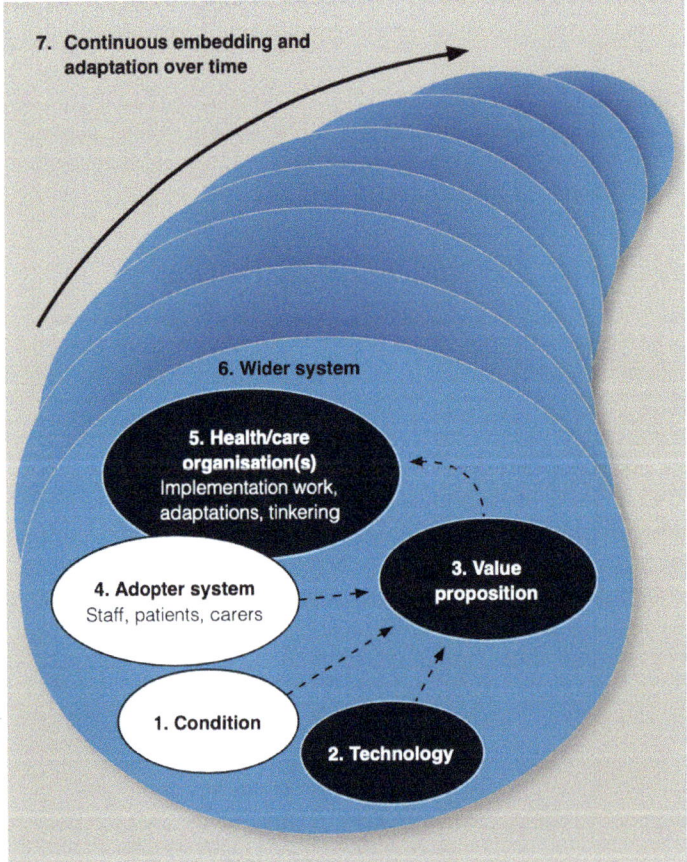

Figure 13.2 The NASSS framework, showing multiple interacting domains affecting the adoption, nonadoption, abandonment, and barriers to scale-up, spread and sustainability of health technologies. Adapted from (Greenhalgh et al., 2017).

technology adoption by individuals (such as the idea of 'innovators' and 'laggards' and an assumed 'tipping point'), or so-called 'technology acceptance models' which centre solely on an individual's decision to adopt a particular technology. They tended to pay much less attention to the dynamic sociotechnical system into which new technologies and care practices must become embedded.

The NASSS framework is designed to identify and explore where complexity (or complexities) lies in a technology project. It has seven interacting domains, described below. Each domain (and the subdomains within it) can be simple (few components, and largely predictable – as in making a sandwich), complicated (multiple components but still largely predictable – as in building a rocket) or complex (dynamic, composed of multiple interacting elements and unpredictable – as in raising a child). This differs per context and innovation.

Complexity in each of the domains of the NASSS framework can be both logistical – relating to such things as scope, scale, deadlines, and resource constraints, or sociopolitical –relating to attitudes, feelings, conflicts of interest or to the particular way a project was set up in the past – for example, who was put in charge and which groups they chose not to consult.

Complexity may also be an emergent feature of a changing system (e.g., a small-to-medium-sized technology provider that responded quickly and flexibly to requests for modifications may be taken over by a large commercial company whose business model is to stick rigidly to contracted transactions).

The Illness or Condition

A simple illness (e.g., sprained ankle) is well characterised and has a clear diagnostic and treatment pathway, so management is predictable and consistent. A complicated illness (e.g., some cancers) requires logistical coordination, but is still predictable to manage. A complex illness (e.g., psychosis, complicated by drug dependency and hepatitis, in an asylum seeker who speaks limited English) is unpredictable and not amenable to management by algorithm. For eHealth technology implementation, this means (for example) that some but not all patients will be able and willing to use the technology as the designers expected – and it may be that as a progressive illness deteriorates, a patient who could initially use the technology becomes unable to.

The Technology

A simple technology (e.g., the traditional stethoscope) is dependable, freestanding, cheap, and substitutable (meaning that if a manufacturer withdrew from the market, you could easily get another one that would do the same job). It is also well designed for the task (including attention to 'human factors'), and it generates data that is easy to interpret and clearly reflects changes in the patient's condition. A complex technology is one that is intended to be widely interoperable across multiple organisations and sectors, or which is less dependable (e.g., keeps crashing) or does not yet exist. And it may generate data that clinicians cannot interpret or do not trust, and/or whose provenance or intellectual property is contested. The implications for health technology implementation are (for example) that a dependable technology with basic functionality is likely to be adopted more widely than one with many 'nice-to-have' features, but which interfaces with multiple other systems, requires advanced training to operate, or only works some of the time.

The Value Proposition

Technologies in development have supply-side value (potential for its developer to make a profit) and demand-side value (benefits to patients and the healthcare provider), also see Chapter 10 on business modelling. A simple value proposition has a robust and well-justified business case and demonstrable benefits in terms of efficacy (it improves survival rates or quality of life), safety (it does not do harm), and cost-effectiveness (the benefits are produced at reasonable cost). In a complex value proposition, the business case for developing the technology is implausible or rests on unverifiable assumptions, and/or the results of research on its efficacy, safety, and cost-effectiveness are unavailable or contested. Those seeking to implement eHealth technologies should produce a clear and plausible business case setting out the anticipated benefits – both financial (e.g., cost savings) and non-financial (e.g., lives saved or improved quality of life).

The Intended Adopters

The most common reason for failure of an eHealth technology is that clinicians do not use it. In a simple situation, intended users (staff and patients/clients and their carers) are able and willing to use the technology and easily trained to do so; using the technology does not upset or threaten them. In a complex situation, intended users lack the capability or willingness to learn to use the technology – perhaps because the technology represents a threat to their professional identity or scope of practice (staff), or symbolises a stigmatising illness (patients/clients). The implication of this domain is that if you want to implement a health technology, you need to find out what people think of it, what their concerns about it are, and whether they believe that it will enhance or diminish their professional role.

The Organisation(s)

In a simple situation, all participating organisations have high capacity to innovate, high tension for change, a good innovation–system fit, formalised links with partner organisations (e.g., an existing subcontract), and a budget that can be allocated to set up and monitor the new technology-supported service. Introducing the technology aligns well with existing work routines, which can be readily adjusted to accommodate them. Things get complex when one or more participating organisations lacks the capacity to innovate, does not wish to change, lacks a partnership agreement, or has no available budget – or when the technology requires significant disruptive changes to hard-wired organisational routines. The implication here is that organisations' capacity to innovate varies and might also differ per innovation, so you should anticipate that things will take longer and require more intensive support in less innovative ones.

The Wider System

The wider system refers to all the forces that are outside the organisation, including other organisations, the economy, the environment, the political and policy context, and public opinion (for example). If this domain is simple, there will be a clear policy push for the technology to be introduced, with relevant levers and incentives. the intended adopter(s) will know and accept that the technology has legal and/or regulatory approval, that it is endorsed by their professional body and that using it is the accepted thing to do. Adopting organisations will share knowledge with other adopting organisations. If the domain is complex, there may be a top-down directive to change, but funding, regulatory or professional bodies may not yet have taken a position on an aspect of the problem, or inter-organisational networking and support may be weak. The implication for eHealth implementation is that if the change is not a policy priority or if regulatory hurdles are not cleared, progress will be slow.

Embedding and Adaptation Over Time

The last domain in the NASSS framework is how things evolve and adapt (or not) over time. In a simple situation, the technology and the care pathway are (to some extent) adaptable and future-proof, and the organisation has a high degree of resilience to external shocks and setbacks. In a complex situation, the technology and service model are implemented rigidly and mechanically by an organisation that lacks resilience. In the latter case, even if a programme is successfully implemented in the short term, its long-term survival (i.e., sustainability) is unlikely. The implication of this domain is that an eHealth technology that is adopted and embedded *today* may become obsolete or less of a priority in a few months or years' time, hence if it's possible to build in potential for adaptation as needs change, you should.

The Added Value of the NASSS Framework

Given that healthcare is inherently complex, how can the NASSS framework help us improve the success of eHealth technology projects?

First, those developing new technologies or seeking to implement them in a healthcare setting should resist the temptation to address an oversimplified version of the problem. Technology developers and those who plan to use technologies need to acknowledge and explore complexity in all seven domains of the NASSS framework. We have developed a NASSS complexity assessment tool (NASSS-CAT) (see ENASS-CAT, 2023) based on the domains above to help generate a narrative of where the key complexities lie (Greenhalgh et al., 2020; Greenhalgh & Papoutsi, 2021).

Second, it is crucial to try to reduce complexity wherever possible. It is important, for example, to carefully consider the trade-off between nice-to-have features, such as interoperability across multiple domains, and the potential knock-on effects of such interoperability in other parts of the system.

Third, remember that complex projects are inherently unpredictable so front-line staff should not be held too rigidly to protocols. Rather, support team members to respond creatively and adaptively to the complexity that emerges in their day-to-day work. Other chapters in this book address interdisciplinary cooperation and teamwork, which are also highly relevant (see Chapter 7).

Box 13.4 gives a worked example of using the NASSS framework.

Box 13.4 Example implementation and spread of technology-based heart failure monitoring.

The NASSS framework underpinned our qualitative process evaluation of a remote monitoring programme aiming to optimise treatment for patients with heart failure in the UK (2016–2018) (Papoutsi et al., 2020). In the context of a clinical trial, patients used networked devices to measure their blood pressure, heart rate and weight, and submitted these measurements along with responses to a daily symptom checker for review by a clinical support team.

NASSS enabled us to surface how various aspects of this technology-based heart failure monitoring programme were complex rather than just simple or complicated. The illness domain highlighted how those with severe heart failure or co-morbidities found it more difficult to engage with the devices. The technology domain pointed to the system described as usable, but occasionally malfunctioning and facing synchronisation issues, which had to be resolved through careful set-up and workarounds. The value proposition remained uncertain in the context of the clinical trial, and trade-offs had to be made between improving functionality and containing cost. Intended adopters, such as some patients, found the system reassuring although it did not always fit in their routines, but healthcare staff had to negotiate new roles and responsibilities in the context of algorithmically driven care. Implementation of technology-based heart failure care across organisations proved variable due to differences in local service models, healthcare team composition, and capacity, among other factors. The wider system was favourable in terms of policy appetite for remote, data-driven care, but underlying infrastructures such as inadequate network coverage limited the scope of the programme. Over time, staffing changes and fluctuations in patients' health status affected the way the system was operationalised.

Informed by the NASSS framework, this analysis complemented the findings of the clinical trial, and extended an understanding of intersecting implementation challenges.

A Reflection on Implementation Frameworks

In this chapter we have introduced a number of key concepts: innovation, improvement and implementation, complexity, spread, scale-up and sustainability. We have also presented three frameworks, each produced at a different time for a slightly different purpose and with a different focus, alongside worked examples. The Diffusion of Innovations framework was originally developed in 2004 in relation to organisational innovation and has been used extensively also in eHealth research Yet, it does not fully account for the specificities of clinical contexts or contemporary digital innovations. The CFIR, originally published in 2009, explicitly adapts and builds on the Diffusion of Innovation framework, incorporating learning from the new discipline of implementation science and the psychology of adoption. The NASSS framework, published in 2017, specifically accounts for complexity in *digital* technology implementation in healthcare, and includes consideration of value proposition -both to innovation users and technology developers.

Each of these frameworks covers a comprehensive range of interacting influences on implementation, spread and scale-up. They can be used in more or less flexible ways, depending on the purpose and methodological approach of each study. They are not static frameworks to be applied prescriptively but act as sensitising devices to help explain complex data and guide thinking around innovation. When using these frameworks, it is important to reflect both on aspects that worked well and aspects that had to be adapted to better suit the study in question.

These are by no means the only frameworks or theoretical models for considering innovation, improvement, spread, scale-up and sustainability. Côté-Boileau et al (2019) described a set of *enabling conditions* for spread, scale-up and sustainability including: innovation adaptability, distributed leadership, reciprocal accountability relations, context receptive to change, iterative timing and pace, empowering management support, and decentralised governance. They and others have identified additional contributing factors including perceived feasibility and added value of the innovation, involvement of champions embedded in local teams or organisational structures; and alignment with organisational priorities and routines (Albury et al., 2020; Côté-Boileau et al., 2019). We developed the PERCS (planning and evaluating remote consultations) framework as a specific adaptation of NASSS to study remote clinical consultations by telephone and video (Greenhalgh et al., 2021).

The point about all these frameworks and theoretical concepts is that innovation and change in healthcare are complex processes which need to be explored through multiple lenses and at multiple levels. We can't just do what Rogers did with the farmers he studied and look at the individual adoption decision, because decisions in healthcare are shaped and constrained by organisational and institutional factors.

Summary

Spread, scale-up and sustainability processes are interlinked and mutually reinforcing. They need to be considered in tandem to ensure innovations implemented across settings are underpinned by the infrastructure required and there is potential for sustained use and measurable outcomes (Papoutsi et al., 2023). The take-home message of this chapter is that these processes cannot be planned neatly and structured from the outset, given the complexity of healthcare. We need to stop thinking mechanistically about *building* innovations (a mechanical metaphor which places too little emphasis on the interaction between the innovation and its context) and place more emphasis on *growing* them organically in particular contexts (Norton & Chambers, 2020).

- Spread, scale-up and sustainability processes are interlinked and mutually reinforcing;
- They need to be considered in tandem to ensure innovations implemented across settings are underpinned by the infrastructure required and there is potential for sustained use and measurable outcomes;

- Given the complexity of healthcare, the introduction, spread and scale-up of eHealth innovations cannot be planned neatly and structured from the outset;
- We need to stop thinking mechanistically about *building* innovations (a mechanical metaphor which places too little emphasis on the interaction between the innovation and its context) and place more emphasis on *growing* them organically in particular contexts.

Key References for Further Reading

Damschroder, L. J., Aron, D. C., Keith, R. E., Kirsh, S. R., Alexander, J. A., & Lowery, J. C. (2009). Fostering implementation of health services research findings into practice: A consolidated framework for advancing implementation science. *Implementation Science*, 4(1), 1–15.

Greenhalgh, T., Robert, G., Macfarlane, F., Bate, P., & Kyriakidou, O. (2004). Diffusion of innovations in service organizations: Systematic review and recommendations. *The Milbank Quarterly*, 82(4), 581–629. https://doi.org/10.1111/j.0887-378X.2004.00325.x

Greenhalgh, T., Wherton, J., Papoutsi, C., Lynch, J., Hughes, G., A'Court, C., Hinder, S., Fahy, N., Procter, R., & Shaw, S. (2017). Beyond adoption: A new framework for theorizing and evaluating nonadoption, abandonment, and challenges to the scale-up, spread, and sustainability of health and care technologies. *J Med Internet Res*, 19(11), e367.

Papoutsi, C., Greenhalgh, T., & Marjanovic, S. (2023). Approaches to sustainability and scaling up in healthcare improvement. In M. Dixon-Woods (Ed.), Great big book of improvement studies. University of Cambridge.

Rogers, E. M. (1995). *Diffusion of innovations*. Free Press.

References

Albury, D., Beresford, T., Dew, S., Horton, T., Illingworth, J., & Langford, K. (2020). Against the odds: Successfully scaling innovation in the NHS. NHS Innovation Unit and Health Foundation. Accessed July 22, 2022 at https://www.health.org.uk/publications/against-the-odds-successfully-scaling-innovation-in-the-nhs.

Barley, S. R. (1986). Technology as an occasion for structuring: Evidence from observations of CT scanners and the social order of radiology departments. *Administrative Science Quarterly*, 78–108.

Birken, S. A., Powell, B. J., Presseau, J., Kirk, M. A., Lorencatto, F., Gould, N. J., Shea, C. M., Weiner, B. J., Francis, J. J., & Yu, Y. (2017). Combined use of the Consolidated Framework for Implementation Research (CFIR) and the Theoretical Domains Framework (TDF): A systematic review. *Implementation Science*, 12(1), 1–14.

Braithwaite, J., Ludlow, K., Testa, L., Herkes, J., Augustsson, H., Lamprell, G., McPherson, E., & Zurynski, Y. (2020). Built to last? The sustainability of healthcare system improvements, programmes and interventions: A systematic integrative review. *BMJ Open,* 10(6), e036453.

Côté-Boileau, É., Denis, J.-L., Callery, B., & Sabean, M. (2019). The unpredictable journeys of spreading, sustaining and scaling healthcare innovations: A scoping review. *Health Research Policy and Systems*, 17(1), 1–26.

Damschroder, L., Reardon, C. M., Widerquist, M. A. O., & Lowery, J. C. (2022). The updated Consolidated Framework for Implementation Research: CFIR 2.0. Preprint available: https://assets.researchsquare.com/files/rs-1581880/v1/556132ae-5de7-4902-9c33-9085ebca9d89.pdf?c=1651077534

Damschroder, L. J., Aron, D. C., Keith, R. E., Kirsh, S. R., Alexander, J. A., & Lowery, J. C. (2009). Fostering implementation of health services research findings into practice: A consolidated framework for advancing implementation science. *Implementation Science*, 4(1), 1–15.

Damschroder, L. J., & Lowery, J. C. (2013). Evaluation of a large-scale weight management program using the consolidated framework for implementation research (CFIR). *Implementation Science*, 8, 1–17.

ENASS-CAT. (2023). Retrieved from https://www.phc.ox.ac.uk/research/interdisciplinary-research-in-health-sciences/enasss-cat/enasss-cat.

Graham, I. D., Logan, J., Harrison, M. B., Straus, S. E., Tetroe, J., Caswell, W., & Robinson, N. (2006). Lost in knowledge translation: Time for a map? *Journal of Continuing Education in the Health Professions*, 26(1), 13–24.

Greenhalgh, T., Macfarlane, F., Barton-Sweeney, C., & Woodard, F. (2012). "If we build it, will it stay?" A case study of the sustainability of whole-system change in London. *Milbank Quarterly*, 90(3), 516–547. https://doi.org/10.1111/j.1468-0009.2012.00673.x

Greenhalgh, T., Maylor, H., Shaw, S., Wherton, J., Papoutsi, C., Betton, V., Nelissen, N., Gremyr, A., Rushforth, A., Koshkouei, M., & Taylor, J. (2020). The NASSS-CAT tools for understanding, guiding, monitoring, and researching technology implementation projects in health and social care: Protocol for an evaluation study in real-world settings. *JMIR Res Protoc*, 9(5), e16861. https://doi.org/10.2196/16861

Greenhalgh, T., & Papoutsi, C. (2018). Studying complexity in health services research: Desperately seeking an overdue paradigm shift. In (Vol. 16, pp. 95): *BioMed Central*.

Greenhalgh, T., & Papoutsi, C. (2021). What are the NASSS-CAT tools? Universiy of Oxford. Accessed July 22, 2022 at https://www.phc.ox.ac.uk/research/interdisciplinary-research-in-health-sciences/enasss-cat/enasss-cat.

Greenhalgh, T., Robert, G., Macfarlane, F., Bate, P., & Kyriakidou, O. (2004). Diffusion of innovations in service organizations: Systematic review and recommendations. *Milbank Quarterly*, 82(4), 581–629. https://doi.org/10.1111/j.0887-378X.2004.00325.x

Greenhalgh, T., Rosen, R., Shaw, S. E., Byng, R., Faulkner, S., Finlay, T., Grundy, E., Husain, L., Hughes, G., Leone, C., Moore, L., Papoutsi, C., Pope, C., Rybczynska-Bunt, S., Rushforth, A., Wherton, J., Wieringa, S., & Wood, G. W. (2021). Planning and evaluating remote consultation services: A new conceptual framework incorporating complexity and practical ethics [hypothesis and theory]. *Frontiers in Digital Health*, 3(103). https://doi.org/10.3389/fdgth.2021.726095

Greenhalgh, T., Wherton, J., Papoutsi, C., Lynch, J., Hughes, G., A'Court, C., Hinder, S., Fahy, N., Procter, R., & Shaw, S. (2017). Beyond adoption: A new framework for theorizing and evaluating nonadoption, abandonment, and challenges to the scale-up, spread, and sustainability of health and care technologies. *J Med Internet Res*, 19(11), e367. https://doi.org/10.2196/jmir.8775

Greenhalgh, T., Wherton, J., Papoutsi, C., Lynch, J., Hughes, G., Hinder, S., Procter, R., & Shaw, S. (2018). Analysing the role of complexity in explaining the fortunes of technology programmes: Empirical application of the NASSS framework. *BMC Medicine*, 16(1), 66.

Grol, R. P., Bosch, M. C., Hulscher, M. E., Eccles, M. P., & Wensing, M. (2007). Planning and studying improvement in patient care: The use of theoretical perspectives. *Milbank Quarterly*, 85(1), 93–138.

Kitson, A., & Straus, S. E. (2010). The knowledge-to-action cycle: Identifying the gaps. *CMAJ*, 182(2), E73–77. https://doi.org/10.1503/cmaj.081231

Leigheb, F., Vanhaecht, K., Sermeus, W., Lodewijckx, C., Deneckere, S., Boonen, S., Boto, P. A. F., Mendes, R. V., & Panella, M. (2012). The effect of care pathways for hip fractures: A systematic review. *Calcified Tissue International*, 91, 1–14.

Lennox, L., Maher, L., & Reed, J. (2018). Navigating the sustainability landscape: A systematic review of sustainability approaches in healthcare. *Implementation Science*, 13(1), 1–17.

Michie, S., Johnston, M., Abraham, C., Lawton, R., Parker, D., & Walker, A. (2005). Making psychological theory useful for implementing evidence based practice: A consensus approach. *BMJ Quality & Safety*, 14(1), 26–33.

Morris, M. E., Haines, T., Hill, A. M., Cameron, I. D., Jones, C., Jazayeri, D., . . . & McPhail, S. M. (2021). Divesting from a scored hospital fall risk assessment tool (FRAT): A cluster randomized non-inferiority trial. *Journal of the American Geriatrics Society*, 69(9), 2598–2604.

Nilsen, P. (2015). Making sense of implementation theories, models and frameworks. *Implement Science*, 10, 53. https://doi.org/10.1186/s13012-015-0242-0

Norton, W. E., & Chambers, D. A. (2020). Unpacking the complexities of de-implementing inappropriate health interventions. *Implementation Science*, 15(1), 1–7.

Papoutsi, C., Greenhalgh, T., & Marjanovic, S. (2023). Approaches to sustainability and scaling up in healthcare improvement. In M. Dixon-Woods (Ed.), *Great big book of improvement studies*. University of Cambridge.

Rogers, E. M. (1995). *Diffusion of innovations*. Free Press.

Sermon, A., Slock, C., Coeckelberghs, E., Seys, D., Panella, M., Bruyneel, L., Nijs, S., Akiki, A., Castillon, P., & Chipperfield, A. (2021). Quality indicators in the treatment of geriatric hip fractures: Literature review and expert consensus. *Archives of Osteoporosis*, 16(1), 152.

14 Sustainable eHealth Implementation

A Practical Perspective

Marcel Pieterse, Annemarie Braakman-Jansen,
Roberto R. Cruz Martinez, & Lisette (J.E.W.C.) van
Gemert-Pijnen

Introduction

Implementation of healthcare innovations is widely acknowledged as a highly complex process involving a variety of factors on multiple levels (Glasgow, Phillips, & Sanchez, 2014; Ross et al., 2016; Greenhalgh et al., 2017; van Gemert-Pijnen, 2022), as is shown in Chapter 13 of this book. Effective implementation entails much more than the mere launch of a self-management app for patients, a patient website, or a multi-user digital platform. It requires thorough and timely systematic attention for the implications of technology-mediated services for individuals, healthcare, and the society at large.

Sustainable implementation of technologies must deal with multiple factors as resources (e.g., time, staff, budget, investment policies), ethical concerns (privacy, security, ownership), governance (policy, accountability, responsibility etc.), and eSkills of users (capabilities, culture, etc.). Although many of these factors apply to healthcare innovations in general, some factors are particularly relevant in the context of eHealth, such as stakeholder involvement, interdisciplinary collaboration, and financial viability.

This chapter discusses eHealth implementation from a practical perspective focussing on factors that play a role when integrating technologies in healthcare practices and upscaling such technologies to the market. IT builds on Chapter 13 and is connected to Chapter 10, on business modelling. After completing this chapter, you will be able to:

- Explain the complexity of eHealth implementation in practice;
- Understand and explain implementation factors that play a role in integrating eHealth in practice and upscaling to the market;
- Identify potential barriers for sustained implementation, in particular related to stakeholder engagement, financing, business modelling, and law and regulations;
- Identify points for improvement of implementation in practice and market.

eHealth Implementation from a Practical Perspective

Implementation has been explained in Chapter 13 as 'the effort put in by individuals, teams and organizations to help the uptake of an innovation or a quality improvement initiative'. In this chapter we focus on process of several planned and guided activities to launch, introduce, and maintain health technologies in practice to innovate or improve healthcare (Pieterse et al., 2018;

DOI: 10.4324/9781003302049-16

van Gemert-Pijnen, 2022). These activities deliver the evidence for adopting and upscaling a technology in healthcare practices. No one size fits all solutions exist, no step-by-step guidelines or protocols can be followed to guarantee success of implementation (Norton & Chambers, 2020 in Chapter 13). However, we can learn from barriers and facilitators experienced in several practices to identify a set of principles to guide the implementation process. The following lessons can be learned from practice.

Implementation entails Value Proposition and Business Modelling

Implementation starts with activities to get insights in the risks and factors that can influence the uptake and adoption. Therefore, systematic attention should be given to the implications for individuals, health care, and society at large. Potential implementation issues such as limited resources (e.g., time, staff, and money), ethics (privacy, security, dependency, cultural diversity), or individual barriers (e.g., lacking skills, or reluctance to change) should be identified. These issues should also be accounted for in the subsequent cycles of development like value proposition, and business modelling (see Chapter 10).

Box 14.1 demonstrates the pitfall of disregarding value proposition and business modelling during the early stage of development, caused by a lack of proper stakeholder involvement.

Box 14.1 Case Study 1: The implementation of an evidence-based smoking cessation app.

A smoking cessation mobile application was developed with a grant from the Dutch National Research funding organization (NWO). The development team consisted of experts from four institutes: Two regional health care organizations (an addiction treatment organization and a local hospital), and two research institutes. The initial goal was to develop the app as an add-on for healthcare organizations' existing smoking cessation services. However, budget limitations did not allow full integration into their digital platforms. Instead, a standalone mobile app was built, targeting individual smokers. The team did not reconsider the stakeholders to be involved, at this stage, though.

The app entails a self-management tool to educate and support smokers in preparing for and during their quitting process, without counsellor guidance. Multiple evidence-based behaviour change techniques (see also Chapter 2) were included to shape knowledge and skills: Psycho-education, self-monitoring, feedback, goal setting, coping planning, habit reversal, peer support, and reward strategies. Complementary to these behavioural techniques, numerous persuasive techniques (see also Chapter 12) to optimize user experience were added, like personalization, reminders, praise, and tunnelling. The app was carefully tested among users in an iterative user-centred design process, in accordance with the CeHRes Roadmap as described in Chapter 7.

The app was released in the app stores and made publicly available for free, without budget dedicated to a pro-active dissemination strategy, the yearly maintenance costs were carried by the four partners. During the years that followed, a study performed in 2020 (Van den Berg et al., 2021) revealed that in total 6400 smokers had downloaded the app, of which about 400 smokers actively used the app during a quit attempt. The app was actively offered to clients by a few organizations at local level. Two of the four partner organizations, e.g., the addiction treatment organization and the hospital, initially used the app as a voluntary part of their smoking cessation service. However, the existing tariff structure for health care providers offering smoking cessation services, as issued by the Dutch national government,

the ones that tell the developers the kind of virtual environments that have to be to be developed, the environments that are relevant for treatment of several diseases. We consider the feasibility of these requests according to the capacity of the current software and hardware, and constantly communicate with the researchers while doing this. By following this approach, we have succeeded in developing complex and detailed interactive environments. It is also important to discuss the limitations in the financial requirements that are necessary to support development and implementation of innovations. It is important to focus on communication, providing clear information about the costs, validity and effectiveness of a VR technology.

Yme Canter Visscher, CleVR (The Netherlands)

Legislation, Regulation, Ethics

When implementing eHealth, compliance to law and regulations for security of data exchange is required. Besides, ethics play a role concerning inclusiveness, diversity, transparency, and unintended patient safety risks due to technology-induced errors or privacy concerns. For example, regarding the privacy of patients online. As case study 3 illustrated, the certification process of AI tools is time demanding as current rules for certification are not sufficiently specified, not directive enough, and require a large number of documents. Laws and regulations could be clearer about requirements for AI models and clearer about what transparency means to ensure privacy, security, and ethics.

In the following example, a dilemma involving the balance between safety and privacy concerns is illustrated.

When safety comes before privacy

Dealing online with patients with depression, our web-based CBT-based platform every now and then required different actions to assess or continue to support the well-being of the programme participants. The platform applied rigorous protocols about how to proceed in every possible scenario. However, in extreme cases sometimes decisions had to be made to, for example, take a more direct approach in reaching possibly suicidal patients that seemed to be at risk and could not be reached through the usual technology channels. This often was not completely consistent with the protocols but was a match with the aim of our platform to look out for the well-being of our users and was appreciated in the end.

Gavin Andrews, University of New South Wales, Sydney (Australia)

Another issue is dealing with data during and after implementation. In the beginning, developers should plan what standards they have to use and how they will store the data gathered by eHealth interventions and determine who can use and re-use the data (according to the Health Data Space Act). The following expert explains what dealing with this issue may entail.

What to do with data?

Long-term storage, archiving and standardization regarding data collected by eHealth technology will be necessary. This also requires funding and regulations to be instituted to allow future generations to make use of the data and knowledge. A decision between close and open access in the case of a technical device or technology could be significant when considering how to deal with data. Open access would mean the data can be freely used by anyone, even in unrelated contexts or fields and sometimes even opposed to the main interests of the creators of such innovation. As long as another party complies with the conditions of use, such as citing the authors, they would not need explicit permission and can make legal use of the data. But imagine, for instance, that data collected by these external parties is used in a harmful way, harming the privacy of the users. The name of the authors of this technology would then be openly linked to this. Therefore, sometimes even the obligation for written permission can be appropriate and required.

Claus-Peter Rückemann, Universität Münster, Unabhängiges Deutsches Institut für Multi-disziplinäre Forschung (DIMF), Leibniz Universität Hannover (Germany)

Chapter 1 of this book pointed out some major ethical issues that should be accounted for during implementation. Practice shows that not all ethical issues are similarly applicable to every eHealth technology, since a wearable might raise other ethical concerns than an online module for depression, or an AI tool to be used for clinical decision making. When implementing eHealth, it is essential to adhere to current rules and regulations. The increasingly demanding regulations also have financial consequences for eHealth implementation, as shown in case study 1: The initial aim to build a smoking cessation app that can be integrated into the highly secured electronic patient environment of addiction treatment providers, was abandoned due to insufficient funding.

Business Modelling and how to Finance eHealth Technology

Implementation of technology often fails due to a lack of a sound business case, and lack of reimbursement by the insurance company. Business modelling with stakeholders to set requirements for financing and investment is needed to overcome these implementation hurdles, see Chapter 10.

Follow the money
You really have to understand how the money flows, and take into account how that will influence the whole development process of your technology. You might have to ask yourself 'Who will pay for this?' and consider the possibility that, at the beginning, no one will. However, that is not necessarily a reason to not do it. In the end, you might have to connect your solution to other products or sources that might have a more immediate monetary value.

Jan Hendrik Croockewit, Nedap N.V. (The Netherlands)

Long-term financing is critical for maintaining and upscaling of a technology. Grants or other ways of funding often lack a sufficient time span to allow innovation to fully mature, as was illustrated in case three on innovative AI. Health care organizations usually are unable to carry such costs. Investments and upscaling therefore require cooperation between hospital, IT supplier, health insurers, and government.

The next example illustrates how to cope with finding funding for an eHealth start-up and shows that a long-term perspective is required.

Perseverance is important
We have learned that our efforts have to be focused on good communication with possible funding parties, providing them with clear information about the costs, validity and effectiveness of our solution. For our platform, this communication is happening on three fronts: with mental health clinics, health insurance companies and the government. Unfortunately, these institutions are part of a system that often doesn't yet allow enough financial support for innovative eHealth technologies. This is a situation that has to be coped with on a higher level rather than something that can be changed by a single firm, so we are aware it might take years of efforts. Hence, together with research partners, we continuously aim to present a case that provides enough evidence about the economic value and advantages of our technology in order to convince potential funders of the importance of investing in eHealth platforms.

Pim Spoor & Oscar van Dijk, MedicineMen (The Netherlands)

In practice, creating long-term value of eHealth is often a complex task, partly because all key stakeholders have to agree on and commit to a plan to create this value, and this is often not the case, as they can have conflicting values. Creating a plan to achieve this value also requires some flexibility on the developers' side.

Another way of creating value is by not merely looking at value from a financial perspective. Value can also be defined in other terms, for example, increased quality of care, or improved well-being of patients. Furthermore, the data that are collected by technologies can be extremely valuable, directly or for later re-use (see the Health Data Space Act), even though at the moment the value of data is not enough to keep a technology sustainable. This is an important issue to keep in mind before, during, and after implementation. The value of data is further explained by an information systems and natural sciences expert in the next case.

Something important to consider is that the real value of data can only truly be established in the long term. For example by revisiting it with new research methods that reveal novel findings, or by accumulating it as part of a global knowledge base. Indeed, data is often the real value, not the application itself. This means, for instance, that data should at least be worth more than the costs that were required to compute it. That's the starting point, and even then, the real value might only be visible after years of use, depending on the context of the project of course. Consequently, in long-term projects, continuity between generations of researchers is important to consider because of this. A consistent idea of the value of data must be transmitted by the heads of research institutes or teams to the rest of the professionals working with them. Long-term storage, archiving and standardization regarding data will be necessary, allowing future generations to make use of the data and knowledge.

Claus-Peter Rückemann, Universität Münster, Unabhängiges Deutsches Institut für Multi-disziplinäre Forschung (DIMF), Leibniz Universität Hannover (Germany)

It can be concluded that it is important to account for financing of an eHealth technology right from the start. Again, several methods can be used to achieve this, and an example that has been proven to be of added value for eHealth development is *business modelling* (see Chapter 10). It assists the development team in determining important matters for implementation such as the intended value of a technology, its customers, resources, cost structures, and potential customers/users.

Towards Sustainable Implementation of eHealth Technology

Several models and frameworks are published to understand the processes and driving factors involved in implementation, and to predict outcomes (Greenhalgh et al., 2017). These frameworks and models have different perspectives. For example, frameworks like, RE-AIM Framework (Glasgow, Vogt, & Boles, 1999), and Consolidated Framework for Implementation Research (Damschröder et al., 2009) were introduced to implement clinical and medical based interventions using evidence from research findings. These frameworks express the acceptance and adoption of research findings in practice. In this view, implementation refers to a set of planned, intentional activities that aim to apply evidence-based practices in real-world services, with the goal to benefit end-users of these services. However, these frameworks yet fail to identify the factors that influence integration of a technology in real-world practice and upscaling it to the market.

Towards a sustainable implementation, integration of the evidence-based advanced frameworks for implementation (Chapter 13) on the one hand, with practice-based know-how on the other, is pivotal. Such integrative knowledge can be translated into dynamic factors to guide the process of implementation. A practical assessment tool that may serve this integrative purpose is currently under construction. This SHTi tool (Stimulate Health Technology implementation; Lindenberg et al., 2022) intends to support stakeholders to make judgements and to set priorities to enable long-term viability and upscaling. For example, in cooperation with relevant stakeholders the SHTi tool can be used to assess and discuss the following factors:

- Project management (ownership, responsibilities for a technology, innovation);
- Infrastructure (is the innovation prepared for a technology, regarding logistics, time, staff, budget, efforts?);
- Value proposition (what are the added values to achieve, form perspective of different stakeholders?);
- System requirements (what is needed considering interoperability, certifications, what are the (technical) risks and ethical considerations regarding a technology?);
- Law and regulations (what are the legal, ethical, and technical considerations regarding implementation of a technology?);
- Business impact (what are the expected effects compared to current practice? What are the costs-benefits for healthcare, staff?);
- Economic aspects (is a technology affordable, sustainable considering stakeholders and market?);
- Effectiveness (what are the effects on healthcare; outcomes, state of the art, research designs, pre-clinical validation etc.?; What are the impacts on market, population size, value proposition, competition?).

The outcomes of the assessment can be reported using data visualization techniques, (e.g., cobweb) to discuss with stakeholders the next steps for implementation.

In the future, similar tools need to be developed to extend the practical validity of the NASSS Framework as presented in Chapter 13.

Summary

This chapter has shown that:

- Effectively planning successful implementation of an eHealth innovation requires an agile and iterative, human-centred development approach that enables early stakeholder involvement, interdisciplinary collaboration, and business modelling;
- Management and maintenance of an eHealth technology requires a long-lasting budget, adequate infrastructure for support, and clear agreements on ownership and responsibilities for a technology;
- eHealth implementation, in particular of complex data-driven systems, goes beyond single organizations, across care domains (hospital, public health, primary care, home care), and this requires interoperability of systems, and alignment with law and regulations. This also makes governance a key factor;
- Implementation is also related to the vision one holds of eHealth technology; some regard this as an innovation, others merely as a device or tool, and nowadays eHealth often refers to a network of interconnected services, to data driven and integrated care systems. This all impacts the approach that is taken towards eHealth implementation.

Acknowledgements

We are very grateful for the contribution of the following expert interviewees to this chapter:

- Claus-Peter Rückemann, Universität Münster, Unabhängiges Deutsches Institut für Multidisziplinäre Forschung (DIMF), Leibniz Universität Hannover (Germany);

- Gavin Andrews, University of New South Wales Sydney (Australia);
- Harry Nienhuis[†] (Menzis (The Netherlands);
- Jan Hendrik Croockewit, Nedap (The Netherlands);
- Pim Spoor & Oscar van Dijk, MedicineMen (The Netherlands);
- Yme Canter Visscher, CleVR (The Netherlands).

Key References for Further Reading

Glasgow, R. E., Phillips, S. M., & Sanchez, M. A. (2014). Implementation science approaches for integrating eHealth research into practice and policy. *International Journal of Medical Informatics*, 83(7), e1–11.

Nilsen, E. R., Stendal, K., & Gullslett, M. K. (2020). Implementation of eHealth technology in community health care: The complexity of stakeholder involvement. *BMC Health Services Research*, 20(1), 395. https://doi.org/10.1186/s12913-020-05287-2

Van Gemert-Pijnen, J. E. W. C. (2022). Implementation of health technology: Directions for research and practice. *Front. Digit. Health*, 4, 1030194. doi: 10.3389/fdgth.2022.1030194

Van Limburg, M., van Gemert-Pijnen, J. E., Nijland, N., Ossebaard, H. C., Hendrix, R. M., & Seydel, E. R. (2011). Why business modeling is crucial in the development of eHealth technologies. *Journal of Medical Internet Research*, 13(4).

Van Woezik, A. F., Braakman-Jansen, L. M., Kulyk, O., Siemons, L., & van Gemert-Pijnen, J. E. (2016). Tackling wicked problems in infection prevention and control: A guideline for co-creation with stakeholders. *Antimicrobial Resistance and Infection Control*, 5, 20. https://doi.org/10.1186/s13756-016-0119-2

References

Cantrell, J., Ganz, O., Ilakkuvan, V., Tacelosky, M., Kreslake, J., Moon-Howard, J., . . . Kirchner, T. R. (2015). Implementation of a multimodal mobile system for point-of-sale surveillance: Lessons learned from case studies in Washington, DC, and New York City. *JMIR Public Health and Surveillance*, 1(2), e20.

Damschroder, L. J., Aron, D. C., Keith, R. E., Kirsh, S. R., Alexander, J. A., & Lowery, J. C., (2009). Fostering implementation of health services research findings into practice: A consolidated framework for advancing implementation science. *Implementation Science*, 4, 50

EU AI Act. (2021). Retrieved from https://www.europarl.europa.eu/RegData/etudes/BRIE/2021/698792/EPRS_BRI(2021)698792_EN.pdf

European General Data Protection Regulation (EU GDPR) 2016/679. (2016). *Official Journal of the European Union (OJ)*. Retrieved from https://gdpr-info.eu/ https://eur-lex.europa.eu/eli/reg/2016/679/oj

European Health Data Space Act. (2023). Retrieved from https://health.ec.europa.eu/ehealth-digital-health-and-care/european-health-data-space_en

European Medical Devices Regulation (EU MDR), Regulation (EU) 2017/745. (2017). *Official Journal of the European Union (OJ)*. Retrieved from https://eur-lex.europa.eu/eli/reg/2017/745/oj

Feldman, S. S., Schooley, L. B., & Bhavsar, P. G. (2014). Health information exchange implementation: Lessons learned and critical success factors from a case study. *JMIR Med Inform*, 2(2), e19.

Glasgow, R. E., Vogt, T. M., & Boles, S. M. (1999). Evaluating the public health impact of health promotion interventions: The RE-AIM framework. *American Journal of Public Health*, 89(9), 1322–1327.

Glasgow, R. E., Phillips, S. M., & Sanchez, M. A. (2014). Implementation science approaches for integrating eHealth research into practice and policy. *International Journal of Medical Informatics*, 83(7), e1–11.

Holden, R. J., Binkheder, S., Patel, J., & Viernes, S. H. P. (2018). Best practices for health informatician involvement in interprofessional health care teams. *Appl Clin Inform*, 09(01), 141–148. doi:10.1055/s-0038-1626724

Lentferink, A., Polstra L., D'Souza A., Oldenhuis H., Velthuijsen H., & van Gemert-Pijnen L. (2020). Creating value with eHealth: Identification of the value proposition with key stakeholders for the resilience navigator app. *BMC Medical Informatics and Decision Making*, 20 (1), art. no. 76.

Lindenberg, M., Van Gemert-Pijnen, L., Nieuwenhuis, B. (2022). Digitalisering in de zorg nader beschouwd. [A closer look at digitalization in health care]. Den Haag: Ministerie van Volksgezondheid, Welzijn en Sport, MEVA. Retrieved from: https://www.utwente.nl/en/techmed/research/research-programmes/sht/projects-and-results/meva/eindrapport-vws-meva-220420.pdf

Mann, M. D., Quintiliani, M. L., Reddy, S., Kitos, R. N., & Weng, M. (2014). Dietary Approaches to Stop Hypertension: Lessons learned from a case study on the development of an mHealth behavior change system. *JMIR mHealth uHealth*, 2(4), e41.

Mitchell, R. K., Agle, B. R., & Wood, D. J. (1997). Toward a theory of stakeholder identification and salience: Defining the principle of who and what really counts. *Acad Manage Rev*, 22, 853–886.

Nancarrow, S. A., Booth, A., Ariss, S., Smith, T., Enderby, P., & Roots, A. (2013). Ten principles of good interdisciplinary team work. *Human Resources for Health*, 11(1), 19.

Nilsen, E. R., Stendal, K., & Gullslett, M. K. (2020). Implementation of eHealth technology in community health care: The complexity of stakeholder involvement. *BMC Health Serv Res*, 20, 395.

Pagliari, C. (2007). Design and evaluation in eHealth: Challenges and implications for an interdisciplinary field. *J Med Internet Res*, 9(2), e15. doi:10.2196/jmir.9.2.e15PMID: 17537718PMCID: PMC1913937

Ross, J., Stevenson, F., Lau, R., & Murray, E. (2016). Factors that influence the implementation of e-health: A systematic review of systematic reviews (an update). *Implementation Science*, 11, 146.

Schmidt, L. B., Falk, T., Siegmund-Schultze, M., & Spangenberg, J. H. (2020). The objectives of stakeholder involvement in transdisciplinary research. A conceptual framework for a reflective and reflexive practise. *Ecological Economics*, 176, 106751. doi:10.1016/j.ecolecon.2020.106751

Van den Berg, S. H. M. P., Pieterse, M. E., & Spook, J. E. (2021). Evaluating a smoking cessation app by involving end-users and health insurance companies: A mixed method approach. Enschede, The Netherlands: published as master's thesis at the University of Twente, department of Health Psychology and Technology, Faculty of Behavioral Management and Social Sciences. Retrieved from https://essay.utwente.nl/88243/1/thesis_1859986_vandenberg.pdf

Van Gemert-Pijnen, J. E. W. C. (2022). Implementation of health technology: Directions for research and practice. *Front. Digit. Health*, 4, 1030194. doi:10.3389/fdgth.2022.1030194

Van Limburg, M., Wentzel, J., Sanderman, R., & van Gemert-Pijnen, L. (2015). Business modeling to implement an eHealth portal for infection control: A reflection on co-creation with stakeholders. *JMIR Res Protoc*, 4(3), e104.

Van Woezik, A. F. G., Braakman-Jansen, L. M. A., Kulyk, O. et al. (2016). Tackling wicked problems in infection prevention and control: A guideline for co-creation with stakeholders. *Antimicrob Resist Infect Control*, 5, 20.

15 Engagement

Saskia M. Kelders & Olga Perski

Introduction

As seen throughout this book, eHealth is a promising way to improve health, well-being, and healthcare. Many examples show that the use of eHealth can, among other things, lead to effective treatments, might save costs, and enhance patient satisfaction. Chapter 5, for example, showed that there are many effective eMental health interventions targeting depression with similar effects as face-to-face interventions. Also, some eMental health interventions have succeeded in reaching different populations than traditional methods of treatment delivery (e.g., students who would not go to their GP for their mental health issues). Chapter 6 has shown many examples from the lifestyle and somatic health areas in which eHealth can play a huge role, for example, preventing disease or complications and empowering patients in taking control over their own health and well-being. Yet, it is also known that there often is a gap between the theoretical promise a technology holds and its actual impact on practice. A big part of that gap may have to do with the extent and manner a technology is experienced and used.

For eHealth technologies to have an effect, and for people to benefit most from what they have to offer, they need to be accepted and used in the intended way. This has proven to be difficult to achieve, see e.g., Kelders et al., 2012. In this chapter, we will go deeper into this issue by first elaborating on three important concepts regarding the use of eHealth technologies, namely acceptance, adoption, and adherence. Second, we will connect these three concepts to engagement – a construct that can be used to explain and increase the effectiveness of eHealth. We will explain what engagement is, what components it entails, and provide a conceptual framework of engagement. Next, we will focus on how to measure engagement, and how the concept of engagement can be applied to increase the effectiveness of eHealth technologies. Last, we will present some directions for future research. After completing this chapter, you will be able to:

- Provide a definition and explain the importance of three key concepts for eHealth: Acceptance, adoption, and adherence;
- Explain the concept, components, and conceptual framework of engagement;
- Name and explain ways of measuring and evaluating engagement;
- Provide examples of how engagement can be used to increase the effectiveness of eHealth technologies;
- Provide an overview of unexplored avenues and future directions for research on engagement with eHealth.

DOI: 10.4324/9781003302049-17

Acceptance

Acceptance is a key concept in eHealth. There are many different definitions of acceptance, but most of them converge on the idea that acceptance captures how people think and feel about a given eHealth technology. It sits at the core of several models that aim to explain why a technology is (not) used, with one of the most well-known being the Technology Acceptance model (TAM) (Davis, 1989). The TAM posits that the decision to use a technology (to accept it), is determined to a large degree by a potential user's attitude towards using that technology. This attitude in turn is influenced by two beliefs: Perceived usefulness and perceived ease of use. So, for example, consider someone who wants to be more active and is thinking about using an app to track their steps. According to the TAM, the actual use of a specific app for that, will be determined largely by this person's intention to use the app, which follows from whether this person believes the app will help them to track their steps, and will be easy to use. In line with this, a recent paper defined acceptability as an emergent property or a 'gut feeling', which arises from the dynamic interplay of affective and cognitive components (Perski & Short, 2021). Acceptance has also been defined as a dynamic process, with perceptions of acceptability formed after learning about a new eHealth intervention but before having had the opportunity to use it ('pre-use acceptability'), during usage ('concurrent acceptability'), and after a period of use ('retrospective acceptability') (Nadal, Sas, & Doherty, 2020). As such, pre-use acceptance is a necessary precondition for the adoption of and long-term use of an eHealth technology since a continuous experience of usage cannot be established if the technology is not accepted in the first place.

Research has shown that acceptance of eHealth technology can be a complex issue. For example, in the area of assistive technologies for older adults, many studies have investigated why many older adults do not use these technologies, despite their many potential advantages, such as helping people to live at home independently for longer (Chen & Chan, 2011; Wrede, Braakman-Jansen, & van Gemert-Pijnen, 2021). Theories about technology acceptance provide some answers to these issues of non-use, but do not seem to paint the full picture (Peek et al., 2014). It has been proposed that precisely what people find acceptable is deeply contextualized and interlinked with prevailing social and cultural norms (Perski & Short, 2021).

Adoption

A second important concept related to the use of technology is adoption. Adoption concerns the decision of the target group to start using a new technology. Adoption and acceptance are related concepts, but acceptance is related to an individual's decision to use a technology, while adoption refers more to a group level. Adoption is a key concept in the Diffusion of Innovations Theory (see also Chapter 4) which aims to explain how, why and at what rate ideas and technologies spread between individuals in social networks (Rogers, 2010). The Diffusion of Innovation theory is often used to explain why technologies do or do not become adopted (e.g., in healthcare settings), even though the benefits of these technologies are apparent. Research has shown that, for example, non-adoption of eHealth technologies by health professionals can be explained with this theory (Greenhalgh, Robert, Macfarlane, Bate, & Kyriakidou, 2004). In addition, the NASSS (non-adoption, abandonment, scale-up, spread, and sustainability) framework (see Chapter 13) proposes seven domains that influence the adoption of eHealth technologies within health and social care organizations: The condition or illness, the technology, the value proposition, the adopter system (including staff, patients, and caregivers), the organization(s), the wider (institutional and societal) context, and the interaction between these domains over time (Greenhalgh et al., 2017). Consequently, adoption is an important factor related to the use of eHealth technologies.

Adherence

Both acceptance and adoption are concepts that relate to the decision to start using a new technology. However, for many eHealth technologies, merely starting to use the technology is not enough. People often need to stick with the technology and use it in the right way to really benefit from it. In the literature, this is called adherence: Whether the technology is used as it is intended by the developers (Christensen, Griffiths, & Farrer, 2009; Sieverink, Kelders, & van Gemert-Pijnen, 2017). Achieving adherence has been found to constitute a major issue in eHealth. Reviews on, for example, web-based interventions have shown that often less than half of the participants adhere to the interventions in the manner intended by the developers. This number decreases even further when the technology is implemented in real life instead of in a research environment (Kelders, Kok, Ossebaard, & van Gemert-Pijnen, 2012).

Consider the following example: Living to the Full is a web-based intervention for people with depressive symptoms. The intervention consists of nine chronological lessons with psycho-education and exercises that participants should complete to get the most out of the intervention. However, even in a research context, only 49% to 73% of the participants completed all nine lessons (Kelders, Bohlmeijer, Pots, & van Gemert-Pijnen, 2015; Pots et al., 2016). Another example is Panic Center, an interactive website to help people who suffer from panic disorder and agoraphobia. Among other things, Panic Center offers a 12-week self-help program with educational text, exercises, and the opportunity to monitor symptoms. An observational study showed that, of the 1161 people who registered for the self-help program across a period of almost two years, only 12 people completed all 12 lessons (Farvolden, Denisoff, Selby, Bagby, & Rudy, 2005). This shows the extent of the adherence issue in both research and real-life implementation of eHealth technologies.

But this begs the question: What is the impact of these low adherence rates for the effectiveness of eHealth technologies? There is a relationship between adherence and effectiveness: If a technology is not used as intended or not at all, then how can it ever be effective? To illustrate this, in the case of Living to the Full, research has shown that, on average, the more lessons a participant completes, the greater the positive effects are (Kelders et al., 2015). This illustrates the dose-response relationship: more usage leads to more effectiveness (Donkin et al., 2011). It is important to note that this is not always the case: Sometimes people who benefit from using a technology quit using it rather quickly, because they don't need it anymore. Or for some people, it might be enough to use a technology once to be able to implement the learned lessons in daily life. Another methodological issue concerning the observed dose-response relationship is that it could be driven by a type of *selection bias* – those who are more motivated or better able to make changes might use the eHealth intervention more frequently and for a longer period. Nonetheless, many researchers agree that it is important to find ways to increase adherence and thereby the chances of eHealth technologies being effective.

Towards a Solution

The concepts of acceptance, adoption, and adherence are central in eHealth, as they contribute to the effectiveness of eHealth technologies. However, as we have seen, improving acceptance, adoption, and adherence is a complex issue. Looking at research that has been conducted in each of the domains gives us some clues as to how to solve this issue, but none of the separate concepts and theories seem to provide the full solution. One solution is to focus on creating a technology that fits the goals and needs of the users, other stakeholders, and is aligned with the context by means of a proper, holistic development process (see Chapter 7). However, even for technologies that are developed in this way, there are differences in both the average (between-subjects) and individual (within-subjects) acceptance, adoption, and adherence. Research has tried to relate these differences to, for example, users' sociodemographic and clinical characteristics. In specific areas, this has led to some insights. For example, in eMental health interventions, being female and having higher treatment expectancies have been shown to predict greater adherence. However, even in this specific context, many factors (e.g., age and severity of complaints) have shown mixed findings, i.e., they do not always and fully predict effectiveness in the same way (Beatty & Binnion, 2016). Based on these kinds of studies, it seems that eHealth technologies need to fit with the characteristics of the users that have to accept, adopt, and adhere to it. Another possibility to increase adherence is to look at the possibilities of the technology itself. As Chapter 12 has shown, persuasive design elements provided a way for the technology itself to become more convincing and thereby reach higher adherence rates (Kelders et al., 2012).

However, the characteristics of users and the technology itself still do not fully explain why people do or do not adhere to eHealth technologies, nor why a technology is effective or not for a given individual. This may also have to do with large individual differences in people's psychological states (e.g., motivation, self-regulation, attitudes), and in processing speeds, memory, learning, etc., required for internalizing the intervention content (e.g., psycho-education, mindfulness exercises). This makes it likely that different people need different doses of the intervention components to reach the same level of a clinical outcome. This makes it very difficult, if not impossible to define a generalizable dose of 'effective' usage which leads to improved outcomes for the majority of participants (Yardley et al., 2016). This is where the concept of engagement comes into play.

Engagement

While engagement is complex to define, it is generally seen as a multifaceted concept that captures not just the extent of usage (e.g., amount, frequency, depth, duration) but also the subjective experience when interacting with the eHealth intervention (Kelders, van Zyl, & Ludden, 2020b; Perski, Blandford, West, & Michie, 2017b). The precise content of this subjective experience with eHealth is not clearcut yet, but a well-known definition characterizes this experience by 'attention, interest and affect' (Perski et al., 2017b). The multifaceted concept of engagement is closely related to the idea of capturing not only *what* the individual does within the intervention (e.g., completing an exercise) but also *how* they process the information (e.g., how much attention and interest they are paying to the exercise). In addition, how an individual feels during the interaction (e.g., how much enjoyment they're experiencing) may on the one hand facilitate that they actually pay attention to the content then and there (contemporaneous relationship). At the same time, it might also be an important predictor of an individual's repeated use and engagement with an intervention at a later time point. The latter phenomenon is referred to as re-engagement after temporal lag. Although still work in progress, the current conceptualization of engagement is closely related to the aim of determining the effect of an intervention for a given individual (Kelders et al., 2020b; Perski et al., 2017b). In other words: engagement seems to be a way to explain why an eHealth intervention works (or does not work) for an individual. Although the above definition is often used in the field, engagement still tends to be operationalized in studies as just the extent of usage, without capturing the subjective experience of attention, interest and affect (Perski et al., 2017b). In other words: Researchers say they study engagement, while actually only looking at usage data, omitting the subjective element. This hampers our understanding of engagement and its role in eHealth effectiveness.

The definition of engagement to eHealth technologies, does not come out of the blue. It is closely related to the concept of user engagement (O'Brien & Toms, 2008). However, there is a need to define engagement specifically for eHealth technologies instead of using the concept user engagement because of the differences in the context where these concepts are used. User engagement is often applied to contexts such as online shopping and searching for information. In these contexts, the goals of the users are quite different from the context of eHealth technologies. For example, in shopping or searching for information online, the goal of the user will be reached (or not) in a reasonably short timeframe, while using the technology. While in an eHealth technology, the goal of the user, such as increasing physical activity, is something that will be reached over a longer period of time, involves behaviour other than the use of the technology, and might be meaningful in a different way than shopping. Others have posited that because of these considerations, engagement with eHealth technologies is also needed at two levels: Engagement with the technology itself, and engagement with the behaviour the technology focuses on (Yardley et al., 2016). These unique aspects warrant a specific definition for engagement with eHealth technologies, instead of borrowing the definition of user engagement.

For this specific definition, there is still a lack of consensus regarding the various components that make up engagement (Kelders, 2015; Kelders et al., 2020b). In fields other than eHealth technologies, such as education (student engagement) (Appleton, Christenson, & Furlong, 2008) and organizations (work engagement) (Bakker, Schaufeli, Leiter, & Taris, 2008), engagement is commonly conceptualized as consisting of behaviour, cognition, and affect. In the context of education, behavioural engagement refers to active participation in classes and displaying positive conduct, while cognitive engagement involves self-regulation and recognizing the value of learning. Affective engagement, on the other hand, encompasses factors such as a feeling of belonging at school and maintaining a positive attitude toward learning. Similarly, within organizational settings (work engagement), behavioural engagement relates to aspects like demonstrating high levels of energy and enthusiasm, whereas cognitive engagement entails being fully absorbed and experiencing a sense of time passing quickly. Affective engagement in the workplace encompasses dedication, a strong involvement in one's work, and the experience of emotions like pride and enthusiasm. Overall, understanding the components of engagement in eHealth remains an ongoing topic of investigation, and the concepts of behaviour, cognition, and affect serve as common frameworks for studying engagement across different domains (Kelders et al., 2020b).

Components of Engagement with eHealth Interventions

To examine how the components of engagement manifest in the specific context of eHealth technologies, a study conducted interviews with engaged health app users to understand their perspectives on engagement (Kelders, 2019). The findings of this study confirmed that, similar to the fields of education and organizations, engagement in the context of eHealth technology can be understood in terms of behaviour, cognition, and affect. It also provided further insights into the operationalizations of each component, which are summarized below.

Behavioural engagement

The primary theme within behavioural engagement is the establishment of a routine around the use of the health intervention. Engaged users integrate the technology seamlessly into their daily lives, perceiving it as a natural part of their behaviours targeted by the technology (e.g., running or having meals). This meant that the distinction between the technology and the target behaviour seemed to blur for them. Another theme in behavioural engagement was the perception of the technology as being user-friendly. Engaged users found using the technology effortless, which facilitated the development of a routine. The final theme was that engaged users reported aligning their technology usage with their personal goals. Their usage of the technology was driven by their intended outcomes. If their goals changed (e.g., from gaining insights into problematic behaviours to actual behaviour change), the intensity of their usage would also adapt. Overall, behavioural engagement was not solely about the extent of usage but rather related to the quality or 'fittingness' of usage.

Cognitive engagement

For engaged users, cognitive engagement was closely linked to the goals they aimed to achieve through the technology. The main themes identified were ability, usefulness, and mental effort. Ability referred to users being engaged because the technology enhanced their capability to reach their goals. For example, a step counter provided them with insights into their activity levels and facilitated behaviour control and change. The second prominent theme was related to users' belief in the usefulness of the technology. They intuitively perceived the technology as motivating and helpful, without necessarily experiencing strong emotions or explicitly stating that it increased their ability. They just felt the technology helped them to achieve their goals. The final theme was mental effort. Engaged users willingly invested mental effort in understanding the data provided by the technology, such as analyzsing their runs, or in using the app itself, such as meticulously entering diet information. This mental effort was not seen as a burden, but quite the contrary: It contributed to goal attainment and served as a motivating activity in itself.

Affective engagement

Within affective engagement, we identified three themes: Enjoyment of using the technology, enjoyment of achieving goals, and identity. Positive emotions played a significant role in the engagement of users. However, these emotions were not solely related to the enjoyment of using the technology but also encompassed positive emotions associated with achieving one's goals, such as reaching a specific step count. Interestingly, negative emotions also emerged as a factor, as not achieving a goal could lead to frustration. However, this was not necessarily detrimental to engagement, as it could increase motivation to strive for the goal in subsequent attempts and thus even increase engagement Identity also played a role within affective engagement. Engaged users seemed to identify themselves in some way with the technology or the goal it represented. They felt a connection and expressed that they would miss the technology if it were no longer available.

In summary, this interview study shed light on the components of engagement within the context of eHealth technologies. Behavioural engagement emphasized the quality of usage rather than just the extent, while cognitive engagement focused on the perception of ability, usefulness, and mental effort. Affective engagement encompassed positive and negative emotions related to both technology use and goal achievement, along with a sense of identity and connection. Although this provides a good starting point, more research is needed to validate these findings in other target groups and technologies, and to provide an even richer understanding of a complex concept as engagement.

Conceptual Framework of Engagement

Besides understanding what engagement entails, it is also important to understand what influences engagement. Researchers have attempted to provide an overview of factors that promote or detract from engagement, aiming to ensure that designers consider these when developing or adapting eHealth technologies. One such attempt involved an interdisciplinary literature review and synthesis of findings from the psychology/health and the computer science/human-computer interaction domains (Perski, Blandford, West, et al., 2017b). It was found that engagement is influenced by aspects of the technology itself (i.e., the specific content and the way in which it is delivered), the context (i.e., the setting in which the technology is used and characteristics of the population using the technology) and the target behaviour. In addition, 'mechanisms of action' of the eHealth technology; that is, the ways in which the technology attempts to change behaviour (e.g., increased motivation as a result of engaging with the technology), was found to influence continued engagement. This implies that being engaged with a technology will change that engagement itself. Therefore, engagement can be usefully considered as a dynamic process: It does not stay constant, but changes over time. It also operates at the within-person level, i.e., these changes are different for each person, making it important to consider engagement of individuals instead of just looking at the average engagement of groups. Lastly, engagement is part of a complex adaptive system in which the eHealth technology, the context of use, the mechanisms of action of the eHealth technology, and the target behaviour all influence each other and may change over time, both within and between individuals (Perski & Short, 2021). An overview of this model can be found in Figure 15.1. Note that this model is based on Digital Behaviour Change Interventions (DBCIs), a specific form of eHealth technology.

Measuring Engagement

If we want to understand more about the role of engagement in eHealth interventions, it is important to have an accepted way of measuring it. However, as there is not yet a clear definition of the concept of engagement with eHealth technologies, you can imagine that there is also not a single generally accepted way of measuring engagement. A paper which aimed to provide a comprehensive overview of measurement options available to assess engagement in eHealth interventions found a variety of measurement methods, ranging from system usage logs to focus groups (Short et al., 2018). The authors highlighted the benefits of using multiple methods and pairing the data in order to gain a more comprehensive understanding of the different components of engagement (i.e., behavioural, cognitive, and affective). However, at the same time, they, and others, noted that to date, most studies in the eHealth and mHealth space primarily rely on system usage data. While

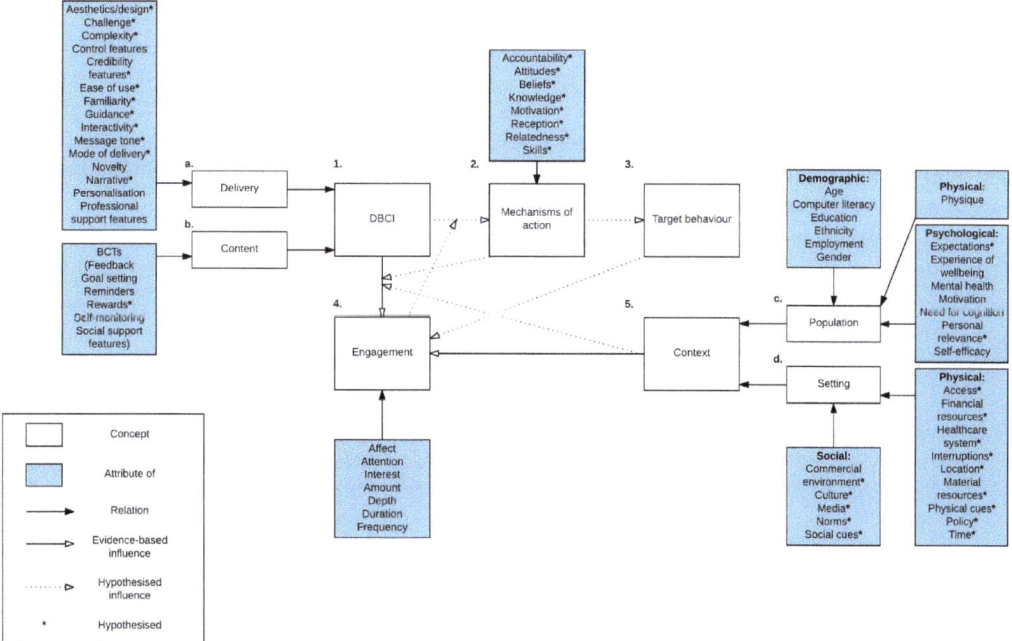

Figure 15.1 A conceptual framework of engagement. Adapted from Perski et al. (2017b). A hypothesised influence or attribute refers to there being no empirical evidence for the specific influence or attribute in question. Instead, such influences or attributes were expected/hypothesised by authors to influence engagement.

valuable, this is not considered a valid measure of engagement on its own, since it only captures objective usage of the technology (see also Bijkerk, Oenema, Geschwind, & Spigt, 2023). Other measures of engagement, such as sensors, social media data, ecological momentary assessment (EMA), and psychophysiological measures such as heartrate were also identified, but limited research has been conducted to explore their use and validity in the digital (health) behaviour change setting. The higher cost, time, and data analysis requirements that are associated with these measures have limited their widespread implementation. Questionnaires were identified as a potential cost-effective approach to assess engagement, but when the overview study was published, there was a lack of validated self-report engagement questionnaires tailored to the eHealth and mHealth context. The authors of the paper emphasized the need for standardized items that cover the breadth of the engagement concept while also enabling cross-comparisons between digital health interventions.

To address this gap, several self-report questionnaires on engagement with eHealth technologies were developed, which are discussed in the next section of this chapter. As you will see, both scales incorporate the behavioural, cognitive, and affective components of engagement. However, for both scales, more research is needed to investigate whether these are useful to paint a clear and complete picture of engagement with eHealth technologies.

Digital Behaviour Change Intervention Engagement Scale (DBCI-ES)

The first scale that we cover is the Digital Behaviour Change Intervention Engagement Scale (DBCI-ES). Two data sources were used to generate a definition of the construct: A literature review and synthesis (discussed in the section 'Conceptual framework of engagement') and a think-aloud and interview study with potential users of smartphone apps for smoking cessation and alcohol reduction (Perski, Blandford, Ubhi, West, & Michie, 2017a). The main outcomes of these studies were that engagement spans two conceptual domains: an experiential domain (with cognitive and emotional facets) and a behavioural domain. Second, engagement has been found to vary within users over time and across eHealth technologies, often as a function of person- (e.g., motivation to change) or technology-specific attributes (e.g., tailoring). Therefore, it was hypothesized that engagement can usefully be defined as a state rather than a trait. Two behavioural indicators and three experiential indicators were identified as particularly important for determining the intensity of the state of engagement: Amount of use, depth of use, attention, interest, and enjoyment. First, spending time on an eHealth technology (i.e., 'amount of use') and accessing at least one of its components (i.e., 'depth of use') were both considered necessary for engagement. These behavioural indicators were hypothesised to be jointly still insufficient for someone to be engaged, as a user may scroll through information on an app without actually paying attention to its content. Therefore, three experiential indicators were also considered necessary for engagement: Paying *attention* to the eHealth technology, feeling *interested* in it and experiencing *enjoyment* whilst using it. It is widely accepted that the process of selective attention helps allocating limited resources to stimuli, and that the function of interest is to direct attention towards important stimuli.

Based on these findings, the DBCI-ES was developed, containing ten items (Table 15.1). The first eight items use a 7-point scale, ranging from 'not at all' (0); 'moderately' (3); 'extremely' (6). The ninth item can be answered in free text, while for the tenth item, the researchers will list the components of the studied technology so the participant can select the ones that they remember using.

To date, the DBCI-ES has been evaluated in two studies, both with the freely available Drink Less app targeting people with the intention to reduce alcohol consumption (Perski et al., 2020; Perski et al., 2019a). Participants were asked to complete the scale immediately after their first app login. Moreover, their app usage was measured. Together, these studies showed that the scale is reliable, but it is difficult to validate the scale because there is no 'gold standard' of engagement.

Table 15.1 Digital Behaviour Change Intervention Engagement Scale (DBCI-ES) (Perski, Blandford, Ubhi, West, & Michie, 2017a).

Item	How strongly did you experience the following?	Construct
1	Interest	Experiental
2	Intrigue	Experiental
3	Focus	Experiental
4	Inattention	Experiental
5	Distraction	Experiental
6	Enjoyment	Experiental
7	Annoyance	Experiental
8	Pleasure	Experiental
9	How much time (in minutes) do you roughly think that you spent on the app?	Behaviour
10	Which of the app's components do you remember visiting?	Behaviour

In the first study, total scale scores were not correlated with the number of subsequent log ins, meaning that higher initial engagement was not related to greater usage of the app over time. However, when looking at the conceptualization of engagement, this would also not be expected (more initial engagement does not necessarily lead to more usage over time). The second study elaborated on this finding and found that the behavioural and experiential subscales of engagement were largely independent. This strengthens the notion that usage in itself may not be engagement but begs the question if and what kind of usage could be part of engagement.

Twente Engagement with Ehealth Technologies Scale (TWEETS)

The second scale that is covered is the TWente Engagement with Ehealth Technologies Scale (TWEETS; Table 15.2) (Kelders, Kip, & Greeff, 2020). This scale is based on the conceptualization of engagement, with the components behaviour, cognition and affect, described earlier in the second section of this chapter. This scale consists of nine items on a 5-point Likert scale, ranging from strongly disagree to strongly agree. Of the nine items, three are aimed at behavioural engagement, three at cognitive engagement, and three at affective engagement. In Table 15.2, the different items of the scale are shown as they can be used to assess engagement with an eHealth technology while participants are using it. The TWEETS can also be adapted to be used very early on in the process of using an eHealth technology, for example after having used the technology for the first time. In this case, the items should be posed as expectations, for example, 'I think using this [technology] can become part of my daily routine'. If the TWEETS is used after the usage of the technology has concluded, it can be used to assess past engagement. In this case items should be posed in past tense, e.g., 'Looking back at using the [technology], I feel that using this [technology] did become part of my daily routine'. Moreover, the scale allows for adaption to the studied technology by adding the technology, the goal, and the behaviour relating to the goal by changing the item's text in [brackets].

The scale has been evaluated on its psychometric properties in a first validation study. In this study, participants were asked to use any step counter app on their smartphones for two weeks and complete questionnaires, including the TWEETS, at four time-points (Kelders et al., 2020a).

The findings of the study show that TWEETS is a reliable scale (engagement). However, the scale was found to consist of a single factor and no evidence was found for the three components being separate subscales. The researchers speculated that this might be due to theoretical overlap between the components, or the small number of items in the scale. Analyses showed moderate positive correlations between engagement at different time points, indicating that engagement may vary over time. This finding aligns with existing models of engagement that suggest engagement

Table 15.2 TWente Engagement with Ehealth Technologies Scale (TWEETS) (Kelders, Kip, & Greeff, 2020a).

Item	Thinking about using [the technology] recently, I feel that:	Construct
1	using this [technology] is part of my daily routine	Behaviour
2	this [technology] takes me little effort to use	Behaviour
3	I'm able to use the [technology] as often as needed (to achieve my goals)	Behaviour
4	this [technology] makes it easier for me to work on [goal of the technology]	Cognition
5	this [technology] motivates me to [goal of the technology]	Cognition
6	this [technology] helps me to get more insight into my [goal of the technology]	Cognition
7	I enjoy using this [technology]	Affect
8	I enjoy seeing the progress I make in this [technology]	Affect
9	this [technology] fits me as a person	Affect

is a dynamic process which changes over the course of an intervention. The study also found that engagement at an earlier time point predicted perceived behaviour change at a later time, serving as an early indication of the relationship between engagement and effectiveness. The TWEETS scale was not correlated with personality factors, supporting the notion that engagement is a distinct construct. The scale was related to involvement and enjoyment measures, which are theoretically related to cognitive and affective engagement, respectively. The scale's correlations with adherence and frequency of use, which are often associated with engagement, were small or nonsignificant. This suggests that engagement is related to usage but to a lesser extent than commonly assumed.

As you have seen, there are two self-report scales that measure engagement. Both scales have their own strong and weak points. The decision on what scale to use in a research project will therefore be mostly related to the conceptualization of engagement that the researchers feel is appropriate for the study. If it seems important to include the three components of engagement (behaviour, cognition, and affect), then either the DBCI-ES or TWEETS scale might be most appropriate. However, if engagement is conceptualized as a momentary state, then the DBCI-ES might be most useful. If the research is focused on engagement over slightly longer temporal scales, then the TWEETS scale might be most appropriate. If the actual usage behaviour is also considered a meaningful component of engagement, the DBCI-ES scale might be most appropriate. Moreover, the choice of a scale depends on what the researchers want to investigate with engagement: When engagement is seen as a concept that is related to the effectiveness of an eHealth intervention, the TWEETS has shown most predictive power in this respect. However, for both scales, more research is needed to understand the validity, robustness, and added value.

Applying Engagement

Until now, in this chapter, we have discussed what the concept of engagement entails and how it might be measured. Now it is time to move towards what we can do with it. In this respect, it is important to note that we assume a few things about (i.e., attributes of) the concept of engagement:

- It is related to clinical outcomes of interest, such as symptoms of depression or health behaviour change;
- It can be measured early on in the process of using an eHealth technology;
- It varies within individuals over time and across different contexts.

Although research supports the assumption that these important attributes hold true, this field is still in its early stages and more work needs to be done to be certain of these attributes. For now, let's consider these attributes to be true, as it gives engagement tremendous application value.

One of the largest issues in intervention research in general, and eHealth intervention research in particular, is that studies are focused on improving and measuring average treatment effects (i.e., between-subjects effects, so the impact an intervention has on a large group of participants). However, research indicates that the average does not really exist in real-world scenarios. When we delve deeper into the effects of an intervention, we find that some individuals experience positive changes, some show no change, and others may even experience deterioration (Andrews & Williams, 2014). Naturally, it is pivotal to ensure that nobody is worse off when utilizing a digital health intervention, so this is something we need to avoid. Moreover, considering the existence of various intervention approaches that have shown to be effective on average (such as positive psychology, Cognitive Behavioural Therapy (CBT), and Acceptance and Commitment Therapy (ACT) for promoting mental health), there might be an effective intervention approach for each individual; we just need to find the right one. To illustrate: while CBT might work best for one person, another might benefit more from mindfulness. The same principle applies to intervention design. For instance, research on the impact of persuasive technology features in general, and gamification specifically, often reveals small effects (Hamari, Koivisto, & Sarsa, 2014; Kelders et al., 2015). This could be attributed, at least in part, to individual differences. While gamification techniques might boost motivation for some individuals, others may perceive it as diminishing the value and seriousness of the intervention. Therefore, it is clear that a one-size-fits-all approach is far from ideal for both the therapeutic content and design of interventions.

However, to date it remains challenging to pre-determine the most appropriate content and design for each individual. For example, studies have shown that consistent characteristics (such as personality age, gender, type of disorder) that predict whether psychotherapy or medication is the best option are yet to be identified (Cuijpers et al., 2012). If a choice between two very different treatment options like medication or psychotherapy cannot even be made based on existing knowledge, his implies that he decision which kind of psychotherapy, or which design of a technological intervention is optimal for an individual is even more complex. This limitation hampers our ability to personalize interventions. However, we might be able to use the concept of engagement to address this issue, without needing the 'a-priori' knowledge of which type of intervention works for whom. Engagement, even when measured early on within an intervention, is related to effectiveness. Also, both the design and therapeutic content of interventions can influence individual engagement (Hyland & Whalley, 2008; Kelders, Sommers-Spijkerman, & Goldberg, 2018; Whalley & Hyland, 2009). Together, this suggests that we can ask people to start using an intervention, measure their engagement and predict the success of this intervention for each individual early on in the process. This prediction could enhance intervention (cost)effectiveness by administering the intervention only to individuals who demonstrate reasonable engagement levels and are likely to benefit from it. If engagement is low, this implies that something needs to be done to increase engagement, i.e., making a change to the intervention.

Technological advancements offer opportunities to create the most suitable intervention to optimally engage a user. It is possible to create multiple versions of an intervention more easily, thus designing interventions not just for a non-existing average but tailored to cater to a diverse target group. An example can be found in how feedback is framed within an eHealth intervention. Some people might like to the point feedback, and don't mind that that can be quite harsh. Others might appreciate a more delicate approach. Developing one intervention that caters to both these groups might be difficult and satisfy neither. But creating multiple versions might allow us to incorporate the wishes of both groups. This allows us to go a step further: not only can we prevent interventions that are likely ineffective for an individual from being administered to that individual, but it also allows us to identify the most suitable version for each individual, by measuring their engagement to different versions of an intervention (see the worked example in Box 15.1). Taking this line of thought even further, engagement can also help us to create adaptive interventions, i.e., interventions that change during their use to suit fluctuating individual needs (also including 'just-in-time adaptive interventions', which aim to provide the right type and dose of support to individuals, at the right time) (Nahum-Shani et al., 2018). When engagement is measured throughout the use of an intervention, preferable real-time, it can signal crucial moments in the process of using and engaging with the intervention. For example, a sudden decrease of engagement may signal that the intervention does not fit the user's goals anymore, prompting a change in the content and/or design of the intervention. However, it is important to note that personalizing and adapting interventions based on individual engagement is still a relatively new and unexplored concept (see for example (Rabbi et al., 2018)). While it holds promise, research should investigate how different groups respond to attempts to enhance their engagement in (near) real-time. Some individuals may exhibit reactance toward such attempts, perceiving them as manipulative. One way to address this concern is by allowing individuals to choose whether or not a suggested change to the intervention should be implemented, or not, thereby increasing their sense of autonomy. Further research is necessary to identify if and how engagement can be used to deliver the most effective interventions for an individual.

Box 15.1 Example of using engagement to personalize an eHealth intervention for people with depressive or anxiety symptoms.

In this box, we provide a worked example of using engagement to personalize an eHealth intervention for people with depressive or anxiety symptoms. For people suffering from these symptoms, various interventions might be useful. These interventions can vary in their content: Cognitive Behavioural Therapy (CBT), Acceptance and Commitment Therapy (ACT), and Positive Psychology (PP) all have shown effectiveness (Bolier & Abello, 2014; Ruiz, 2012). Even though they were all found to be effective, different individuals may respond better to different approaches. According to the Motivational Concordance Theory, the approach that aligns most closely with an individual's personal values and beliefs is likely to be the most effective for that individual (Hyland & Whalley, 2008; Whalley & Hyland, 2009). Second, in an online intervention, the manner in which feedback is provided is likely to impact individual engagement and the effectiveness of the intervention. Research suggests that individuals are engaged differently when feedback is given in different ways (Kelders et al., 2015; Talbot, 2012). Finally, various design approaches, such as gamification, are likely to have an impact on engagement, and this influence is likely to vary among individuals (Hamari et al., 2014). Table 15.3 offers an overview of the factors mentioned (content, feedback, design) along with three potential options for an eHealth intervention. Naturally, there are many other factors and choices that could be considered, but these have been selected to demonstrate how a personalization approach could function in practice.

By considering these three factors, each with three levels, a total of 27 (i.e., $3{\times}3{\times}3$) different versions of an intervention can be created. Although this might initially seem challenging, technological tools make this feasible. The current example was developed within the Twente Intervention and Interaction Machine (TIIM), which is system created at the University of Twente. It allows researchers to create their own mobile interventions without the need to code. The system works similar to online survey tools as e.g., Qualtrics or Survey Monkey. In essence, the researchers created different modules that together form an intervention. These modules consist of short texts, questions and/or videos. This allows for the creation of different versions of interventions. Figure 15.2 provides three screenshots of a basic intervention as displayed to a user. By adding different images, it is also possible to create a more elaborate version that may increase engagement. For example, Figure 15.3

shows the same content, but this time, gamification aspects and a virtual coach are included (thus varying the 'design' aspect as shown in Table 15.3). This way 27 version of the intervention can, and have been, created.

The subsequent step would involve determining the most appropriate version of the intervention for each individual. One approach is to have participants go through a setup phase, where they try out the different versions of various aspects step-by-step. For example, each participant first reads the descriptions of different content approaches and complete an exercise. After that, their engagement is measured. If for example this participant's engagement was highest for the ACT intervention, this approach will be selected for this individual. Second, the participant receives feedback in the three different ways. Again, engagement

Table 15.3 Intervention and technology factors that can be used for personalisation.

Factor	Option
Content	*Intervention can be based on*: a. Cognitive Behavioural Therapy b. Acceptance and Commitment Therapy c. Positive Psychology
Feedback	*Feedback on completed exercises*: a. in text b. by a counsellor in a pre-recorded video c. in text given by a virtual agent
Design	*Intervention can*: a. be gamified competitively (points, levels, and achievements) b. be gamified non-competitively (story line, personal challenges, and rewards) c. not be gamified

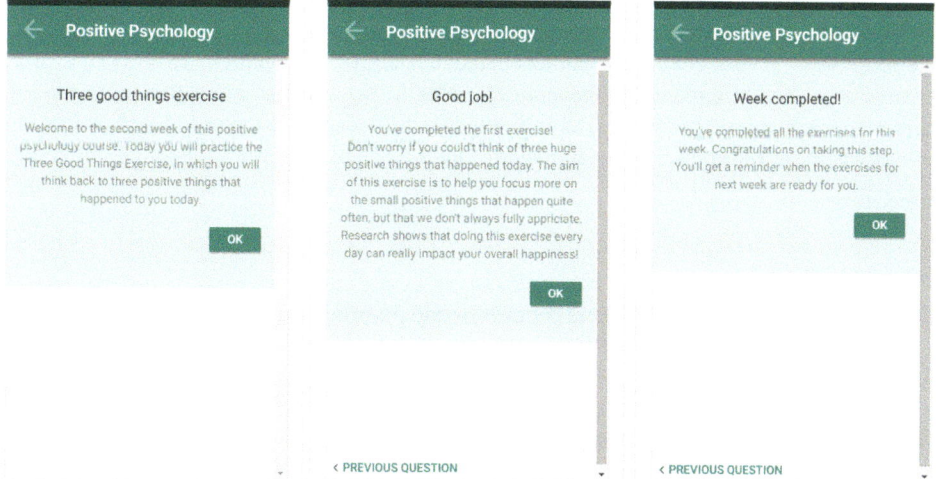

Figure 15.2 Basic mobile positive psychology intervention, created with TIIM.

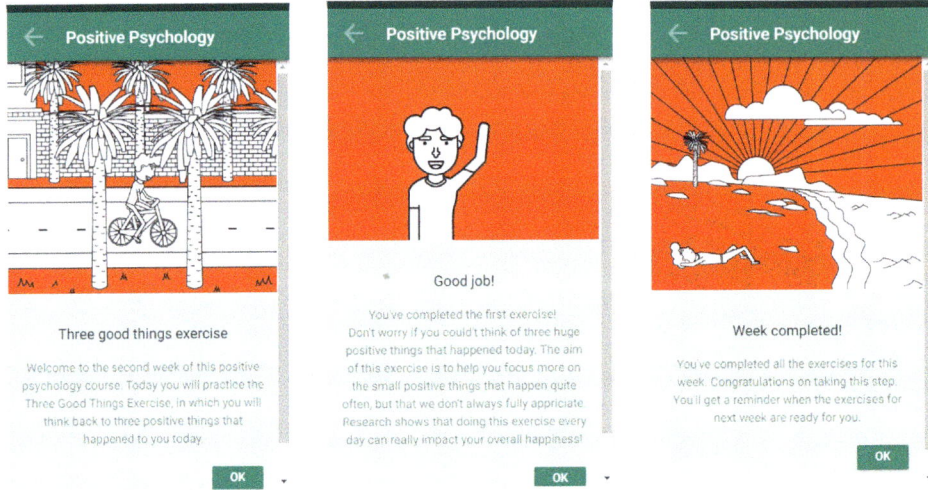

Figure 15.3 More elaborately designed mobile positive psychology intervention, created with TIIM.

is measured and the feedback option with the highest engagement score is selected. The same can be done with the different design options together, these steps enable us to predict the most appropriate version out of the 27 interventions for each individual, allowing for personalized interventions.

Future Research

As we have seen in this chapter, a comprehensive view of engagement is emerging, together with ways to measure and apply the concept. But to be able to make the most out of this important concept, much more research is needed. In this section, we would like to address three directions of future research that are needed to lay the foundation for a thorough understanding of engagement.

Engagement Over Time

Engagement is often seen as a dynamic process, made up of a sequence of states over time within individuals (Kelders et al., 2020b). However, measuring engagement is often done at a fixed point in time, often only once. This does not give us insight into how engagement might fluctuate over time, which hampers our ability to say whether a certain amount of engagement is good enough, or if it warrants adaptation of the intervention. Studies exploring if and how engagement changes over time, are needed to gain insight into this (Perski et al., 2019b). But to do this, other ways of measuring engagement are also needed. Longer self-report scales are not ideal to measure engagement more often, and near real-time. Experience sampling methods, or unobtrusive methods using the technology of interventions might provide a way to do this. But much more research is needed on what these measures and methods might be.

Optimal Engagement

Second, at the moment, it is often assumed that more engagement is always better. But this is still an assumption that needs to be investigated. As engagement itself is a complex concept, consisting of multiple dimensions, it may very well be that optimal engagement is more of a balance between the different dimensions than solely a 'high score'. For example, the total engagement score of person A and person B might be similar. Yet, for person A this is solely in the form of behavioural engagement. This means that they may quickly become disengaged when something breaks their routine. Person B, on the contrary, has a less strong behavioural engagement and has stronger cognitive or affective engagement. They might be quicker to miss a day of usage due to lower behavioural engagement but be inclined to stay engaged due to the larger cognitive or affective engagement which might motivate a renewed engagement. Gaining insights into the optimal engagement patterns can assist us in designing more effective interventions tailored to these patterns and in guiding users toward these optimal patterns.

Engagement between People and Technologies

Last, it is probable that both the aspects we have just discussed – the engagement process and optimal engagement – vary among individuals and across different eHealth technologies. Gaining insight into these variations may aid our understanding of why a particular approach is effective for some individuals in certain contexts but not for others. Keeping an eye on these differences does not mean we cannot learn from what others are studying, on the contrary, it allows us to put our findings into perspective and build on each other's work.

Summary

In this chapter, we have focused on an important mechanism of the effectiveness of eHealth interventions: Engagement. Engagement is related to concepts as acceptance, adoption, and adherence, yet is a different concept. It is more about how an individual experiences an eHealth intervention, and it is more directly related to the effectiveness of eHealth interventions. Engagement is seen as a multifaceted concept that captures the quality or extent of usage, but also the subjective experience when interacting with the eHealth intervention. It seems to consist of behavioural, cognitive, and affective components which have been explored more in depth in this chapter. There are some ways of measuring engagement – of which self-report questionnaires have received most attention – but these are still in the early phases of development. More research is needed to gain an in depth understanding of engagement: Of the components, the process over time, and the differences between individuals and technologies. Based on those insights, our measurements also need to be refined. When we achieve more in-depth knowledge and measurement of engagement, there are a lot of opportunities to improve the effectiveness of eHealth interventions, most prominently due to the power of engagement to personalize and adapt interventions to an individual's needs. The take home messages for this chapter are:

- eHealth technologies can only have an impact when they are used in an effective manner, and taking engagement into account is key in getting people to use them in such a way;
- Although they are important and related aspects, acceptance, adoption, and adherence are not sufficient to explain eHealth effectiveness or engagement;
- Engagement is a multifaceted concept, which includes a behavioural, cognitive, and affective component;
- As engagement is more than the usage of eHealth technology, usage data is not a sufficient measure of engagement. Rather, questionnaires can be a good option, and there are two relatively new validated engagement questionnaires.

Key References for Further Reading

Kelders, S. M., Kip, H., & Greeff, J. (2020). Psychometric evaluation of the Twente Engagement with Ehealth Technologies Scale (TWEETS): Evaluation study. *Journal of Medical Internet Research*, 22(10), e17757.

Kelders, S. M., Van Zyl, L. E., & Ludden, G. D. (2020). The concept and components of engagement in different domains applied to ehealth: A systematic scoping review. *Frontiers in Psychology*, 11, 926.

Perski, O., Blandford, A., West, R., & Michie, S. (2017). Conceptualising engagement with digital behaviour change interventions: A systematic review using principles from critical interpretive synthesis. *Translational Behavioural Medicine*, 7(2), 254–267.

Perski, O., Lumsden, J., Garnett, C., Blandford, A., West, R., & Michie, S. (2019). Assessing the psychometric properties of the digital behaviour change intervention engagement scale in users of an app for reducing alcohol consumption: Evaluation study. *Journal of Medical Internet Research*, 21(11), e16197.

Short, C. E., DeSmet, A., Woods, C., Williams, S. L., Maher, C., Middelweerd, A., ... & Crutzen, R. (2018). Measuring engagement in eHealth and mHealth behaviour change interventions: Viewpoint of methodologies. *Journal of Medical Internet Research*, 20(11), e292.

References

Andrews, G., & Williams, A. D. (2014). Internet psychotherapy and the future of personalized treatment. *Depress Anxiety*, 31(11), 912–915. doi:10.1002/da.22302

Appleton, J., Christenson, S., & Furlong, M. (2008). Student engagement with school: Critical conceptual and methodological issues of the construct. *Psychology in the Schools*, 45, 369–386. doi:10.1002/pits.20303

Bakker, A. B., Schaufeli, W. B., Leiter, M. P., & Taris, T. W. (2008). Work engagement: An emerging concept in occupational health psychology. *Work & Stress*, 22(3), 187–200. doi:10.1080/02678370802393649

Beatty, L., & Binnion, C. (2016). A systematic review of predictors of, and reasons for, adherence to online psychological interventions. *International Journal of Behavioral Medicine*, 23(6), 776–794.

Bijkerk, L. E., Oenema, A., Geschwind, N., & Spigt, M. (2023). Measuring engagement with mental health and behavior change interventions: An integrative review of methods and instruments. *Int J Behav Med*, 30(2), 155–166. doi:10.1007/s12529-022-10086-6

Bolier, L., & Abello, K. (2014). Online positive psychological interventions: State of the art and future directions. In: *The Wiley-Blackwell handbook of positive psychological interventions* (pp. 286–309), Wiley-Blackwell.

Chen, K., & Chan, A. H. (2011). A review of technology acceptance by older adults. *Gerontechnology*, 10(1), 1–12.

Christensen, H., Griffiths, K. M., & Farrer, L. (2009). Adherence in internet interventions for anxiety and depression: Systematic review. *Journal of Medical Internet Research*, 11(2), e13.

Cuijpers, P., Reynolds, C. F., 3rd, Donker, T., Li, J., Andersson, G., & Beekman, A. (2012). Personalized treatment of adult depression: Medication, psychotherapy, or both? A systematic review. *Depress Anxiety*, 29(10), 855–864. doi:10.1002/da.21985

Davis, F. D. (1989). Perceived usefulness, perceived ease of use, and user acceptance of information technology. *MIS Quarterly*, 13(3), 319–340. doi:10.2307/249008

Donkin, L., Christensen, H., Naismith, S. L., Neal, B., Hickie, I. B., & Glozier, N. (2011). A systematic review of the impact of adherence on the effectiveness of e-therapies. *Journal of Medical Internet Research*, 13(3), e52.

Farvolden, P., Denisoff, E., Selby, P., Bagby, R. M., & Rudy, L. (2005). Usage and longitudinal effectiveness of a Web-based self-help cognitive behavioral therapy program for panic disorder. *Journal of Medical Internet Research*, 7(1), e7.

Greenhalgh, T., Robert, G., Macfarlane, F., Bate, P., & Kyriakidou, O. (2004). Diffusion of innovations in service organizations: Systematic review and recommendations. *Milbank Quarterly*, 82(4), 581–629.

Greenhalgh, T., Wherton, J., Papoutsi, C., Lynch, J., Hughes, G., A'Court, C., . . . Shaw, S. (2017). Beyond adoption: A new framework for theorizing and evaluating nonadoption, abandonment, and challenges to the scale-up, spread, and sustainability of health and care technologies. *J Med Internet Res*, 19(11), e367. doi:10.2196/jmir.8775

Hamari, J., Koivisto, J., & Sarsa, H. (2014, 6–9 Jan. 2014). Does gamification work? — A literature review of empirical studies on gamification. Paper presented at the 2014 47th Hawaii International Conference on System Sciences.

Hyland, M. E., & Whalley, B. (2008). Motivational concordance: An important mechanism in self-help therapeutic rituals involving inert (placebo) substances. *J Psychosom Res*, 65(5), 405–413. doi:10.1016/j.jpsychores.2008.02.006

Kelders, S. (2019). Design for engagement of online positive psychology interventions. In: *Positive psychological intervention design and protocols for multi-cultural contexts* (pp. 297–313). Springer.

Kelders, S. (2015). *Involvement as a working mechanism for Persuasive Technology* (pp. 3–14). Springer International Publishing.

Kelders, S. M., Bohlmeijer, E. T., Pots, W. T., & van Gemert-Pijnen, J. E. (2015). Comparing human and automated support for depression: Fractional factorial randomized controlled trial. *Behaviour Research and Therapy*, 72, 72–80.

Kelders, S. M., Kip, H., & Greeff, J. (2020a). Psychometric evaluation of the TWente Engagement with Ehealth Technologies Scale (TWEETS): Evaluation study. *J Med Internet Res*, 22(10), e17757. doi:10.2196/17757

Kelders, S. M., Kok, R. N., Ossebaard, H. C., & van Gemert-Pijnen, J. E. (2012). Persuasive system design does matter: A systematic review of adherence to web-based interventions. *Journal of Medical Internet Research*, 14(6), e152.

Kelders, S. M., Sommers-Spijkerman, M., & Goldberg, J. (2018). Investigating the direct impact of a gamified versus nongamified well-being intervention: An exploratory experiment. *J Med Internet Res*, 20(7), e247. doi:10.2196/jmir.9923

Kelders, S. M., van Zyl, L. E., & Ludden, G. D. S. (2020b). The concept and components of engagement in different domains applied to eHealth: A systematic scoping review. *Frontiers in Psychology*, 11. doi:10.3389/fpsyg.2020.00926

Nadal, C., Sas, C., & Doherty, G. (2020). Technology acceptance in mobile health: Scoping review of definitions, models, and measurement. *J Med Internet Res*, 22(7), e17256. doi:10.2196/17256

Nahum-Shani, I., Smith, S. N., Spring, B. J., Collins, L. M., Witkiewitz, K., Tewari, A., & Murphy, S. A. (2018). Just-in-Time Adaptive Interventions (JITAIs) in mobile health: Key components and design principles for ongoing health behavior support. *Ann Behav Med*, 52(6), 446–462. doi:10.1007/s12160-016-9830-8

O'Brien, H., & Toms, E. (2008). What is user engagement? A conceptual framework for defining user engagement with technology. *JASIST*, 59, 938–955. doi:10.1002/asi.20801

Peek, S. T., Wouters, E. J., van Hoof, J., Luijkx, K. G., Boeije, H. R., & Vrijhoef, H. J. (2014). Factors influencing acceptance of technology for aging in place: A systematic review. *International Journal of Medical Informatics*, 83(4), 235–248.

Perski, O., Blandford, A., Garnett, C., Crane, D., West, R., & Michie, S. (2020). A self-report measure of engagement with digital behavior change interventions (DBCIs): Development and psychometric evaluation of the "DBCI Engagement Scale". *Transl Behav Med*, 10(1), 267–277. doi:10.1093/tbm/ibz039

Perski, O., Blandford, A., Ubhi, H. K., West, R., & Michie, S. (2017a). Smokers' and drinkers' choice of smartphone applications and expectations of engagement: A think aloud and interview study. *BMC Med Inform Decis Mak*, 17(1), 25. doi:10.1186/s12911-017-0422-8

Perski, O., Blandford, A., West, R., & Michie, S. (2017b). Conceptualising engagement with digital behaviour change interventions: A systematic review using principles from critical interpretive synthesis. *Transl Behav Med*, 7(2), 254–267. doi:10.1007/s13142-016-0453-1

Perski, O., Lumsden, J., Garnett, C., Blandford, A., West, R., & Michie, S. (2019). Assessing the psychometric properties of the digital behavior change intervention engagement scale in users of an app for reducing alcohol consumption: Evaluation study. *J Med Internet Res*, 21(11), e16197. doi:10.2196/16197

Perski, O., Naughton, F., Garnett, C., Blandford, A., Beard, E., West, R., & Michie, S. (2019). Do daily fluctuations in psychological and app-related variables predict engagement with an alcohol reduction app? A series of N-Of-1 studies. *JMIR Mhealth Uhealth*, 7(10), e14098. doi:10.2196/14098

Perski, O., & Short, C. E. (2021). Acceptability of digital health interventions: Embracing the complexity. *Transl Behav Med*, 11(7), 1473–1480. doi:10.1093/tbm/ibab048

Pots, W. T., Fledderus, M., Meulenbeek, P. A., Peter, M., Schreurs, K. M., & Bohlmeijer, E. T. (2016). Acceptance and commitment therapy as a web-based intervention for depressive symptoms: Randomised controlled trial. *The British Journal of Psychiatry*, 208(1), 69–77.

Rabbi, M., Philyaw Kotov, M., Cunningham, R., Bonar, E. E., Nahum-Shani, I., Klasnja, P., . . . Murphy, S. (2018). Toward increasing engagement in substance use data collection: Development of the substance abuse research assistant app and protocol for a microrandomized trial using adolescents and emerging adults. *JMIR Res Protoc*, 7(7), e166. doi:10.2196/resprot.9850

Rogers, E. M. (2010). *Diffusion of innovations*: Simon and Schuster.

Ruiz, F. (2012). Acceptance and commitment therapy versus traditional cognitive behavioral therapy: A systematic review and meta-analysis of current empirical evidence. *International Journal of Psychology and Psychological Therapy*, 12, 333–357.

Short, C. E., DeSmet, A., Woods, C., Williams, S. L., Maher, C., Middelweerd, A., . . . Crutzen, R. (2018). Measuring engagement in eHealth and mHealth behavior change interventions: Viewpoint of methodologies. *J Med Internet Res*, 20(11), e292. doi:10.2196/jmir.9397

Sieverink, F., Kelders, S. M., & van Gemert-Pijnen, J. E. (2017). Clarifying the concept of adherence to eHealth technology: Systematic review on when usage becomes adherence. *J Med Internet Res*, 19(12), e402. doi:10.2196/jmir.8578

Talbot, F. (2012a). Client contact in self-help therapy for anxiety and depression: Necessary but can take a variety of forms beside therapist contact. *Behaviour Change*, 29. doi:10.1017/bec.2012.4

Whalley, B., & Hyland, M. E. (2009). One size does not fit all: Motivational predictors of contextual benefits of therapy. *Psychol Psychother*, 82(Pt 3), 291–303. doi:10.1348/147608309x413275

Wrede, C., Braakman-Jansen, A., & van Gemert-Pijnen, L. (2021). Requirements for unobtrusive monitoring to support home-based dementia care: Qualitative study among formal and informal caregivers. *JMIR Aging*, 4(2), e26875. doi:10.2196/26875

Yardley, L., Spring, B. J., Riper, H., Morrison, L. G., Crane, D. H., Curtis, K., . . . Blandford, A. (2016). Understanding and promoting effective engagement with digital behavior change interventions. *Am J Prev Med*, 51(5), 833–842. doi:10.1016/j.amepre.2016.06.015

16 Evaluating eHealth

Hanneke Kip, Iris ten Klooster, Julia Keizer,
Lisa Klein Haneveld, Tessa Dekkers, & Saskia M. Kelders

Introduction

Imagine you have developed a technology to support self-management in patients with chronic diseases and you want to know if it really has added value for your target group. Therefore, you have set up an evaluation study. Before patients start to use the technology, you ask them to complete questionnaires to assess how they feel. After they have been using the technology for a while, you ask them again to complete the same questionnaires. Now you might know a bit more about what the effects of the technology might be on, for example, the users' quality of life. But there is a lot more that you do not know. For instance, how cost-effective is the technology? What are the experiences of the patients? Do healthcare providers like the technology as well? Was the technology used at all, and how can we improve its usage? The goal of this chapter is to explain how to answer these types of questions by explaining the why and what of eHealth evaluations. Multiple types of evaluation approaches and research methods that are suitable for eHealth will be presented. However, – as is the case in any activity related to eHealth – the exact evaluation process will differ per technology, context, and research team.

This chapter is divided into two parts. The first part is focused on the why of eHealth evaluation. We dive into the current state of affairs and provide some overarching frameworks that can be used to shape evaluation processes. The second part of this chapter is focused on specific methodologies that can be used for evaluation. After completing this chapter, you will be able to.

- Provide several reasons for the importance of multi-method, iterative eHealth evaluation processes;
- Explain why eHealth can be seen as a black box and what the pitfalls of only conducting one experimental study are;
- Explain how holistic, multi-method evaluations can contribute to opening the black box of eHealth;
- Explain the goals and phases of different types of evaluation frameworks: MOST-design, realist evaluation, and process evaluation;
- Name and explain several methods for the evaluation of effectiveness, efficiency and adherence and engagement: RCTs, fractional factorial designs, Single-Case Experimental Designs (SCEDs), log data analysis, mixed-methods research, and Health Technology Assessment (HTA).

DOI: 10.4324/9781003302049-18

Part 1: Evaluation – What and Why?

What is Evaluation?

In short, evaluation can be defined as the systematic collection, interpretation, and presentation of information in order to determine value and results of a specific product. This is a rather general description, but a bit more concretely, the purpose of eHealth evaluation is to systematically obtain information that can be used to determine the overall effectiveness of an eHealth technology. The results of evaluation studies are not just used to assess whether the goals of the technology have been met, but also to improve its design, implementation, adoption, and usage. eHealth evaluation encompasses more than determining the effectiveness of a single technology: Different evaluations of different technologies can be used to form a scientific base about what works, for whom, and why. For example, if we know from previous research what type of feedback is effective for a certain target group, this can be incorporated in new interventions to increase their chances of effectiveness. Finally, it is important to note the difference between efficacy and effectiveness. These terms are often used interchangeably, but they are two different concepts. Efficacy is focused on how well an eHealth technology works under ideal, controlled conditions, such as in lab settings or highly controlled clinical trials. Effectiveness, on the other hand, refers to how well an eHealth technology performs in the real world, under uncontrolled conditions, often after it's been implemented in practice. In other words: Efficacy refers to assessing clinically measurable effects under ideal circumstances, while effectiveness focuses on measuring intended health results under normal or usual circumstances. For clarity purposes, we will use the term effectiveness in this chapter, but when thinking of evaluation, it is important to consider if the study is focused on efficacy or effectiveness.

Why Perform Evaluation?

The most commonly known reason for evaluation is to test the effectiveness of an eHealth technology, or in other words, to know if (and how) it reaches its intended goals. However, there are several more reasons to evaluate eHealth technologies in different phases of the development (Bonten et al., 2020; Lilford, Foster, & Pringle, 2009). Already in early phases of development, evaluation studies can be conducted to find (technical) problems with an eHealth technology. In the CeHRes Roadmap, this is referred to as formative evaluation (see Chapter 7). A broad range of points of improvement or potentially negative effects can be identified to ensure that no harm will be inflicted and to create the best possible technology for the end-users. These types of formative evaluations enable immediate improvements of the technology or can even result in a discontinuation of development before further investments are required. In turn, this increases the likelihood of developing a successful technology that is accepted by stakeholders and by financers such as healthcare insurers.

Evaluation can facilitate the integration of the perspectives of a broad range of stakeholders in the eHealth technology. As described in Chapter 7, eHealth development and implementation should take the needs, wishes, and goals of end-users and other stakeholders into account. Imagine the example we mentioned at the beginning of this chapter. The users of a technology to support self-management can be considered the most important stakeholders. However, there are more stakeholders involved in the care for patients with chronic diseases. For example, caregivers (who want the technology to be of added value in daily care routines), healthcare insurance companies (who want the technology to be cost-effective), or policy makers (who want the technology to fit within the existing regulations and guidelines). To evaluate whether all goals of the technology have been met, the perspectives of all of these stakeholders should thus be accounted for during the evaluation. Also, including stakeholders in evaluation can result in a better adoption and long-term implementation of the technology. Moreover, by conducting viable evaluations of eHealth technologies, and thus providing a strong foundation for the effectiveness and efficiency, the technology will be more likely to be perceived as trustworthy: Evidence-based technologies are more likely to be adopted in practice and reimbursed by e.g., healthcare insurers. Finally, evaluation provides a basis for identifying promising approaches or features that can be used and combined in other (new) technologies.

The Goals of eHealth Evaluation

Roughly speaking, a distinction can be made between four types of evaluations of eHealth: Formative evaluation, evaluation of impact, evaluation of uptake, and evaluation of working mechanisms. These types are explained in more detail below.

Formative Evaluation

Formative evaluation refers to the continuous collection of information to improve eHealth technologies, using an iterative approach in which constant adaptations to the technology can be made. As described in Chapter 7, these continuous, formative evaluations are already relevant from the start of the development process, and they are intertwined throughout all further phases. This type of evaluation has two main goals. First, it can be conducted as a backward evaluation, which occurs at the end of a specific development phase, to check whether the goals as set at the start of that phase have been reached and have been accounted for. For example, in the operationalization phase, a multi-method study can be conducted to investigate whether the initially set implementation objectives have been met. Second, forward formative evaluations provide information on the current state of the development process and how to make improvements before moving on to the next phase (forward evaluation). An example of this is a usability test, in which a prototype of a technology is presented to its users, who provide feedback and points for improvements that can be accounted for in a next prototype or the 'final' version of a technology (also see Chapter 11). The results of these formative evaluations can be used to improve the technology's design, activities, or performance, and to make sure that the technology fits the users, other stakeholders, and the context. Therefore, evaluation during eHealth development and operationalization is a way of 'creating by evaluating'.

Evaluation of Impact

Evaluation of impact is conducted to determine what has been achieved at a specific point in time, mostly after the technology is ready to be used and/or implemented in practice for a while. However, impact evaluations can also be conducted with eHealth technologies that are not yet implemented in practice. For example, an app that is developed for a vulnerable target group such as people with severe mental illness can first be evaluated with students to investigate if it actually works and if no unintended, negative consequences arise, before implementing and using it in psychiatric practice. Different types of outcomes can be assessed in an evaluation of impact, but these outcomes should be related to the objectives that have been set at the start of the development process. Of course, new, unexpected outcomes can arise as well, requiring a flexible mindset from researchers. Examples of outcomes include:

- **Clinical outcomes**: Improvements in the health status of the users, for example, blood pressure, quality of life, depressive symptoms, or blood glucose levels;

- **Behavioural outcomes**: Changes in behaviour, such as prescription behaviour or levels of physical activity;
- **Organizational outcomes**: Changes in the context in which the technology is used, for example cost-reductions in healthcare or more efficient working routines.

In line with a holistic approach, attention must be paid to outcomes related to the end-user (e.g., patients), but also the technology's impact on other stakeholders (healthcare providers, managers) and the organizational and wider context (e.g., cost-effectiveness). This type of evaluation is mostly focused on if a technology works, but in itself does not provide answers regarding why, how and for whom it is (not) effective.

Evaluation of Uptake

Evaluation of uptake refers to the way in which a technology is used in practice. This type of evaluation is conducted to explain (lack of) effects found in impact evaluation, and/or to identify points of improvement for is usage. For example, if a technology is shown to be ineffective, an explanation might be that it is not used at all in most participating organizations, or users might only use one element of it (e.g., information about a disease), and skip the elements that are expected to contribute most to its effectiveness (e.g., feedback, goal setting). Also, if elements of a technology were not used, this implicates that changes in design or content are required. There are different types of questions that are related to evaluation of uptake. Some examples are:

- By how many users was the technology used?
- How often did the users log in and for how long did they use the technology?
- Which elements of the technology were (not) used and in what combination?
- How often and by whom was the technology used over time?
- By how many organizations/teams/countries was the technology used?
- Who were the active users, and who were the dropouts?

While there are many ways to study if and how a technology was used, it is important to combine this information with results on its impact and working mechanisms to paint a complete picture of the technology's effectiveness.

Evaluation of Working Mechanisms

Evaluation of working mechanisms is conducted to gain insights into why a technology is (not) effective. These types of evaluations result in outcomes that are often more generalizable and contribute to theory-building regarding eHealth in general – especially if the findings of multiple types of these studies are combined.

There are different types of explanations for (in)effectiveness that can be used in eHealth evaluation, of which some examples are:

- **Adherence**. Adherence refers to the extent to which a technology is used as intended by its developers. To put it (very) bluntly: If a technology is not used (in the right way), it will probably not be effective. Indeed, a dose-response relationship is sometimes observed, in which more usage is related to higher effectiveness. However, this is not always the case – it might also be that users stop using a technology once they've experienced enough benefits;
- **Engagement**. Engagement refers to the behavioural, cognitive, and affective experience of users with technology and can be used to assess whether the technology is useful to them.

Engagement is not the same as adherence, but has a more subjective element to it, and can be a predictor of the effectiveness of eHealth interventions;

- **Behaviour change techniques**. Many studies have focused on investigating if and how (sets of) behaviour change techniques such as feedback, personalization, or goal setting are related to the effectiveness of (eHealth) interventions. However, this can be difficult to study since papers do not always report on which techniques were used and how they were operationalized;
- **Socio-demographic characteristics of users**. A relatively straightforward way of gaining insight into why a technology does (not) work for a specific group is to examine if variables such as demographic variables (age, gender), social characteristics (e.g., socio-economic status), or personality traits (e.g., conscientiousness, neuroticism) are related to effectiveness. While this might yield some interesting results, it is important to note that these types of outcomes are difficult to account for in design of eHealth;
- **Domain-specific working mechanisms**. An example of this is mindfulness: By increasing mindfulness via for example a mobile app, depressive complaints can decrease. In other words, first, mindfulness has to increase before depression can improve, making mindfulness into the working mechanism.

There are more types of variables that can be used as explanations for why eHealth works. As is the case with any type of evaluation, it is important to link this to the outcomes of e.g., impact and uptake evaluation.

As you might have noticed, it is not always possible to make a clear distinction between these four types of evaluation. For example, outcomes of uptake or impact evaluations can be used to further improve an intervention, and in that way, can also be viewed as formative evaluations. Furthermore, in order to identify working mechanisms, impact evaluations are always necessary because researchers have to analyse whether proposed working mechanisms predict the outcomes of an intervention. This again underlines that evaluation is a multi-method, iterative process, and not one single activity.

Evaluation Approaches and Frameworks

As seen before, there are a lot of different objectives that can be reached with evaluation. Ideally, most are met in an overarching evaluation process, using multiple methods. There are different types of frameworks that can be used to guide these processes. In the following section, we will describe three of such frameworks: Multiphase Optimization Strategy (MOST), realist evaluations, and process evaluations. However, to explain the importance of viewing evaluation as a multi-method process as opposed to a single post-implementation activity, we will first explain the possibilities and pitfalls of a randomized controlled trial (RCT) – often viewed as the 'gold standard' for evaluations of (behavioural) interventions.

RCTs as the 'Gold Standard' for eHealth Evaluation?

Often, experimental studies, such as *randomized controlled trials (RCTs)* are viewed as the best (or only) way to conduct evaluation research on eHealth. By means of RCTs, the effects of an intervention on pre-specified health outcomes are assessed. In short, these studies are used to find an answer to the question: 'Does it work?' (Oakley et al., 2006). An RCT is a study design in which participants are randomly assigned to an experimental group or a control group. The experimental group receives the therapy that is the subject of the evaluation, which can either be a drug, a behavioural (eHealth) intervention, or something else. The control group receives the usual care, an adjusted version of the therapy, a placebo (a product without any therapeutic effect)

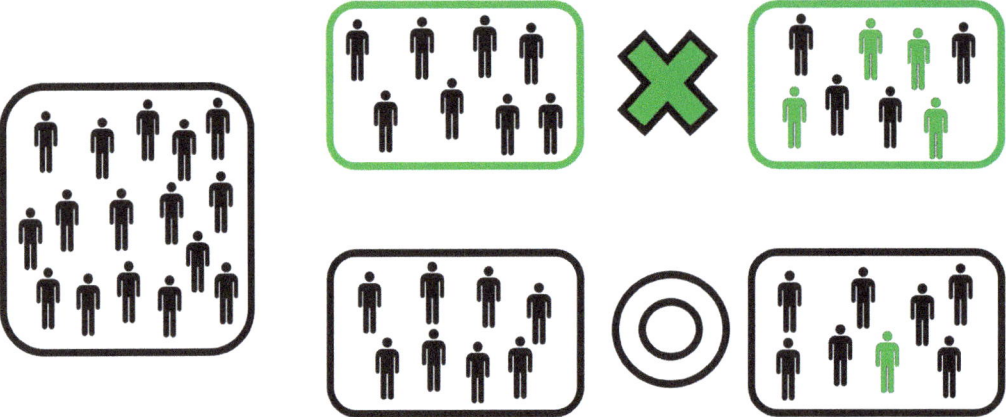

Figure 16.1 A visualization of a randomized controlled trial.

or is placed on a waiting list. It is also possible to conduct an RCT with more than two conditions (e.g., two version of an intervention), but in any case, a control group has to be used. Before receiving the therapy, included participants are assessed on predetermined outcomes to establish the effects of the experimental therapy (e.g., heart rate, blood pressure, quality of life, depression). After receiving the therapy for a predetermined period of time, all participants undergo the same assessments again. If the therapy was effective, the therapy group should have significantly better outcomes than the control group, meaning that statistical analyses show that differences between groups in changes over time are not coincidental. This process is visualized in Figure 16.1, where the X represents the therapy and the O represents the control group condition. The green blocks refer to the group that received the therapy, and the green figures represent the participants with improved outcomes.

Box 16.1 An example of a randomized controlled trial.

In close cooperation with partners of cancer patients, the *web-based intervention 'Hold on, for each other'* was developed (Köhle et al., 2015). The aim of this eHealth intervention is to prevent and decrease stress, psychological and physical health problems in people whose partner has cancer.(Li, Mak, & Loke, 2013) The content of the intervention is based on approaches from positive psychology; Acceptance and Commitment Therapy (ACT), and self-compassion. A randomized controlled trial with three groups was conducted to evaluate its effectiveness. A total of 203 partners of cancer patients with mild to moderate distress were randomized to three conditions: the intervention with personal feedback (*n* = 67); the intervention with automated feedback (*n* = 70), and a waiting list control condition without any intervention (*n* = 66). All participants completed validated questionnaires before and after the intervention. Participants of the two feedback conditions also completed all questionnaires at a six-month follow-up.

Results revealed that 'Hold on, for each other' has the potential to reduce partners' psychological distress. The automated feedback condition was more effective in reducing distress when compared to the waiting list control condition in the short term. However, in the long term, the personal feedback condition seemed to be more effective. It was not clear why this was the case, nor for which participants the intervention was (not) effective, and what the main points of improvements for its design were. Future research with other methods such as interviews or log data analysis was necessary (Köhle, 2016).

Added Value and Limitations of RCTs

As was pointed out before, RCTs are often considered as the gold standard for comparing different conditions for almost any intervention. In healthcare, RCTs were initially mostly used for effectiveness research on medication. However, as shown in the example in the previous paragraph, RCTs also bear several limitations – partly because eHealth interventions are profoundly different from e.g., drugs for hypertension or diabetes. There are several reasons for this (see e.g., (Bonten et al., 2020; Glasgow, 2007)):

First of all, (quasi)-experimental methods such as RCTs mostly provide insight into if an intervention works, and not into how, why and for whom the intervention is effective. Pre- and post-measurements provide evidence on, for example, health outcomes, satisfaction and adoption rates at different, fixed cut-off points. However, such measurements provide limited insights into the interaction process between the user and the technology, and how the technology supported the user in for example healthier living. Also, many outcome measures, such as well-being, blood pressure, and technology usage, change over time and are dynamic processes, so by only assessing them twice, fluctuations over time might be overlooked. Furthermore, RCTs often only contain quantitative data, and while those are useful for identifying significant effects, they do not provide insight into user experiences. Also, analyses are often conducted for the entire group of participants, overlooking individual differences.

Second, RCTs are suitable for evaluating 'fixed' entities such as medication, partly since the 'content' of a drug does not change over time. However, the content and design of an eHealth intervention should be continuously adapted and improved. When the technology is adjusted during this intervention period, it might remain unclear whether the effects are found despite or thanks to these adjustments. If the intervention is not changed and remains the same, it is often changed after the study is completed, which raises questions about whether the effects identified in the RCT are still found for the adapted version. In line with this, in experimental studies, there often are strict protocols for using the intervention (e.g., instructions for healthcare providers, or external rewards to ensure that participants continue to use the intervention). However, this is often not ecologically valid, which might mean that the results of an RCT are not generalizable to clinical practice – in which the eHealth intervention is probably used in a different, less structured way. Not changing an eHealth intervention at all might be a solution to overcome this, but a characteristic of technology is its constant evolution, so when a technology does not move with new developments, they have the chance to become obsolete – however evidence-based they might be.

Third, eHealth often consists of multiple components. Examples are different lessons in an internet-based intervention, multiple components in a personal health record, or even different, tailored versions of an intervention. These components can or cannot be used and can also be used in different compositions or in different orders by different users. Furthermore, as opposed to e.g., face-to-face interventions delivered by a healthcare professional, eHealth interventions can be used in many different ways in terms of the elements that are used, and the frequency, time, and place of use. Experimental study designs mostly provide insight into outcomes at fixed time points and treat technologies as a singular entity. Therefore, too little attention is paid to process outcomes, such as how the use of the different components of the technology has contributed to healthier living, improved well-being, or a user's ability to conduct daily tasks.

Finally, it takes a lot of time and money to conduct an RCT, especially in clinical practice. Especially in projects with limited budget, an RCT will take up most of the available resources. Consequently, especially considering the fast pace of technological change, it might be more efficient to conduct more smaller evaluation studies instead of one very large experimental trial. Additionally, because planning, executing and publishing the results of an RCT takes up a lot of time, it might be that a technology is already obsolete once the study results are available to others. Less time-consuming studies – of which the outcomes can be shared with other interested researchers sooner – can be more suitable.

While an RCT can be very useful to answer specific research questions, it is important to note that evaluation should encompass more than this one specific type of outcome evaluation in order to open the black box of eHealth – which is explained in Box 16.2.

Box 16.2 The Black Box of eHealth further explained.

Different to many in-person therapies, one of the main characteristics of eHealth is that individuals can use the same technology in many different ways. For example, one person can use the technology more often than another, can use different elements of the technology, or can complete an entire technology while another does not finish it. By only looking at the effectiveness of a technology for the whole user group, we do not know how or what parts of the technology were effective and for whom. In this way, eHealth can be seen as a black box where it is unknown what happens inside (Kelders, Oinas-Kukkonen, Oörni, & van Gemert-Pijnen, 2016; Resnicow et al., 2010; Sieverink, 2017). A visualized explanation of the Black Box phenomenon is depicted below.

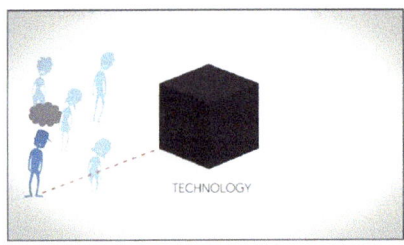

This is Pete, a man who suffers from mild depressive feelings. He wants to start using an eHealth intervention to address his complaints.

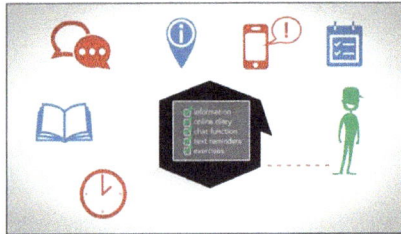

Pete regularly used several features of the technology. For example, he kept an online diary and he has used the chat function to stay in touch with his therapist. Furthermore, he also chose to receive text message reminders to keep him motivated. He completed all the exercises as well. This resulted in a significant decrease of his depressive complaints.

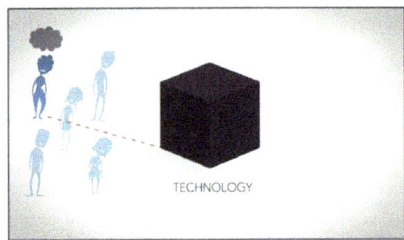

And this is Mary, a woman experiencing depressive feelings. She has heard about the eHealth technology and wants to try it as well.

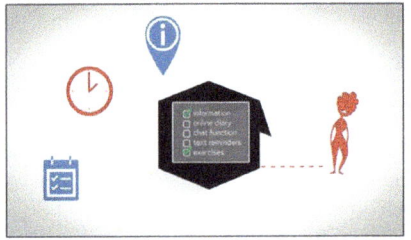

Mary logged in frequently and used some features of the technology. For example, she read all the information, completed most exercises, but she decided that she did not want to receive the text message reminders with motivational texts. The program did not help to improve her complaints.

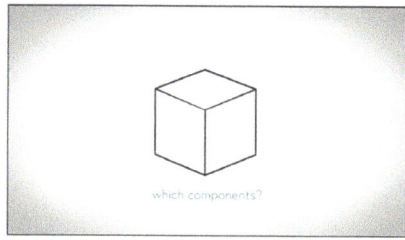

When we just would have looked at the impact of the technology, we would only have been able to see whether it was effective or not, without recognizing the differences between the usage patterns of Pete and Mary.

However, by collecting information on the usage, we are able to evaluate the uptake as well. For example, we can figure out how the use of the different elements, patterns, and the frequency of use have contributed to the effects and for whom. We can use this information to improve the technology or develop different versions of it for different types of users.

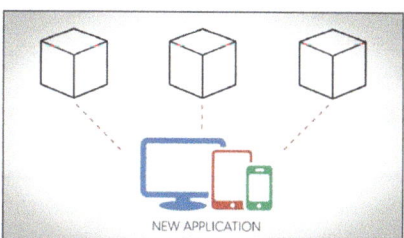

Also, we can use the knowledge we gain by opening the black boxes of other technologies as well. We can combine effective elements to create a new technology.

Over the past years, the field of eHealth has paid more attention to ways to open this black box. In general, it has become clear that eHealth evaluation is not one single activity, to be performed once a technology is completed. Just as development and implementation, it is an iterative process in which multiple methods are used to gain as much insight as possible into different outcomes and points of improvement. In order to shape these processes, there are different approaches that can be used. Below, three frameworks that can provide useful tools to guide eHealth evaluation processes are explained: Multiphase Optimization Strategy (MOST), realist evaluation, and process evaluation.

Multiphase Optimization Strategy (MOST)

Imagine that you want to evaluate a multi-component app-based intervention for people with depressive complaints. Based on previous research, you have decided that the intervention can consist of different components that might contribute to its effectiveness, such as feedback on exercises, guided meditation in VR, and a diary-app asking about positive experiences. However, there are some questions as to whether the feedback should be provided by a therapist, or if automated AI-generated messages might suffice. Also, it is not clear if the guided meditation exercises will be of added value for your intended users and providing them to all users via VR would cost a lot of time and money, so you want to know if they actually add to the effectiveness of the whole intervention. Finally, you are not sure how many reminders the app should send throughout the day since previous research did not report on this. To answer these questions and thus to compile and evaluate the most optimal version of your intervention, the Multiphase Optimization Strategy (MOST) framework can be used (see Figure 16.2). This interdisciplinary framework is grounded in behavioural sciences and based on engineering principles. It aids researchers in determining the most efficient and effective version of an intervention by means of multiple evaluation studies (Collins,

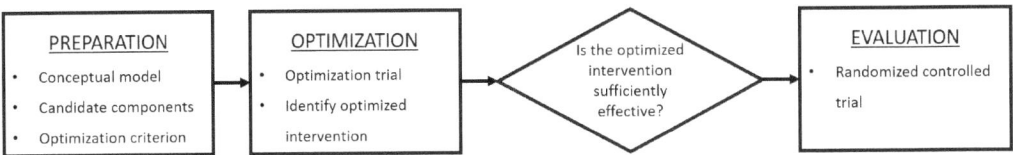

Figure 16.2 A visualization of the Multiphase Optimization Strategy (MOST) framework (Guastaferro, Strayhorn, & Collins, 2021).

Murphy, & Strecher, 2007). It is especially suitable for complex, multi-component interventions, such as those aimed at changing behaviour. MOST is not a research method, but a framework with three phases, for which researchers have to select the most suitable research methods. The three phases are preparation, optimization, and evaluation.

Preparation

In the preparation phase, the researchers select the intervention components they want to examine, ideally based on previous research, such as systematic reviews on effective intervention components. In this phase, a conceptual model of why and how the intervention works should be developed, based on e.g., previous research, theories and frameworks. In the example provided before, examples of components are feedback, guided meditation and a diary-app. These can be operationalized and pilot-tested to ensure that they are usable by the participants. Researchers also have to decide on criteria that can be used to assess whether to keep different components of an intervention (optimization criteria) to ensure that decisions on whether to keep an element are based on transparent criteria. Examples of these criteria are efficiency criteria (e.g., removing components that are not related to effectiveness), cost criteria (e.g., including only components up to a certain cost per user), or time criteria (e.g., including only the effective components that cost less than a specific number of minutes to complete).

Optimization

In the optimization phase, the most optimal version of the intervention is established. Using different types of research methods, the set of components that comprise the most effective version of the intervention are identified and combined into the final intervention. In this phase, the effects of separate components can be tested to identify if and how much they contribute to the effectiveness of the intervention, using experimental designs such as (fractional) factorial designs (which are described in more detail later in this chapter). In the example study at the beginning of this paragraph, researchers could investigate whether there is a difference in effectiveness between therapist-generated and automated feedback. If no difference is observed, it might be advantageous to choose automatically generated feedback because it is the cheaper option (cost criterion). A version of the intervention with and without the VR-guided meditation exercises could be studied to determine if it is of added value (effectiveness criteria). Furthermore, you could test two versions of the diary-app: One with three daily reminders and one version with only one, to see which version leads to better results.

Besides these quantitative methods, a more qualitative approach might be useful as well to create the most optimal version of an intervention. Examples include usability testing, log data analysis, or interviews. These types of methods can help researchers to gain insight into how end-users use and experience the different intervention-components, and what points of improvement are according to them. For example, if there are no differences in effectiveness regarding the number of reminders in the diary-app, what version do the users prefer? In any case, it is important to identify if a component contributes to the intervention – if it is not of added value, it can and should be removed to make the most effective and efficient version of an intervention. The previously set criteria should be used to make sure the decision on whether it is included in the 'final' version of an intervention is made in a well-informed manner.

Evaluation

In this final phase, the entire intervention is evaluated as a whole. Ideally, this is the most optimal version of the intervention, as was established in the previous phase. For example, a version of the intervention with automated feedback, no guided meditation in VR, and a diary-app with only one daily reminder. The evaluation can be done via, for example, a randomized controlled trial (RCT). As explained before, RCTs have pitfalls, but within the context of the MOST framework, it is important to note that questions about effective elements have been identified in the previous phase – addressing some of the previously mentioned concerns about 'opening the black box of eHealth'. Nonetheless, attention for questions about for whom the intervention is (not) effective, what its main points of improvement are, is pivotal, so other methods besides an RCT can of course also be used to gain insight into effectiveness.

Realist Evaluation

A pitfall of many studies on eHealth-effectiveness is that they are conducted in a non-realistic setting. For example, many studies are conducted with students. Not because they are the intended users of the intervention, but simply because they can easily be reached and included by researchers. Furthermore, if interventions are studied in practice, a researcher is often actively involved. Imagine a study in which VR is evaluated in addiction care. Following the 'RCT-paradigm', the researcher is actively involved in motivating therapists and patients to complete the intervention. Additionally, a strict, elaborate protocol for using the intervention in treatment is developed to ensure that it is used exactly as intended. However, after the study is completed, clinicians often use the intervention as they see fit and create their own habits in working with the intervention, which are often not in line with the strict guidelines of a clinical trial. Regardless of the lack of ecological validity, results of such studies that are *not* set in the real-world are often directly applied to the real-world, or even generalized to other settings and other target groups, which does not account for the differences in context and participants. Realist approaches account for this. This type of methodology is based on the assumption that the same intervention will not work everywhere and for everyone, so the focus lies on 'what works, for whom, why, under what circumstances, and how'? (Nielsen & Miraglia, 2016; Pawson & Tilley, 1997; Salter & Kothari, 2014) This approach is especially suitable for the evaluation of complex interventions, particularly those that show mixed results regarding effectiveness, to better understand how and why these differential outcomes occur. Realist evaluations are built around the idea that interventions do not work in isolation but are influenced by specific contexts. This also implies that this approach can only be used for interventions that are already used in practice, and not lab-based evaluations, or evaluations in which the researcher exercises a high level of control over the process, since this is not 'realistic'. While different methods can be used, realist evaluations are built on the assumption that three concepts should be considered: Context, mechanisms, and outcomes. This information is used to build Context-Mechanism-Outcome (CMO) configurations, which explain how a particular context triggers specific mechanisms, leading to particular outcomes. CMO-configurations seek to answer questions like: What is it about this context that makes this intervention (not) work for this outcome, and in what way does this happen? In order to develop and test these configurations, a more detailed overview of the context, mechanisms and outcomes is necessary.

Context

The context refers to the specific conditions, settings, and circumstances in which the intervention is implemented. Examples are environmental factors, cultural aspects, and available resources. In the VR-example provide above, different contexts will probably lead to different results. Imagine if an intervention for substance abuse is used in an outpatient setting with generally highly educated patients who have ample opportunity to practice the skills they acquired in VR in real life. The clinicians are very enthusiastic and skilled in using VR, and managers provide them with a lot of time to work with new technologies. Now imagine the use of this same intervention in an inpatient clinic with patients with intellectual disabilities and limited opportunities to practice with their new skills due to their lack of freedom to go outside. Therapists are overworked, not motivated to use VR, and managers are mostly focused on saving costs. It is highly likely that the exact same intervention will be less successful when faced with the second set of contextual factors than the first. Therefore, these types of contextual factors need to be taken into account when evaluating an intervention. Overlooking them will result in a limited view of why the intervention is (not) effective. Contextual factors can be mapped using a plethora of methods, such as desk research, interviews, or focus groups (also see Chapter 8 on the contextual inquiry).

Mechanism

Mechanisms refer to the underlying processes that represent the 'how' and 'why' of intervention effectiveness within a specific context. They are the underlying entities, processes, or structures which operate in particular contexts to generate outcomes of interest. In other words: they help to explain why an intervention is effective within a specific context. (Nielsen & Miraglia, 2016). They can be seen as contextualized working mechanisms. The assumption is that these mechanisms need the right context to work and thus cannot be viewed as independent from the context in which the intervention is used. Mechanisms can be psychological or social in nature. In the previous example, several mechanisms that are related to intervention effectiveness within a specific context can be identified. For example, skill-training in VR could be an important mechanism, especially for inpatients because of the limited opportunity they have for dealing with temptation. This mechanism might be less relevant for outpatients because they have more contact with the 'outside world', highlighting the influence of the context on the extent to which a working mechanism is effective.

Outcome

Outcomes are the results or changes that are produced by the intervention. These can be intended, in other words: Planned in advance by the researcher and specifically measured with e.g., validated questionnaires. In the VR-example, this can be e.g., the number of consummated alcoholic beverages and experienced craving. However, especially when doing research in context, unintended effects can occur. It might be that using VR results in more efficient treatment sessions because therapists can 'get to the core' sooner. On the other hand, VR might also cost more time in some clinics due to limited training possibilities, again highlighting the importance of accounting for the context. Another advantage of using the intervention might be increased confidence in resisting temptation, or improved treatment motivation due to the use of VR – but again, this might not be relevant or true for all patients, depending on their experiences with the technology. This highlights the importance of not only setting concrete objectives related to the expected outcome of an intervention in a specific context, but also conducting explorative research and looking for unexpected, context-specific effects.

As is the case with all evaluation processes, realist evaluations rely on iterative processes, in which CMO-configurations are generated, evaluated, improved, et cetera. Furthermore, it is important to note that there is no single correct way to conduct a realist evaluation, many ways can be appropriate, as long as the underlying principles are taken into account. The most essential underpinning of this type of evaluation is that interventions do not work in isolation, but are influenced by specific contexts, and what works in one context, may not work in another.

Process Evaluation

RCTs provide insight into if an intervention work, i.e., the focus lies on the outcomes of an intervention. However, terms such as effect sizes do not provide concrete input for e.g., policy makers on how an intervention might be used within their specific context, or how the outcomes of an RCT can be reproduced in real life (Moore et al., 2015). To answer these types of questions, process evaluation can be used as an addition to impact evaluation. The Medical Research Council (MRC) guideline towards conducting process evaluations of complex health interventions (Figure 16.3) emphasises the relationship between context, implementation, and mechanisms of impact, and their influence on the actual outcomes of the intervention. As is the case for the two previously described approaches, multiple methods can be used within this framework, all with the goal of understanding why an intervention works, how it might be replicated in a different context, or whether trial outcomes will be reproduced. For example, interviews can be used to identify how the context might explain findings, how it shaped how the intervention worked, or how effectiveness was related to implementation. In this way, information that is necessary to implement effective interventions in practice can be identified. It is specifically suitable for complex interventions – i.e., those that consist of various interconnecting elements (e.g., a mobile app with a diary function, feedback, psycho-education and videos). Within this framework, it is important to specify what the underlying causal assumptions about how the intervention will work are, since this will help researchers and policy makers identify if and how an intervention can be evaluated and implemented. The MRC process evaluation model emphasizes the relationships between implementation, the context, and mechanisms of impact. Since the relationship between these components is central, they cannot be viewed and studied separately, but for overview purposes, the three elements are described separately below.

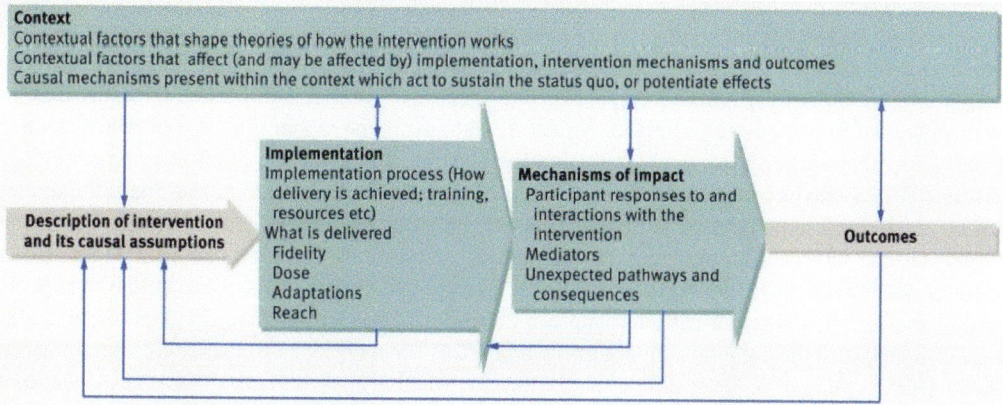

Figure 16.3 The Medical Research Council (MRC) process evaluation model (Moore et al., 2015).

Implementation

Implementation refers to the activities that are undertaken to realize the adoption, dissemination, and long-term use of the eHealth technology in its intended context (see Chapter 13). Gaining insight in how implementation was done and received is pivotal for process evaluation for multiple reasons. First of all, even a very well-designed intervention might not be effective because it is not properly implemented. To be able to gain insight into what works, a first step in process evaluation is to determine how the intervention was actually used in practice. Implementation outcomes such as the fidelity (whether the intervention was delivered as intended) and dose (the 'quantity' of the intervention that was implemented, or how often it was used by participants) can be used to assess this. This is an important step to take since when interventions are implemented in a context, they are often adapted in some way, e.g., several parts might not be introduced to patients by healthcare providers due to time constraints. By accounting for such adaptations in evaluation, researchers can gain insight into whether it was suitable, or if it undermined the intervention fidelity and effectiveness. Furthermore, implementation evaluation is also important to be able to learn about how the eHealth technology was delivered. This can provide policy makers with vital information about how it might be used in different contexts and might even result in generalizable knowledge on how to implement these types of eHealth technologies. Finally, especially in eHealth, it is important to study the reach of an intervention, since it is often not directly visible who comes in contact with the intervention.

It is important to point out that implementation can be studied in multiple ways (see Chapters 13 and 14), but it is recommended to use a mixed-methods approach to paint a complete picture of the uptake of a technology (Kip, Sieverink, van Gemert-Pijnen, Bouman, & Kelders, 2020). To summarize: According to this framework, implementation and evaluation cannot be viewed as separate activities, because the (in)effectiveness of an eHealth technology is often dependent on if and how it was delivered and used.

Mechanisms of Impact

A mechanism of impact links the intervention (components) to the outcome of an evaluation. It is about how the user responds to and interacts with the intervention. It is important to note that participants do not passively receive interventions, but actively interact with complex interventions and exercise agency. This means that the intervention will never work exactly the same for each individual. Therefore, it is important to explore these mechanisms, since they provide an explanation for why an eHealth technology was effective for an individual and what is required to ensure that it is also effective when it is implemented in other settings, with other individuals. When adaptations are made to tailor the intervention to a specific context, it is important to ensure that the mechanisms of impact are not affected. An additional advantage is that this type of research often brings generalizable knowledge, meaning that insights into a mechanism of impact in one eHealth technology can also be integrated into other technologies. In process evaluations, quantitative data can be used to test hypothesised pathways between intervention components, the expected mechanism, and the intervention outcome, but qualitative, exploratory research can also be conducted to better understand these pathways or to identify unexpected mechanisms. An example of a mechanism of impact that is specifically relevant for eHealth, is engagement (see Chapter 15). It can be used to investigate the behavioural, cognitive and affective experience of users with (components of) an eHealth technology and can be used to assess whether they perceive it as useful (Kelders, van Zyl, & Ludden, 2020). In that way, engagement can explain why the eHealth technology is (not) effective for a user: a user with low engagement probably does not respond well to the technology, while this might be the case of a highly engaged user, resulting in increased outcome measures. This mechanism can be applied to many types of interventions. It can also be used in practice to assess whether the users are engaged. If this is not the case, changes to the way an intervention is delivered might be necessary.

Context

Within process evaluation, the context is a very broad concept which refers to anything that is external to the intervention that may be a barrier or facilitator to its effectiveness, implementation, or even a mechanism of impact. An eHealth technology can be used in different ways within different contexts. For example, an internet-based intervention can be used as part of a blended treatment for people with depression, but it might just as well be used as a stand-alone intervention by a general practitioner. Because of these different contexts, the same intervention may have different effects in different situations. The mechanism(s) of impact should fit within the specific context, regardless of the specific problem that is targeted, which might differ from one context to the other. Consequently, to fully understand the (in)effectiveness of an intervention and to adequately interpret the findings, it is important to understand the context (also see Chapter 8 on the contextual inquiry). Also, in order to know what knowledge can (not) be generalized, it is important to identify the influence that a specific context has on the effectiveness. There are many different ways to achieve this, but in any case, it is essential to focus on the role of the context when evaluating interventions within a process evaluation framework.

Part 2: Research Methods

Different Research Methods for eHealth Evaluation

As can be seen in the previous sections, there are many different approaches to conduct eHealth evaluations. The frameworks described before do not provide instructions about which methods to use at which phase in the process, which means that this has to be determined by researchers. The selection of such a method should always depend on the main question(s) they want to address, practical preconditions such as a limited budget for a research project, the phase in the evaluation process, and characteristics of the intended participants (such as limited time, low literacy levels, or heterogeneity of the target group). It is important to note that while an RCT has its limitations, it is still a useful method to answer specific types of research questions – especially if it is combined with other types of data. In Table 16.1 below, a short (non-exhaustive) overview of research methods that can be used in eHealth evaluation is provided, partly based on Bonten et al. (2020).

As can be seen, there are many different methods that can be used. Below, several methods that are suitable for eHealth evaluation are described to further illustrate how different types of methods can be applied. This does not mean that these methods are 'the best', they merely are illustrative examples of methods that can be used to answer questions about why, when and for whom interventions work. The following methods are described: (fractional) Factorial designs, Single-Case Experimental Designs, mixed-methods research, Health Technology Assessment, and log data analysis.

(Fractional) Factorial Designs

As explained before, an RCT often treats technologies as singular entities. However, eHealth technologies usually are complex interventions, consisting of multiple components, including the intervention content (e.g., the topics in different lessons or a diary), features that promote adherence (e.g., reminders or rewards), and other features, such as features aimed at improving intervention fidelity (e.g., delivering the intervention as it was intended by, for instance, enhanced training of

Table 16.1 An overview of several Research Methods that can be used for eHealth Evaluation.

Method	Definition
Factorial designs	An experimental design in which multiple components of an intervention are varied within a group of participants to study their individual effects on outcomes.
Action research	A systematic and collaborative approach in which researchers and practitioners work together to identify and address real-world problems or challenges in a practical and iterative way,
Case series study	A type of observational research design in which a collection of participants with similar characteristics is monitored over a period of time to describe their experiences, outcomes, or responses to an intervention, typically without a control group for comparison.
Randomized controlled trial (RCT)	An experimental design in which participants are randomly assigned to an experimental condition (with the intervention) or control condition (without the intervention), after which between group comparisons are made.
Cluster RCT	In a cluster RCT, randomization does not take place on individual, but on cluster-level, e.g., groups of individuals, schools, or hospitals.
Micro-RCT	An experimental design in which individuals are randomly assigned to different intervention conditions at multiple, closely spaced time points (e.g., daily).
Pragmatic RCT (PRT)	An experimental design that aims to evaluate an intervention under real-world conditions, with practical outcomes, involving a broader, more heterogeneous range of participants, settings, and circumstances than a regular RCT.
Sequential Multiple Assignment RCT (SMART)	An experimental research design that involves multiple stages of randomization and decision points to determine the most effective intervention strategies for individuals over time, adapting interventions based on their responses.
Non-randomized controlled trial	A study in which participants are assigned to different groups, such as treatment and control, without random allocation, often based on factors like participant choice or clinical judgement.
Trial of intervention principles	A type of RCT in which not a 'locked down' version of an intervention, but its underlying core principles are evaluated, allowing for evaluation of personalized and continuously improved interventions.
Pretest-post-test design	A non-experimental design in which only one group receives the intervention and is assessed before and after the introduction of the intervention.
Cohort study	An observational design in which individuals who share a common characteristic or experience (the cohort) is followed over time to compare outcomes.
Cost-effectiveness analysis	An approach in which the efficiency of different interventions is compared by assessing the ratio of their costs to the achieved health or economic outcomes.
Cross-sectional study	An observational design in which data are collected from participants at one single point in time, mostly to analyse characteristics or assess prevalence of a phenomenon.
Mixed-methods research	A research approach in which the outcomes of both qualitative and quantitative methods are integrated within a single study.
Interviews	A qualitative design in which (semi-)structured conversations with an individual are conducted by a researcher to gain in-depth information on individual perspectives.
Focus groups	A qualitative design in which structured discussions with a small group of participants on a pre-specified topic are led by a researcher to gain insights into individual perspectives.
Survey methods	A survey is a method used to collect data through structured, often validated, questionnaires or open-ended questions from a sample of individuals to gather insight into specific topics.

counsellors). To create the optimal intervention, you have to know the individual and combined effects of the different components. This way, you can create the most effective intervention (that includes all the components that add to the effectiveness), or you can create the most effective intervention that can be completed within a certain amount of time or with a certain maximum of costs. A (fractional) factorial design is aimed at doing just that: It is an experimental research design in which the effects of multiple intervention components are investigated (Collins, Dziak, Kugler, & Trail, 2014).

Consider the following example: You are interested in investigating the effects of four complementary components in a physical activity intervention:

1. Keeping an emotion diary related to physical activity;
2. Using an activity tracker;
3. Weekly group activities;
4. Daily email reminders.

For each of these components, you want to know whether they add to the effectiveness of the intervention. Based on the outcomes, you will decide for each of the components whether or not to include them in the optimal intervention. In a factorial experiment, each of the components that you wish to investigate is manipulated experimentally, thus each of them becomes an independent variable. In this case, there are four factors (the components) each with two levels (yes, the component is added; or no, the component is not added). This is a 2^4, or $2 \times 2 \times 2 \times 2$ factorial design and will have 16 different experimental groups (Table 16.2). Each experimental group represents a different treatment protocol. To investigate the main effect of a component, you compare the mean of all groups including that particular component (all the rows with 'yes' on that component in the table) with the mean of all groups not including that component (all the rows with 'no' on that component in the table). For keeping an emotion diary, this means comparing conditions 1 to 8 with 9 to 16. Note that this is very different from a RCT with 16 arms!

A fractional factorial experiment (or study with a fractional factorial design) includes a simple fraction (e.g., ½, ¼) of the conditions of the full factorial experiment. Furthermore, the design should be balanced, meaning that there are an equal number of groups for each level of each component. As an example, for the physical activity intervention, you could carry out ½ of the conditions as shown in Table 2. You could use either the white or the grey conditions. How to get from a full factorial design to a fractional factorial design is beyond the scope of this chapter, but more information can be found elsewhere (Collins, Dziak, & Li, 2009).

Table 16.2 An example of the conditions in a factorial design.

Group	Component			
	Emotion diary	Activity tracker	Group activities	Daily email
1	No	No	No	No
2	No	No	No	Yes
3	No	No	Yes	No
4	No	No	Yes	Yes
5	No	Yes	No	No
6	No	Yes	No	Yes
7	No	Yes	Yes	No
8	No	Yes	Yes	Yes
9	Yes	No	No	No
10	Yes	No	No	Yes
11	Yes	No	Yes	No
12	Yes	No	Yes	Yes
13	Yes	Yes	No	No
14	Yes	Yes	No	Yes
15	Yes	Yes	Yes	No
16	Yes	Yes	Yes	Yes

Possible Research Questions

Factorial designs can provide insight into what the effects of individual components within an intervention are. In the example above, the research question would be: What are the effects of an emotion diary, an activity tracker, weekly group activities, and weekly phone reminders within an intervention to improve physical activity? Overall, example research questions are:

- Does adding a certain component in an intervention increase the effectiveness on outcomes such as depression, physical activity, or diabetes self-management?
- Which version of a component (e.g., reminders once a week vs three times a week, or psychoeducation through animations vs in text) adds most to the effectiveness of an intervention?
- Which component increases adherence or engagement most?
- Are there interaction effects between the components, e.g., does one component work better when a different component is also present?
- Do all envisioned components add to the effectiveness of the intervention?

Added Value and Limitations

To explain the added value of (fractional) factorial designs, it is helpful to compare these designs to an often-used design, the RCT. Consider the example of the physical activity intervention. Often when assessing the effectiveness of such an intervention, an RCT would be used to compare the full intervention (including the emotion diary, the activity tracker, and the weekly group activities) with a control condition.

This is of course a perfectly valid research design to answer the question whether this intervention as a whole is effective in improving physical activity. What it does not provide, is insight into the effectiveness of its individual components. Thus, it is not helpful in optimizing the intervention. Two other research designs could answer these questions: You could conduct four separate RCTs in which the intervention (including only one of these features) is compared to a control condition; or you could conduct one larger RCT with five conditions, one condition for each of the components and a control condition. However, these research designs have two important drawbacks: First, the number of participants needed in both designs to have adequate power is quite large. In the separate RCT design, you have a total of $4 \times 2 = 8$ conditions, or RCT arms. In the larger RCT design, you have 5 conditions. Considering you need at least 100 participants in each condition to have sufficient power to detect a difference of a medium effect size (and often you would like to be able to detect smaller effects than this) this would mean needing at least 500 to 800 participants. However, when using a factorial design, each component is 'active' in half of the experimental groups.

So, to assess the effects of a component, all experimental groups, and all participants are used in the analysis. In other words: None of the efforts (and data) go to waste. For this example, effectively, you would only have two 'conditions', resulting in 200 needed participants. However, there is a trade-off: For this factorial design, you do need to develop and implement 16 different interventions, which might pose a challenge. This is where the fractional factorial design might be useful, as it allows you to lessen the number of interventions (experimental groups), while keeping the number of participants and the power the same. But, of course, there is trade-off: When choosing a fractional factorial design, you lose some of the opportunities to investigate more in depth whether and which components work well together: The so-called interaction effects. In a full factorial design, you can investigate all of these interaction effects, while in a fractional factorial design, you can only study some, or even none at all. Whether this trade-off is worthwhile depends on the available knowledge and context of the precise context. In (eHealth) intervention research, there is often no empirical or theoretical reason to believe that these (higher order) interactions are substantial, which makes fractional factorial designs a valid option to consider (Kelders, Bohlmeijer, Pots, & van Gemert-Pijnen, 2015).

(Fractional) Factorial Designs: An Example

An example of a fractional factorial design in the context of an eHealth intervention is the study of Strecher et al. (2008). This study investigated the effects of five components of a web-based smoking cessation intervention: High- versus low-depth tailored success story, outcome expectation, and efficacy expectation messages; high- versus low personalized source; and multiple versus single exposure to the intervention components. The study employed a 16 experimental group design with 1866 participants. Due to the large number of participants, the study was powered to find relatively small effects. The study found that high-depth tailored success stories and a high personalized message source were effective components in this web-based intervention.

Single-Case Experimental Design (SCED)

Single-Case Experimental Designs (SCEDs) are a group of high-quality experimental research methods in which individuals serve as both the intervention group and their own control group. In a SCED, an intervention is systematically introduced – and dependent on the type of design, withdrawn – across multiple phases, while outcome variables are frequently and repeatedly measured, often at multiple points during the day (Tate et al., 2016). Data can be collected automatically through, for example, wearables, observed by the researcher or healthcare practitioner, or collected through experience sampling, a kind of 'diary', often an app, in which a participant reports multiple times a day on the outcome of interest. SCEDs are experimental research methods and can therefore be used to discover causal relationships between the intervention and outcome measures.

There are several forms of SCEDs. A first example is an introduction-withdrawal design (see Figure 16.4). In this type of design, an intervention is not used on certain days (phase A) and is applied on other days (phase B), after which it is again withdrawn. This happens at least two times and provides insight into what happens when an intervention is (not) used (Krasny-Pacini & Evans, 2018). In a so-called ABAB-design, an intervention can be considered effective when the outcome improves (or reduces, depending on the intervention goal) at the introduction phases (B), compared to the withdrawal phases (A). Next, the changes in outcome are expected to revert (close) to original levels when the intervention is withdrawn in the second withdrawal phase A and to improve again during the second introduction phase B (Smith, 2012). An important advantage is that not many participants have to be used; only three can suffice.

Another example of a SCED is a multiple baseline design (see Figure 16.5), which is a step-wise approach, where the intervention starts at different, randomized times for various participants (Barger-Anderson, Domaracki, Kearney-Vakulick, & Kubina, 2004). This varied introduction of the intervention ensures that the results can be attributed to the intervention rather than external factors. For example, think of a physical activity app that is expected to increase the steps per

	Phase A	**Phase B**	**Phase A**	**Phase B**
Participant 1	No intervention	Intervention	No intervention	Intervention
Participant 2	No intervention	Intervention	No intervention	Intervention
Participant 3	No intervention	Intervention	No intervention	Intervention

Figure 16.4 Overview of introduction-withdrawal design with three participants.

Participant 1	Baseline	Intervention	Intervention	Intervention	Intervention	Follow-up
Participant 2	Baseline	Baseline	Intervention	Intervention	Intervention	Follow-up
Participant 3	Baseline	Baseline	Baseline	Intervention	Intervention	Follow-up

Figure 16.5 Overview of multiple baseline design with three participants.

day. However, this might be influenced by other factors, such as the weather, so if all participants start using the app at the same time (e.g., within a week with bad weather), this might influence the results. The multiple baseline design has several benefits. It can be applied when effects of the intervention are not likely to revert (e.g., in educational interventions) or when withdrawal of the intervention would not be ethical or appropriate (Smith, 2012). However, the design also requires that the intervention is initially withheld to some participants which, depending on the intervention, may be both impractical as well as unethical.

Other SCED designs are the alternating design, the changing criterion design, and the mixed design. These designs are used to explore comparative effectiveness of interventions, demonstrate gradual change, or to embed the SCED in other research designs (e.g., in a RCT), respectively (Smith, 2012). Discussing them is beyond the scope of this chapter, but all of them have in common that they all involve some kind of experimental manipulation. In line with this, it is important to note the distinction with regular case studies, amongst other things due to the manipulation of the different conditions and randomization of participants to a specific condition (Smith, 2012; Tate et al., 2016).

Possible Research Questions

SCEDs can be conducted to answer research questions regarding the effectiveness of an eHealth technology on specific outcomes, for example:

- To what extent can an improvement be seen in e.g., stress, self-efficacy, engagement, or physiological arousal on days that the technology is being used, versus days that the intervention is not being used?
- How long are the effects of the technology noticeable on e.g., well-being?
- To what extent does the introduction of the technology lead to an improvement in e.g., anger, stress, or well-being?
- What is the relationship between implementing the technology and an improvement in e.g., anger, stress, well-being in different healthcare settings, e.g., general practitioner's office, rehabilitation centre, or hospital?
- To what extent do participant characteristics such as age, gender, or knowledge moderate the effect of a technology?

Added Value and Limitations

For a SCED, only a small number of participants (one to three) are required to assess the effectiveness of an intervention, because the patient serves as their own control condition (Krasny-Pacini & Evans, 2018). The power for the analyses does not come from the total number of participants, but from the high number of measurement points from a single participant (Kratochwill et al., 2012).

A known challenge in research involving complex populations is the difficulty of including large, homogeneous groups in studies, which is often a requirement for methods like randomized controlled trials (RCTs). Because SCEDs can be conducted with relatively few participants, this type of effectiveness research is more feasible, as it is easier to involve enough participants. Additionally, SCEDs can be used in a heterogeneous population, as patients function as their own control condition. This makes it possible to include a diverse group of participants (Dallery, Cassidy, & Raiff, 2013). Finally, SCEDs provide better answers to questions like 'why does an intervention work (or not) and when', because more data is collected about an individual. To further explore such questions, SCEDs can also easily be combined with qualitative methods.

The focus on individuals instead of a group is not just an advantage, but can also be seen as a limitation, mostly because it raises questions on external validity (Alnahdi, 2015). External validity or 'generalizability' is related to the extent to which an observed causal relationship could be generalized across different persons and settings. However, this limitation can be resolved by repeatedly testing experimental effects across a variety of settings and participants (Horner et al., 2005).

Single-Case Experimental Design: An Example

In a recent study on the effectiveness of the virtual reality biofeedback game DEEP for forensic psychiatric inpatients, an ABAB introduction-withdrawal SCED was conducted. In this SCED, six patients all received four sessions with DEEP (B-phase). Between these sessions, there were two days without DEEP sessions, but data was still collected (A-phase). During the study, participants wore an Empatica E4 wristband that measured their heart rate variability (HRV) and skin conductance throughout the day. They also rated their experienced tension, stress, and anger three times a day via an experience sampling app, and completed validated questionnaires on stress, anxiety, depression, and aggression three times in total as well. The participating patients and healthcare professionals were also interviewed to gather their experiences with DEEP. The SCED showed that DEEP could reduce user HRV directly after using DEEP, indicating a decrease in tension, although this effect was not consistent for every patient or session. Furthermore, two patients experienced a significant reduction in self-reported stress during the SCED, and one of them also showed a significant decline in tension and anger. Significant changes were not identified in the other four patients, showing that the intervention does not seem to be effective for all.

Mixed-methods Designs

Many eHealth evaluation methods are quantitative, meaning that numerical data from e.g., questionnaires is collected and then analyzed using inferential statistics to find significant effects on predetermined outcome measures. However, if only quantitative data are used to investigate the added value of an eHealth technology, much information might be missed. Imagine if an Internet-based intervention for depression is evaluated via an RCT, but is found not to be effective. The researchers have no idea why it is not – it has been studied before in different settings and has been shown to lead to improved outcomes in other populations. When asking the specific target group, it becomes clear that they have difficulty reading and writing and that they simply did not understand many of the intervention's texts and exercises. On the other hand, if only (qualitative) interviews are used, only 'subjective' information is collected, and reliable conclusions about whether an effect is actually observed and does not rely on coincidence or the participants' perception cannot be drawn. It can be difficult for end-users to identify if and how a technology helped them. This highlights the importance of complementing these two types of data and shows the relevance of mixed-methods approaches that help researchers gain a deeper and more holistic understanding of the impact, effectiveness, and underlying mechanisms of an eHealth intervention (Sieverink, 2017).

In a mixed-methods study, both quantitative and qualitative data are collected and 'mixed'; in other words, merged or integrated (Creswell & Plano Clark, 2018; Venkatesh, Brown, & Sullivan, 2016). Triangulation is applied, in which different types of data sources are combined in one study. It is important to make the distinction with multi-method research, in which several only qualitative, or several only quantitative sources can be used, as opposed to a mixed-methods study, in which qualitative and quantitative data should always be combined. Besides triangulation, another key component of mixed-methods research is that these quantitative and qualitative data are merged, meaning that they have to be actively integrated. If this is not done and analysis takes place separately, a study is not mixed-methods, but again multi-method. The merging of data can happen at different stages in the process, for example during data analysis, e.g., the topics of questionnaires are used to code the qualitative data (e.g., depression, anxiety, self-control). Merging data can also take place after data analysis. For example, first questionnaire data are analyzed, qualitative data is coded inductively – meaning that researchers identify new codes from the interview data using a bottom-up approach. Next, the codes that are identified in the interviews are used to search for reasons for (non)-effectiveness. Furthermore, there are different types of research designs that can be used (also see Figure 16.6):

- Concurrent designs: Data are collected within the same design, for example, directly after an RCT, interviews are conducted, or open-ended questions about context are asked via an experience sampling app during the use of an activity tracker, allowing for a combination of qualitative data on context, and quantitative data on physical activity;

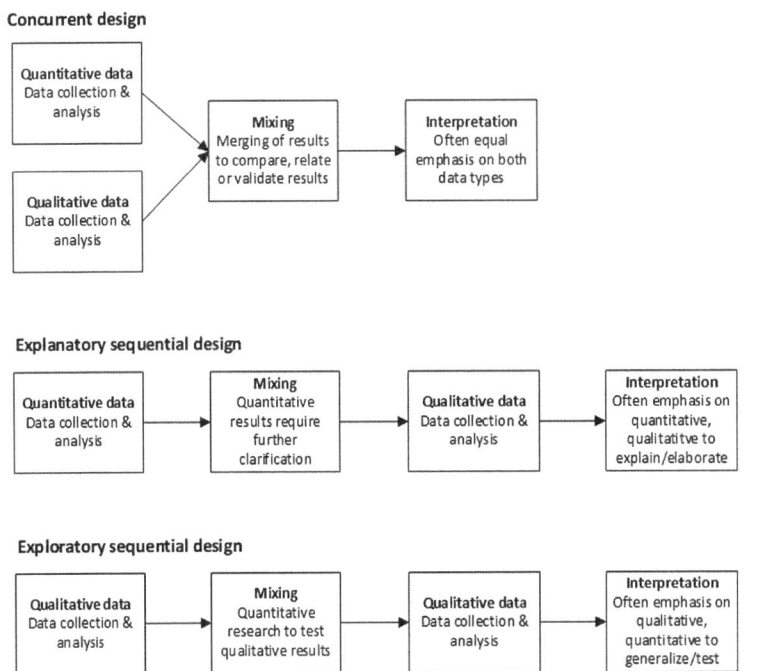

Figure 16.6 An overview of different types of mixed-methods designs.

- Sequential design: Data are collected separately, and only after analysis, integration takes place. Two types of sequential designs can be identified:
  - Explanatory sequential designs: First, quantitative data are collected (e.g., log data), and qualitative data (e.g., interviews) are collected to explain the outcomes of this analysis;
  - Exploratory sequential designs: First, qualitative data is collected (e.g., interviews on expected outcomes of an eHealth technology), after which quantitative data is used to explore whether these outcomes are also observed quantitatively.

However, there are more ways to conduct mixed-methods research, as long as triangulation of qualitative and quantitative methods are used and data are merged in a separate step of analysis.

Possible Research Questions

Mixed-methods studies are very broad and can be used for a wide range of research questions – not just for evaluation, but also for development and implementation. Some possible types of research questions for eHealth evaluation are:

- To what extent does an intervention improve outcomes such as anxiety, depression, and well-being, according to validated questionnaires and participants themselves?
- What elements of the eHealth intervention are used most and how are they experienced by users?
- How does the eHealth intervention compare to an existing face-to-face intervention in terms of effectiveness and experienced benefits?
- Which type of users experience the most effect and what are the main reasons for this?
- How do users explain the (lack of) effectiveness of a specific method?

Added Value and Limitations

The main benefit of mixed-methods research is that it can paint a more comprehensive picture of the impact, uptake, and working mechanisms of an eHealth intervention. Combining 'objective' quantitative data with 'subjective' qualitative data allows for integration of the stakeholder perspective, but also prevents a one-sided picture. An important barrier is that mixed-methods research is of course more complex than conducting a single-method study. The merging of data is especially complex and the way in which this should be done can differ per study. It is important to carefully plan this in advance. Furthermore, it might be that data contradict each other, e.g., participants might indicate that they experience effects on well-being, but this might not be reflected in the questionnaire data, which can make interpretation complex – while this of course also raises interesting questions about the validity of selected quantitative outcome measures. Finally, mixed-methods research is often time- and resource intensive and should be conducted by a research team with ample expertise in not just qualitative and quantitative research, but also the specific mixed-methods approach.

Mixed-Methods: An Example

In a sequential explanatory mixed-methods study, the effect of a self-modelled video-feedback parent-child interaction intervention programme on infant sleep was studied (Keys, Benzies, Kirk, & Duffett-Leger, 2022). After an RCT was conducted, interviews were conducted to explain the results. Data were coded inductively, and a compare-and-contrast method was used to compare themes between groups (intervention and control). Themes were also compared between families with the least and most improvements in infant sleep to look for explanations for (non)effectiveness. Amongst other things, the intervention was effective in reducing reported duration of infant nocturnal wakefulness. Parents from the intervention group who experienced the greatest improvements in their infant's sleep, reported in interviews that individualized video feedback on infant cues increased their confidence, showing a possible explanation for its effectiveness. However, non-significant results were found as well, e.g., on the number of awakenings. Interviews showed that the lack of effectiveness could be partly explained by a suboptimal number and timing of sessions, warranting the need for further improvement of the intervention. This example shows the added value of using qualitative data to explain quantitative outcomes.

Health Technology Assessment (HTA)

Health Technology Assessment (HTA) is a multidisciplinary evaluation method that summarizes information about clinical, economic, social, organizational, ethical, and legal aspects of health technologies and interventions. The main goal of a HTA is to inform policy- and decision making in healthcare, with a prominent role for questions of 'value for money' and 'limited resource allocation' (WHO, 2015). Given the cost-saving and efficiency-increasing potential of eHealth, economic evaluations are of central importance to HTA for eHealth. Therefore, this section focuses specifically on economic evaluations.

In an economic evaluation, alternatives are compared in terms of input (costs) and output (consequences) as shown in Figure 16.7. For a new eHealth technology, this means that costs and consequences of the technology are compared with costs and consequences of conventional care,

based on the following ratio: $\left(\dfrac{\Delta\text{costs}}{\Delta\text{consequences}} \right)$.

Possible outcomes of the economic evaluation are shown in Figure 16.7. Quadrant I and IV are dominant outcomes; a negative evaluation occurs if eHealth costs more, but gives worse consequences than conventional care (I) and a positive evaluation occurs if eHealth costs less with better consequences (IV). For quadrants II and III, one should consider if the increase in costs is worth the better consequences (II) or if the cost-saving is worth the worsening of consequences (III).

Within economic evaluations, there are three prominent analysis techniques (also see Chapter 10): Cost-benefit analysis (CBA), cost-effectiveness analysis (CEA), and cost-utility analysis (CUA). All techniques follow the process in Figure 16.7, but they differ in the handling of consequences (see Figure 16.8).

- **A cost-benefit analysis** (CBA) identifies different consequences, not necessarily the same for each alternative, but translates them into monetary units, resulting in a net cost/benefit ratio (or net monetary benefit);

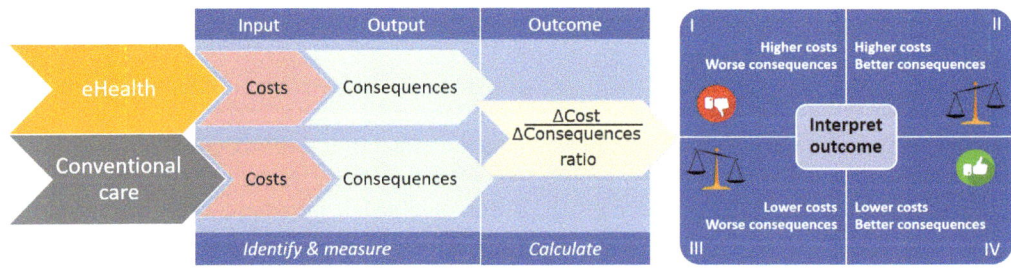

Figure 16.7 Economic evaluation process and possible outcomes (Drummond, 2015).

Analysis technique	Costs	Consequence identification	Consequence measurement	Result evaluation ($\frac{\Delta costs}{\Delta consequences}$)
Cost-benefit analysis (CBA)	Monetary units	Single/multiple effects, not necessarily common to both alternatives.	Monetary units	Net Monetary Benefit (NMB)
Cost-effectiveness analysis (CEA)	Monetary units	Single effect of interest, common to both alternatives, but achieved to different degrees.	Natural units (e.g. life-years gained, clinical values)	Incremental Cost-Effectiveness Ratio (ICER)
Cost-utility analysis (CUA)	Monetary units	Single/multiple effects, not necessarily common to both alternatives.	Quality-adjusted life years (QALYs)	Incremental Cost-Utility Ratio (ICUR)

Figure 16.8 Characteristics of CBA, CEA, and CUA.

- **A cost-effectiveness analysis** (CEA) measures consequences in terms of natural units common to both alternatives (e.g., life years gained (LYG) or clinical effects), resulting in costs per effect change (ICER).
- **A cost-utility analysis** (CUA) identifies different consequences, which don't necessarily have to be the same for both alternatives but translates them into one utility measure of the health outcome produced, resulting in costs per utility measure. The most common utility measure is the Quality Adjusted Life Year (QALY), which incorporates both survival time (extra life-years) and quality of life (expressed as a utility value on a scale of 0 – death to 1 – total health). Result of the CUA is expressed in costs per QALY change (ICUR).

Various perspectives can be used in economic evaluations (e.g., societal, insurance, healthcare provider, patient perspective). The perspective determines which costs and consequences are included and thus for whom the outcome is relevant. Furthermore, informed and preferably evidence-based assumptions about costs and consequences have to be made in economic evaluations. The general principle of 'garbage in is garbage out' is very important for economic evaluations. An uncertainty analysis should always be part of economic evaluation.

Possible Research Questions

CBA:

- Do the benefits of an eHealth technology exceed the costs?

CEA/CUA:

- Is the improvement in effect/utility of the eHealth technology worth its costs?
- Is the improvement in effect/utility that is realizable given the budget sufficient?

Added Value and Limitations

The cost-effectiveness of eHealth is often unproven (Black et al., 2011). Therefore, economic evaluations of eHealth are important to prove value for money, to support decision making, and to develop new business models, so that financial support for large-scale uptake can be facilitated (Bergmo, 2015). A limitation of economic evaluations is the possibly limited generalizability of the outcomes, caused by varieties in eHealth (e.g., technology used, medical field, service provided, and local context) that determine which costs and consequences should be included (Bergmo, 2015). Another limitation is that, traditionally, benefits other than health-outcomes are not included in economic evaluations (Drummond et al., 2014). However, eHealth is known for (and sometimes primarily focused on) creating non-health–outcome value as well, such as improvements in the healthcare process and improved self-confidence, perceived life control, knowledge about one's health, and social support. The possibility to include these benefits in analyses as well is still being studied (Benning et al., 2015).

Health Technology Assessment: An Example

Loohuis et al. (2022) studied the cost-effectiveness of an app-based treatment for women with urinary incontinence compared with care-as-usual in Dutch primary care. Costs, cost-effectiveness, and cost-utility were studied from a societal perspective, based on incontinence impact adjusted life years (IIALY), QALYs and medical, non-medical, and productivity costs. The gained effects and utilities were comparable between both groups after one year, but costs were lower for app-based treatment with € −161 per year (i.e., between quadrants III and IV in Figure 16.7). Thus, the app-based treatment is a cost-effective alternative for care-as-usual for women with urinary incontinence in Dutch primary care.

Log Data Analysis

As stated earlier, many experimental evaluation methods do not account for the main characteristics of technology, for example, its constant development and the high likelihood that not all participants use the technology in the same way. As mentioned before, when only using the more traditional experimental evaluation methods, no insights can be obtained on process outcomes, meaning how the use of the different components of the technology has contributed to healthier living, improved well-being, or a user's ability to conduct daily tasks. Log data can provide continuous and objective insights into the actual usage of the different components of the technology and thus has the potential to open the Black Box of eHealth (see the example in Box 16.2).

   Log data are anonymous records of real-time actions performed by a user of a technology (Han, 2011). In general, log data contains information of every action of the users of a technology, including an (anonymous) identification of the user, the date and time of the action, and an identification of the action (Figure 16.9), e.g., which elements of the technology are used.

   Log data analysis is a promising approach to explain the identified effects of a technology (e.g., in an RCT). It can provide insight into the navigation process of a user in daily life (Sieverink, Kelders, Poel, & van Gemert-Pijnen, 2017) on the level of seconds to minutes (e.g., transitions between pages), on the level of minutes to hours (e.g., combinations of functionalities used within a session), and on the level of hours to days (e.g., similarities in user patterns) (ten Klooster, Noordzij, & Kelders, 2020). This knowledge can result in concrete points of improvement for the technology to help the user better navigate through the system.

User	Time Stamp	Action
1	January 12; 01:14 p.m.	Login
1	January 12; 01:21 p.m.	Login
2	January 12; 01:20 p.m.	Login
2	January 12; 01:22 p.m.	Opening monitoring
2	January 12; 01:47 p.m.	Adding monitoring value
3	January 21; 10:11 a.m.	Login
3	January 21; 10:12 a.m.	Opening mailbox
3	January 21; 10:13 a.m.	Opening monitoring
3	January 21; 10:13 a.m.	Opening mailbox
3	January 21; 10:21 a.m.	Send message
1	January 23; 10:11 a.m.	Login
1	January 23; 10:13 a.m.	Opening mailbox
1	January 23; 10:15 a.m.	Send message

Figure 16.9 A fictional example of log data.

Possible Research Questions

Log data can be used to answer research questions related to how the eHealth technology works, such as:

- What usage patterns emerge when users navigate through the technology?
- What groups of similar user patterns appear and to what extent do users show similar usage patterns over time?
- Which (combinations of) elements of the technology are used?
- How do users respond to behaviour change strategies and persuasive triggers?
- How do users use the technology in order to complete an intervention or to achieve their health-related goals in terms of frequency or combinations of elements they use?
- How did these usage patterns contribute to the (clinical, behavioural, and organizational) impact?

Added Value and Limitations

We have already established that many experimental evaluation methods do not account for the characteristics of a technology, and log data analyses can help to provide more insight into how a technology is used, addressing the 'black box' problem. Another common problem in (eHealth) research is that participants often drop out from the evaluation study because they find it too time-consuming and labour-intensive to complete questionnaires at different time points or to participate in an interview or focus group. An important advantage of log data is that it is always available and easy to collect, without requiring any extra effort from the participants (Sieverink et al., 2017).

An important limitation is that the results of the log data analyses do not indicate why certain usage patterns occur. It is therefore important to combine the analyses with additional research via interviews, usability tests, or other quantitative and qualitative research methods to gain more precise insights into what users experience. The insights obtained from the log file analyses can be used to form hypotheses about, for example, usability problems. These hypotheses can then be used to inform the design of the additional research (ten Klooster, Kelders, & Noordzij, 2020).

Finally, it is not always possible to collect log data, so the function to retrieve these data should be built into the technology from the start – which might require additional knowledge and resources.

Log Data Analysis: An Example

Epic's MyChart is an outpatient portal for pregnant individuals with various functionalities, such as sending and receiving messages to healthcare providers, gaining insight into personal health information, and managing appointments (Morgan, Schnell, Singh, & Fareed, 2022). In their study, the proportion in which users used the functionalities of Epic's MyChart were used to find similar groups of users. They carried out a cluster analysis, which means that users who are in the same cluster share similar proportions of use, whereas users in other clusters show different proportions of use. The results showed that there were four groups of similar users for all pregnant individuals, namely 'Schedulers', 'Resulters', 'Intense Digital Engagers', and 'Average Users'. Thus, different patterns appeared among participants, showing that not all participants used the technology in the same way. By taking into account this heterogeneity among users, we gain insight into the 'Black Box' of technology use.

Another example of a log data analysis can be found in the example of Pot et al. (Pot et al., 2020), who performed a dose-response analysis of a web-based Human Papillomavirus Vaccination (HPV) intervention. They investigated to what extent users visited all web pages of the intervention, and the time that participants spent in the HPV intervention. This usage information was used to determine the effects on HPV vaccination uptake and other secondary outcomes. They concluded that intervention usage had a significant effect on various outcome measures. While a traditional RCT could have provided insights into whether or not using the intervention improved the outcomes, this study shows how log data analysis can provide a more detailed understanding of the use that is needed to experience certain effects.

Summary

When looking back at this chapter, there are several aspects to keep in mind when evaluating eHealth. First, it is important to realize that there is no single gold standard or one step-by-step approach for all eHealth evaluations. The selection of evaluation methods depends on the goals of the study, the nature of the studied eHealth technology, practical preconditions such as available time and money, and participant characteristics. Ideally, evaluations are conducted to gain more insight into the points of improvement, impact, uptake, and working mechanisms of an eHealth technology. To paint a complete picture of the added value of a technology, a holistic approach is again advised, in which attention is paid to the people, context, and technology itself. The overview of frameworks and methods in this chapter are not exhaustive: There are many more suitable frameworks, and many more suitable methods that can be used. Additionally, attention should be paid to new technological developments and their implications for evaluation. Examples are artificial intelligence and machine learning, which can be useful to conduct evaluation studies with large data sets and gain more (and even real-time) insights into working mechanisms. Furthermore, new technologies might require new evaluation methods. For example, how to optimally measure a sense of presence in VR and relate it to its effectiveness? And in what ways can we measure real-time experiences with technology in a continuous way, such as engagement or experienced effectiveness? The unique characteristics of technology require (and provide opportunities for) unique ways of doing research. The take-home messages of this chapter are:

- There is not one main objective to conduct eHealth evaluation: It can be focused on determining the impact, uptake, working mechanisms, and points of improvement of the eHealth technology;

- Evaluation is not a post-implementation activity, but already begins from the start of the development and is never really finished;
- eHealth is not a separate thing or tool and thus should not be evaluated as such: A holistic approach in which sufficient attention is paid to the role of and impact on the different stakeholders, the context, and technology is pivotal;
- There is not one gold standard for evaluation: Ideally, different research methods are combined into a coherent, iterative evaluation process;
- A mixed-methods approach in which quantitative and qualitative data are combined often provides more insight into the effectiveness of an eHealth technology than using only one method.

Key References for Further Reading

Bonten, T. N., Rauwerdink, A., Wyatt, J. C., Kasteleyn, M. J., Witkamp, L., Riper, H., ... & eHealth Evaluation Research Group. (2020). Online guide for electronic health evaluation approaches: Systematic scoping review and concept mapping study. *Journal of Medical Internet Research*, 22(8), e17774.

Collins, L. M., Murphy, S. A., & Strecher, V. (2007). The multiphase optimization strategy (MOST) and the sequential multiple assignment randomized trial (SMART): New methods for more potent eHealth interventions. *American Journal of Preventive Medicine*, 32(5), S112–S118.

Moore, G. F., Audrey, S., Barker, M., Bond, L., Bonell, C., Hardeman, W., Moore, L., O'Cathain, A., Tinati, T., Wight, D., & Baird, J. (2015). Process evaluation of complex interventions: Medical Research Council guidance. *BMJ* (Clinical research ed.), 350, h1258. https://doi.org/10.1136/bmj.h1258

Pawson, R., & Tilley, N. (1997). An introduction to scientific realist evaluation. In E. Chelimsky & W. R. Shadish (Eds.), *Evaluation for the 21st century: A handbook* (pp. 405–418). Sage Publications, Inc. https://doi.org/10.4135/9781483348896.n29

Sieverink, F. (2017). Opening the black box of eHealth [doctoral dissertation]. Twente: Universiteit van Twente.

References

Alnahdi, G. H. (2015). Single-subject designs in special education: Advantages and limitations. *Journal of Research in Special Educational Needs*, 15(4), 257–265. doi:https://doi.org/10.1111/1471-3802.12039

Barger-Anderson, R., Domaracki, J. W., Kearney-Vakulick, N., & Kubina, R. M. (2004). Multiple baseline designs: The use of a single-case experimental design in literacy research. *Reading Improvement*, 41, 217.

Benning, T. M., Alayli-Goebbels, A. F. G., Aarts, M.-J., Stolk, E., de Wit, G. A., Prenger, R., ... Evers, S. M. A. A. (2015). Exploring outcomes to consider in economic evaluations of health promotion programs: What broader non-health outcomes matter most? *BMC Health Services Research*, 15(1), 266. doi:10.1186/s12913-015-0908-y

Bergmo, T. S. (2015). How to measure costs and benefits of eHealth interventions: An overview of methods and frameworks. *J Med Internet Res*, 17(11), e254. doi:10.2196/jmir.4521

Black, A. D., Car, J., Pagliari, C., Anandan, C., Cresswell, K., Bokun, T., ... Sheikh, A. (2011). The impact of eHealth on the quality and safety of health care: A systematic overview. *PLoS Med*, 8(1), e1000387. doi:10.1371/journal.pmed.1000387

Bonten, T. N., Rauwerdink, A., Wyatt, J. C., Kasteleyn, M. J., Witkamp, L., Riper, H., ... Chavannes, N. H. (2020). Online guide for electronic health evaluation approaches: Systematic scoping review and concept mapping study. *J Med Internet Res*, 22(8), e17774. doi:10.2196/17774

Collins, L. M., Dziak, J. J., Kugler, K. C., & Trail, J. B. (2014). Factorial experiments: Efficient tools for evaluation of intervention components. *Am J Prev Med*, 47(4), 498–504. doi:10.1016/j.amepre.2014.06.021

Collins, L. M., Dziak, J. J., & Li, R. (2009). Design of experiments with multiple independent variables: A resource management perspective on complete and reduced factorial designs. *Psychol Methods*, 14(3), 202–224. doi:10.1037/a0015826

Collins, L. M., Murphy, S. A., & Strecher, V. (2007). The multiphase optimization strategy (MOST) and the sequential multiple assignment randomized trial (SMART): New methods for more potent eHealth interventions. *American Journal of Preventive Medicine*, 32(5), S112–S118.

Creswell, J. W., & Plano Clark, V. L. (2018). *Designing and conducting mixed methods research* (Third edition ed.). Thousand Oaks, California: SAGE.

Dallery, J., Cassidy, R. N., & Raiff, B. R. (2013). Single-case experimental designs to evaluate novel technology-based health interventions. *J Med Internet Res*, 15(2), e22. doi:10.2196/jmir.2227

Drummond, M. (2015). *Methods for the economic evaluation of health care programmes* (Fourth edition ed.). Oxford, United Kingdom: Oxford University Press.

Glasgow, R. (2007). eHealth evaluation and dissemination research. *American Journal of Preventive Medicine*, 32, S119–126. doi:10.1016/j.amepre.2007.01.023

Guastaferro, K., Strayhorn, J. C., & Collins, L. M. (2021). The multiphase optimization strategy (MOST) in child maltreatment prevention research. *Journal of Child and Family Studies*, 30(10), 2481–2491. doi:10.1007/s10826-021-02062-7

Han, J. Y. (2011). Transaction logfile analysis in health communication research: Challenges and opportunities. *Patient Education and Counseling*, 82(3), 307–312. doi:https://doi.org/10.1016/j.pec.2010.12.018

Horner, R., Carr, E., Halle, J., McGee, G., Odom, S., & Wolery, M. (2005). The use of single-subject research to identify evidence-based practice in special education. *Exceptional Children*, 71, 165–179. doi:10.1177/001440290507100203

Kelders, S. M., Bohlmeijer, E. T., Pots, W. T., & van Gemert-Pijnen, J. E. (2015). Comparing human and automated support for depression: Fractional factorial randomized controlled trial. *Behav Res Ther*, 72, 72–80. doi:10.1016/j.brat.2015.06.014

Kelders, S. M., Oinas-Kukkonen, H., Oörni, A., & van Gemert-Pijnen, J. E. W. C. (2016). Health behavior change support systems as a research discipline; A viewpoint. *International Journal of Medical Informatics*, 96, 3–10. doi:http://dx.doi.org/10.1016/j.ijmedinf.2016.06.022

Kelders, S. M., van Zyl, L. E., & Ludden, G. D. S. (2020). The concept and components of engagement in different domains applied to eHealth: A systematic scoping review. *Frontiers in Psychology*, 11. doi:10.3389/fpsyg.2020.00926

Keys, E. M., Benzies, K. M., Kirk, V. G., & Duffett-Leger, L. (2022). Effect of Play2Sleep on mother-reported and father-reported infant sleep: A sequential explanatory mixed-methods study of a randomized controlled trial. *J Clin Sleep Med*, 18(2), 439–452. doi:10.5664/jcsm.9618

Kip, H., Sieverink, F., van Gemert-Pijnen, L. J. E. W. C., Bouman, Y. H. A., & Kelders, S. M. (2020). Integrating people, context, and technology in the implementation of a web-based intervention in forensic mental health care: Mixed-methods study. *J Med Internet Res*, 22(5), e16906. doi:10.2196/16906

Köhle, N. (2016). *Hold on, for each other: Supporting partners of cancer patients via eHealth and positive psychology*. Universiteit Twente.

Köhle, N., Drossaert, C., Schreurs, K., Hagedoorn, M., Verdonck-de Leeuw, I., & Bohlmeijer, E. (2015). A web-based self-help intervention for partners of cancer patients based on Acceptance and Commitment Therapy: A protocol of a randomized controlled trial. *BMC Public Health*, 15(1), 1–13. doi:10.1186/s12889-015-1656-y

Krasny-Pacini, A., & Evans, J. (2018). Single-case experimental designs to assess intervention effectiveness in rehabilitation: A practical guide. *Ann Phys Rehabil Med*, 61(3), 164–179. doi:10.1016/j.rehab.2017.12.002

Kratochwill, T. R., Hitchcock, J. H., Horner, R. H., Levin, J. R., Odom, S. L., Rindskopf, D. M., & Shadish, W. R. (2012). Single-case intervention research design standards. *Remedial and Special Education*, 34(1), 26–38. doi:10.1177/0741932512452794

Li, Q., Mak, Y., & Loke, A. (2013). Spouses' experience of caregiving for cancer patients: A literature review. *International Nursing Review*, 60(2), 178–187.

Lilford, R. J., Foster, J., & Pringle, M. (2009). Evaluating eHealth: How to make evaluation more methodologically robust. *PLoS Med*, 6(11), e1000186. doi:10.1371/journal.pmed.1000186

Loohuis, A. M. M., Van Der Worp, H., Wessels, N. J., Dekker, J. H., Slieker-Ten Hove, M. C. P., Berger, M. Y., . . . Blanker, M. H. (2022). Cost-effectiveness of an app-based treatment for urinary incontinence in comparison with care-as-usual in Dutch general practice: A pragmatic randomised controlled trial over 12 months. *BJOG*, 129(9), 1538–1545. doi:10.1111/1471-0528.17191

Moore, G. F., Audrey, S., Barker, M., Bond, L., Bonell, C., Hardeman, W., . . . Baird, J. (2015). Process evaluation of complex interventions: Medical Research Council guidance. *BMJ: British Medical Journal*, 350, h1258. doi:10.1136/bmj.h1258

Morgan, E., Schnell, P., Singh, P., & Fareed, N. (2022). Outpatient portal use among pregnant individuals: Cross-sectional, temporal, and cluster analysis of use. *Digit Health*, 8, 20552076221109553. doi:10.1177/20552076221109553

Nielsen, K., & Miraglia, M. (2016). What works for whom in which circumstances? On the need to move beyond the 'what works?' question in organizational intervention research. *Human Relations*, 70(1), 40–62. doi:10.1177/0018726716670226

Oakley, A., Strange, V., Bonell, C., Allen, E., Stephenson, J., & Team, R. S. (2006). Health services research: Process evaluation in randomised controlled trials of complex interventions. *BMJ: British Medical Journal*, 332(7538), 413.

Pawson, R., & Tilley, N. (1997). An introduction to scientific realist evaluation. In *Evaluation for the 21st century: A handbook.* (pp. 405–418). Thousand Oaks, CA, US: Sage Publications, Inc.

Pot, M., Paulussen, T. G., Ruiter, R. A., Mollema, L., Hofstra, M., & Van Keulen, H. M. (2020). Dose-response relationship of a web-based tailored intervention promoting human papillomavirus vaccination: Process evaluation of a randomized controlled trial. *J Med Internet Res*, 22(7), e14822. doi:10.2196/14822

Resnicow, K., Strecher, V., Couper, M., Chua, H., Little, R., Nair, V., . . . Atienza, A. A. (2010). Methodologic and design issues in patient-centered e-Health research. *American Journal of Preventive Medicine*, 38(1), 98–102. doi:http://dx.doi.org/10.1016/j.amepre.2009.09.034

Salter, K. L., & Kothari, A. (2014). Using realist evaluation to open the black box of knowledge translation: A state-of-the-art review. *Implementation Science*, 9(1), 115. doi:10.1186/s13012-014-0115-y

Sieverink, F. (2017). *Opening the black box of eHealth: A mixed methods approach for the evaluation of personal health records.* University of Twente.

Sieverink, F., Kelders, S., Poel, M., & van Gemert-Pijnen, L. (2017). Opening the black box of electronic health: Collecting, analyzing, and interpreting log data. *JMIR Res Protoc*, 6(8), e156. doi:10.2196/resprot.6452

Smith, J. D. (2012). Single-case experimental designs: A systematic review of published research and current standards. *Psychol Methods*, 17(4), 510–550. doi:10.1037/a0029312

Strecher, V. J., McClure, J. B., Alexander, G. L., Chakraborty, B., Nair, V. N., Konkel, J. M., . . . Pomerleau, O. F. (2008). Web-based smoking-cessation programs: Results of a randomized trial. *Am J Prev Med*, 34(5), 373–381. doi:10.1016/j.amepre.2007.12.024

Tate, R. L., Perdices, M., Rosenkoetter, U., Shadish, W., Vohra, S., Barlow, D. H., . . . Wilson, B. (2016). The Single-Case Reporting guideline In BEhavioural interventions (SCRIBE) 2016 statement. *Remedial and Special Education*, 37(6), 370–380. doi:10.1177/0741932516652893

ten Klooster, I., Noordzij, M. L., & Kelders, S. M. (2020). Exploring how professionals within agile health care informatics perceive visualizations of log file analyses: Observational study followed by a focus group interview. *JMIR Hum Factors*, 7(1), e14424. doi:10.2196/14424

Venkatesh, V., Brown, S. A., & Sullivan, Y. W. (2016). Guidelines for conducting mixed-methods research: An extension and illustration. *Journal of the Association for Information Systems*, 17, 435–495. doi:10.17705/1jais.00433

WHO. (2015). Health technology assessment. Retrieved from https://www.who.int/teams/health-product-policy-and-standards/assistive-and-medical-technology/medical-devices/assessment

Key Terms

Key Term	Definition
Acceptance and Commitment Therapy	A type of behavioural therapy that teaches clients to accept matters that are under their direct control, such as their own behaviour, instead of trying to control experiences that are not directly influenceable.
Acceptance of technology	The decision of members of the target group on if, how, and when they would use the technology.
Adherence to technology	Whether the technology is used as it is intended by the developers.
Adoption of technology	Key concept in the Diffusion of Innovations Theory which aims to explain how, why, and at what rate ideas and technologies spread.
Affective engagement	A component of engagement that is seen as a combination of enjoying the technology, enjoying progress, and identity.
Agile	A method of project management, used especially for software development, which is characterized by the division of tasks into short phases of work and frequent adaptation of plans.
Agile Software Development	A vision on software development based on values as collaborative development, a 'lean' mentality, active stakeholder involvement, and acceptance of uncertainty which encourages rapid and flexible response to change.
Application Programming Interface (API)	An API is a set of rules and protocols that allows different software applications to communicate and interact with each other.
Applied research	Applied research uses scientific theories, findings, and methods to address practical issues, e.g., via the development of products.
Artificial intelligence	AI is a multidisciplinary field of computer science that focuses on creating machines or systems capable of emulating human-like intelligence and decision-making processes.
Augmented reality	In AR, an additional layer of virtual, non-existing elements is added to reality.
Behaviour change interventions	Interventions designed to intentionally affect the actions that individuals take with regard to their health.
Behaviour change taxonomy	A scheme of classifying behaviour change techniques.
Behaviour Change Technique (BCT)	A systematic, observable procedure derived from theory included as an element or active component of an intervention designed to change behaviour.

Behaviour change theories	Behaviour change theories aim to explain and predict why behaviours change, often via a set of related factors on, e.g., cognition or environment.
Behaviour Change Wheel (BCW)	An overarching framework of behaviour change that supports intervention developers in adding theory-based behaviour change techniques to their interventions.
Behavioural design thinking approach	An approach that uses an innovative framework that synthesises and leverages behavioural science and design thinking processes to optimise digital health interventions by maximising user engagement.
Behavioural engagement	A component of engagement that emphasizes the importance of routine, no effort, and active periods as qualities of engaged behaviour.
Behavioural medicine	The interdisciplinary field concerned with the development and integration of behavioural, psychosocial, and biomedical science knowledge and techniques relevant to the understanding of health and illness, and the application of this knowledge and these techniques to prevention, diagnosis, treatment, and rehabilitation.
Behavioural model by Fogg	A behavioural model which assumes that three factors together determine if a behaviour occurs: Motivation, ability, and a prompt (the latter of which can be delivered through a technology).
Big data	Data sets that are so voluminous and complex that traditional data processing application software are inadequate to deal with them.
Binary code	The language that computers use to communicate internally; a system of representing data with two symbols: 0 and 1.
Biopsychosocial model	A broad view on health that attributes disease to an interaction between biological factors (e.g., genetic, biochemical), psychological factors (e.g., personality, behaviour), and social factors (e.g., culture, family).
Black box of eHealth	A term that represents the lack of insight into the active ingredients and working mechanisms of eHealth interventions, even after conducting evaluation studies.
Blended Care	The combination of face-to-face services with technological treatment elements in an effort to improve the efficacy, efficiency, or reduce the cost of health services.
Business model	A model that defines how an organization creates and delivers value to customers, and then converts payments received into profit.
Business Model Canvas	A methodology for creating business models, making use of a canvas consisting of interdependent elements that are influencing the business model of a product or service.
CeHRes Roadmap	An interdisciplinary framework for the planning, coordination, and execution of holistic, iterative, and participatory development, implementation, and evaluation processes of eHealth technology.
Channels	An element of business modelling that that refers to the way products and services are delivered to customers.
Chatbot	A chatbot or conversational agent is a system that can converse and interact with users using spoken, written, and visual language.
Chronic disease	Chronic diseases persist for a long time, often defined as three months or more. Chronic diseases generally cannot be prevented by vaccines or completely cured by medication.

Chronic Care Model	A model explaining the organization of care for people with a chronic disease. It suggests six elements for high-quality care: The community, the health system, self-management support, delivery system design, decision support, and clinical information systems.
Cognitive bias modification	A technique that targets cognitive biases by directly retraining them via simple computer tasks.
Cognitive engagement	A component of engagement that emphasizes ability, usefulness, and mental effort; which shows that engagement should always be seen in the context of the goals of the users.
Cognitive walkthrough	A type of usability testing in which experts on content or design use a technology in a structured, task-oriented way, guided by tasks that a user would want to perform with a system.
Cognitive work analysis	A work-centred conceptual framework that aims to analyze the cognitive work of actors by evaluating the systems already in place, and developing recommendations for design accordingly.
Cognitive task analysis	A conceptual framework to dissect mental work into more manageable, smaller constructs that shed light on a specific problem.
Cognitive Behavioural Therapy	A widely used and evidence-based form of psychological treatment that focuses on the links between one's thoughts, behaviours, and emotions, and primarily aims to teach a patient skills to be able to change one's thinking in order to improve one's feelings and actions.
Computer vision	Computer vision empowers computers to interpret and understand visual information from the world, much like humans do with their eyes and brains.
Conversational agent	A chatbot or conversational agent is a system that can converse and interact with users using spoken, written, and visual language.
Consolidated Framework for Implementation Research (CFIR)	A model based on reviews which organizes a total of 39 determinants of implementation outcomes into 5 larger domains: characteristics of the innovation, outer setting, inner setting, characteristics of the intervention, process of implementation.
Co-design	An approach in which the importance of actively involving relevant persons throughout the development of technologies is central.
Conceptual investigations	A term within Value Sensitive Design; investigations to identify both the direct and indirect stakeholders affected by the eHealth technology, define the values implicated by its use, and prioritize competing values.
Context	The tangible and intangible environment in which a technology is intended to be used, consisting of multiple elements such as the physical surroundings, the people and their perspectives, the existing processes and routines, and the rules and regulations.
Contextual inquiry phase	A development phase of the CeHRes Roadmap in which activities are undertaken in order to get a good grasp of the context and its stakeholders, the main points of improvements within a specific context, and ways in which technology can contribute to resolving identified issues.
Cost-benefit analysis (CBA)	A methodology for the assessment of future policies (project-alternatives) that are compared to the situation without new policies (null-alternatives).
Cost structure	An element of business modelling that describes how costs are distributed across the internal and external activities of an organization.

Customer relationship	An element of business modelling that describes the relationship of an organization with its customers.
Customer segments	An element of business modelling that refers to a set of customers with common needs and interests that could benefit from the value proposition.
Customer profile	An element of the Value Proposition Canvas that maps the customer's needs by looking at the jobs-to-be-done, the pains, and gains of the customer.
Define-phase	A phase within the human-centred design process in which a problem statement that describes the main challenge the design will tackle is formulated and accompanying requirements are defined.
Deliver-phase	A phase within the human-centred design process in which prototypes are tested with users and further developed based on outcomes.
Delphi study	Creating consensus among experts on a certain topic through asking questions, reflecting upon the answers of others, and potentially adjusting one's opinion until consensus is reached, in multiple consecutive rounds.
Design phase	A development phase of the CeHRes Roadmap and in HCD in which a functioning version of an eHealth technology is created iteratively via prototyping, usability testing, and the addition of persuasive elements and behaviour change techniques.
Design with intent	A design approach intended to influence or result in certain user behaviour. To achieve this, it draws from insights from a multitude of disciplines to offer cross-domain guidance for designers.
Desk research	Collecting material in a non-systematic way in order to help the development team to learn as much as possible about the context.
Development process	The entire, iterative process of the creation of an eHealth technology that can be used in practice.
Dialogue support	Dialogue support facilitates the interaction between a system and the user by providing persuasive features that aim to motivate and engage the user to achieve desired goals with the system. The dialogue is incentive-driven to motivate users in a positive way, so that the technology takes a social role, for example, an avatar that guides you through exercises.
Diary study	The keeping of an (electronic) diary by an individual of certain events on a regular basis.
Diffusion	Diffusion refers to the spread of new practices or products.
Diffusion of innovation theory	A theory that seeks to explain how, why, and what rate innovations such as new technologies spread within a context.
Digital prototype	A way of prototyping in which the interface of a technology is represented in a simple way, using specific prototyping programmes.
Digital revolution	The very fast and impactful changes brought about by digital computing and communication technology.
Discover-phase	A phase in the human-centred design process during which designers aim to understand what the main problem is according to the people who are affected by it.
Dissemination	The active spread of new knowledge or practices to a target population using planned strategies.

Double Diamond Model	A visualization of the design process that visualizes the phases of divergence and convergence that are common in design.
Ecological momentary assessment (EMA)	Collecting real-time (and continuous) data from people's everyday lives (e.g., using an experience sampling app).
Effectiveness	The extent to which the technology actually produces the decided, decisive, or desired effects in the real world.
Efficacy	The extent to which an intervention leads to specific outcomes within controlled, ideal conditions.
Efficiency	The efficiency of a technology refers to whether the same or even better outcomes may be achieved with fewer resources, such as money or time.
eHealth	The use of technology to support health, well-being, and healthcare.
eHealth intervention	An intervention that is delivered through or supported by technology in an existing context by changing behaviour and/or cognitions.
eHealth technology	The actual technological instrument via which health, well-being, and healthcare is supported, often information or communication technology.
Elaboration Likelihood Model (ELM)	A behaviour change theory which states that there are two routes for persuading people: The central route underscores reason and argument, and the peripheral route builds upon social cues and often on the way arguments are provided.
eMental health	The use of technology for the prevention and treatment of mental disorders and the promotion of positive mental health.
Empirical investigations	A term within Value Sensitive Design; investigations of stakeholders' understandings, context, and experiences in relation to the eHealth technology and implicated values.
End-user	The person or group of people for whom the eHealth technology is designed.
Engagement	A multifaceted concept that captures not just the extent of usage but also the subjective experience when interacting with the eHealth intervention. Commonly, it is seen to consist of behaviour, cognition, and affect.
Evaluation	The systematic collection, interpretation, and presentation of information in order to determine value and results of a product.
Expanded Chronic Care Model	Expansion of the CCM, encompassing eHealth technologies. It consists of several elements that can contribute to successful care: Self-management support, delivery system design, clinical decision support, clinical information system, and eHealth education.
Expert-based usability testing	A form of usability testing in which experts on design or the subject of a technology are involved.
Explainable AI	Explainable AI is all about making AI systems transparent and interpretable.
Factorial designs	An experimental design in which multiple components of an intervention are varied within a group of participants to study their individual effects on outcomes.

Field test	An evaluation study in which a technology is close to being finished and can be used by end-users (also referred to as pilot test), focused on identifying how people are using the technology and what points of improvement are.
Flow	The performance of an activity while fully immersed in a feeling of energized focus, full involvement, and enjoyment in the process of the activity.
Focus group	Collecting qualitative data among a small number of stakeholders in a group discussion, 'focused' around a particular topic or set of issues.
Formative evaluation	Continuous activities throughout the entire development process that provide ongoing information on how to improve the eHealth technology and development process.
Fractional Factorial Design	Gaining insight into components that contribute to effectiveness in order to create the most effective intervention (that includes all the components that add to the effectiveness), or, for instance, create the most effective intervention that can be completed within a certain amount of time or with a certain maximum of costs.
Fundamental research	Fundamental research aims to create or improve abstract scientific theories for understanding, predicting, or changing phenomena.
Gamification	The application of gaming principles, such as points, levels, achievements, in non-game contexts.
Generative design	A form of co-design in which users make (generate) artefacts to help reflect on their experiences or preferences regarding a design.
Graphical User Interface (GUI)	A GUI is a visual interface that allows users to interact with software or devices through graphical elements like windows, buttons, and icons, rather than text-based commands.
Health	According to an influential paper by Huber et al. (2011), health should be seen as the ability to adapt and self-manage.
Healthcare systems	The complex interdependent system of amongst others, healthcare organizations, healthcare providers, and insurance companies in a country.
Health promotion	Health promotion enables people to increase control over and improve their own health via focusing on a wide range of social and environmental interventions.
Health psychology	The aggregate of the specific educational, scientific, and professional contribution of the discipline of psychology to the promotion and maintenance of health, the promotion and treatment of illness and related dysfunction.
Health Technology Assessment (HTA)	The evaluation of technologies in terms of (un)intended/(in)direct short- and long-term consequences, considering clinical, economic, social, organizational, ethical, and legal aspects. Informing policy- and decision making in healthcare, with a prominent role for questions of 'value for money' and 'limited resource allocation'.
Heuristic	A heuristic is a rule-of-thumb or method that helps people, often experts, investigate or solve problems efficiently.
Heuristic evaluation	A type of evaluation in which usability experts review a prototype or a completed design using pre-determined heuristics, often via a checklist to remind them of key usability problems to look out for.

Holistic approach	The notion that eHealth is a complex system and all elements such as technology, people, and context are interrelated and interdependent, indicating that separate analysis of these parts should be avoided.
Human-centred design	A framework and value system in which the user is the most important partner in design and is involved in co-designing a technology via iterative cycles of data collection in which the human perspective is actively involved.
Human-media interaction	A field of study focusing on how people interact with and are influenced by information technology.
Immersion	Immersion refers to the perception of actually being present in a non-physical, virtual world.
Impact evaluation	The assessment of whether the intended effects of an eHealth intervention were reached in clinical, organizational, and behavioural terms at a given point in time.
Implementation	The activities that are undertaken to realize the adoption, dissemination, and long-term use of a product in its intended context.
Implementation barrier	Obstacles, challenges, or other factors that hinder the successful integration of a product into real-world contexts.
Implementation strategy	Specific activities that are tailored to stakeholders and target groups to facilitate the integration of a product into a specific context.
Implementation science	A relatively new paradigm in which methods and strategies for effectively integrating evidence-based practices into real-world settings are studied.
Information and Communication Technologies (ICTs)	ICT is a broad term that encompasses technologies and systems used to manage and process information, as well as facilitate communication. ICT encompasses a wide range of hardware, software, networks, and applications that are used to store, transmit, and manipulate data and enable people to communicate with each other effectively.
Interdisciplinary	In an interdisciplinary approach, experts from multiple disciplines work on a topic with the goal to integrate and synthesize knowledge from different fields, aiming to bridge gaps between disciplines.
Intervention Mapping	Intervention Mapping is presented as a planning approach which uses theory and evidence as foundations for taking an ecological approach to intervening in health problems.
Interviews	A method in which questions are asked to a participant in a structured, semi-structured, or unstructured way to obtain insights into perspectives from a (group of) individual(s).
Involvement	The importance of a product (or eHealth technology) to the individual.
Iterative design	A design methodology based on a cyclic process of prototyping, testing, analyzing, and refining a product, during which changes and refinements are made to the product based on the outcomes of the most recent iteration of a design process.
Key activities	An element of business modelling that refers to activities that are carried out by the organization itself to create value.
Key partners	An element of business modelling that refers to other organizations that offer intermediate products and services to the organization.
Key resources	An element of business modelling that refers to the resources that are needed by an organization to conduct its key activities to create value.

Key stakeholders	Stakeholders who have a greater influence on or may be more influenced by the technology than other stakeholders.
Literature review	Gaining insight in the current status quo of scientific literature in a certain broad field of study by means of a systematic search of literature.
Log data	Objective registration of an event that can be recorded on an individual basis, e.g., logging in, entering a room, sending a message, performing a certain action, and a 'timestamp'.
Log data analysis	The use of data that logs certain behaviour on a system or in daily life to analyze patterns.
Machine Learning	A subset of AI that focuses on developing algorithms and models capable of learning from data and making predictions or decisions without being explicitly programmed.
mHealth	A specific form of eHealth making use of mobile technologies such as apps.
Mixed-methods study	A research approach in which the outcomes of both qualitative and quantitative methods are integrated within a single study.
Mobile applications	Software programs designed to run on mobile devices such as smartphones or tablets.
Mock-ups	A prototype that provides a medium-fidelity representation of a design, including elements such as colours, images, and texts.
Modality	In human-centred design, modality typically refers to the sensory modality that will interact with the user. Modalities are visual, auditory, tactile, and kinaesthetic.
Multidisciplinary	In a multidisciplinary approach, multiple separate disciplines are working on a topic, but each discipline maintains its own methods, theories, and approaches, without significant integration between the disciplines.
Multi-method approach	The use of different types of methods (quantitative and/or qualitative) without actively integrating the outcomes.
Multiphase Optimization Strategy (MOST)	A systematic approach for optimizing and refining interventions by breaking them down into their constituent components, testing these components in a phased and efficient manner, and identifying the most effective combination for achieving the desired outcomes in three phases (preparation, optimization, and evaluation).
NASSS Framework	The Nonadoption, Abandonment, Scale-up, Spread and Sustainability (NASSS) framework, with seven main categories: The condition, technology, value proposition, adopters, organization, wider system, and embedding and adaptation over time.
Natural language processing (NLP)	NLP enables machines to understand, interpret, and generate human language in a way that is both meaningful and contextually relevant.
Nudging	Nudging is concept in behavioural science, political theory, and economics which proposes positive reinforcement and indirect suggestions to try to achieve non-forced compliance to influence the motives, incentives, and decision making of groups and individuals.
Observations	Observing an event of interest while it occurs by a researcher, direct or technology-mediated.
Operationalization phase	A phase of the CeHRes Roadmap in which plans for the implementation of an eHealth technology in the intended context are developed and rolled out in practice.

Paper prototype	A prototype of an interface that is created with materials such as paper, pencils, paints, or cards.
Participatory Development	An approach in which the importance of actively involving relevant persons throughout the development of technologies is central.
Patient engagement	A patient's personal commitment to his or her own healthcare.
Patient-centred care	Providing care that is respectful of, and responsive to, individual patient preferences, needs, and values, and ensuring that patient values guide all clinical decisions.
Patient journey mapping	A HCD-method that is used to create a graphic representation of a health service and its procedure from the patient perspective, including feelings and interactions.
Perceived persuasiveness	A construct that measures how far a system is perceived as persuasive by its users.
Performance test	A performance test is a test with a prototype that is as close as possible to the eventual product and compares the user performance to some level of benchmark performance, often using statistical analyses.
Persona	Specific, concrete representations of fictitious persons that represent the target group and are used to put a face on the user throughout the (human-centred) design process.
Personal health record	A PHR is an electronic application through which individuals can access, manage, and share their health information and that of others for whom they are authorized, in a private, secure, and confidential environment.
Personalisation	The adapting of an eHealth intervention to the characteristics of an individual.
Person-based approach	The person-based approach involves in-depth qualitative research conducted with the users before the digital intervention is developed, which is used to develop 'guiding principles' that state the key intervention design objectives and describe the key features of the intervention required to achieve each objective.
Persuadability	A score that measures the tendency of a person to comply with the different persuasive strategies.
Persuasive communication	Communication that intends to describe, explain, and predict the factors that contribute to change attitudes and behaviours.
Persuasive features	Concrete ways of translating abstract design principles into aspects of a technology that contribute to its persuasiveness.
Persuasive Systems Design model	The PSD model aims to make technologies more persuasive, via persuasive features which are categorized into four categories: Primary task support, dialogue support, credibility support, and social support.
Persuasive technology	Technology that aims to reinforce, change, shape, or influence behaviour and attitudes by being compelling and without being coercive or deceptive.
Positive psychology	The scientific study of positive human functioning and flourishing on multiple levels that include the biological, personal, relational, institutional, cultural, and global dimensions of life.
Prevention	Prevention, or preventive healthcare, consists of measures taken for disease prevention, as opposed to disease treatment.
Primary prevention	The prevention of disease before it ever occurs.

Primary task support	Primary task support facilitates the performance of the user in carrying out the primary activities to reach the goal of the intervention (e.g., decrease depressive symptoms, improve self-management of diabetes). The purpose of these features is to facilitate to the user the friendliness and understandability of the information, by presenting it in personalized and small steps, reduced to tiny behaviours to achieve their goals, as well as to provide monitoring strategies of users' performance and progress towards such goals.
Project team	A team consisting of stakeholders and experts from multiple disciplines that manages the development, implementation, and evaluation process and outcomes.
Process evaluation	A type of evaluation that is focused on providing information on how an intervention is effective and usable within a specific context, emphasizing the relationship between context, implementation, mechanisms of impact, and their influence on outcomes.
Programming language	Programming languages are intermediary tools that allow humans to communicate with computers. They consist of human-readable syntax and semantics that represent the underlying complex binary code.
Prototype	A representation of a technology that can be a raw and more sketch-like (low fidelity/lo-fi) or can resemble the to-be-developed technology more closely (high fidelity/hi-fi).
Psychology	The scientific study of mental and behavioural functioning. More specifically, psychology aims to describe, explain, predict and, where possible, intervene to modify behavioural and cognitive processes.
Public health	A domain that promotes and protects the health of people and the communities where they live, learn, work, and play.
Quality adjusted life years (QALY)	The number of gained life years corrected for quality of life.
Questionnaire	Collecting quantitative or qualitative data by asking participants to fill out open- or closed-ended questions, either online or on paper.
Randomized controlled trial (RCT)	An experimental design in which participants are randomly assigned to an experimental condition (with the intervention) or control condition (without the intervention), after which between-group comparisons are made.
Reach	The absolute number, proportion, and representativeness of individuals who are willing to participate in an intervention.
RE-AIM framework	A process theory describing the stages in intervention development, among which is the stage of implementation. RE-AIM refers to five steps in the process of translating research findings into practice: Reach, effectiveness, adoption, implementation, and maintenance.
Realist evaluations	An approach to assessing and understanding the effectiveness of interventions by examining the underlying mechanisms and contexts that lead to particular outcomes, aiming to uncover how, why, and for whom a programme works or doesn't work, based on the presumptions that interventions do not work in isolation, but are influenced by specific contexts.

Remote patient monitoring	Patients' vital signs, such as heart rate or blood pressure, are (continuously) monitored using wireless sensing devices such as blood pressure monitors and pulse oximeters. Data is shared with the patient itself and/or healthcare professionals, who are at another location.
Remote interviews	Interviews in which the researcher and participant are not at the same location, facilitated via technologies such as videoconferencing services.
Remote usability testing	A way of usability testing in which users interact with a prototype from a distance, e.g., via screensharing or eye-tracking through webcams.
Requirements	Requirements state what is required of a technology: They describe what a technology should do, what data it should store or retrieve, what content it should display, and what kind of user experience it should provide.
Revenue streams	An element of business modelling that refers to the way in which the organization is paid for its efforts to the customers.
Robotics	Robotics in healthcare involves the use of automated machines to assist, diagnose, or treat patients and enhance medical procedures.
Scenario	In human-centred design, a scenario describes the envisioned use of an eHealth technology by the designated end-user.
Scoping review	A type of literature review that is conducted to gain insight into the current status quo of scientific literature within a certain broad field of study by means of a systematic literature search, without paying too much attention to the quality of studies.
Scrum software development framework	A form of agile development where developers work in teams and break up their work in short cycles, called sprints.
Secondary prevention	Secondary prevention refers to the early detection, optimal treatment, and reduction of the impact of diseases.
Self-care and prevention technologies	In these types of technologies, the patient or health consumer is put in the lead: Technology can be used to foster self-management in an easy and convenient way.
Self-management	The individual's ability to manage the symptoms, treatment, physical, and psychosocial consequences, as well as the lifestyle changes inherent in living with a chronic condition.
Self-monitoring	Self-monitoring is the ability to both observe and evaluate one's behaviour.
Sense of presence	The sensation of 'being there', referring to physical and digital/virtual environments, and the interaction with a technology.
Sequential multiple assignment randomization trial (SMART)	Yielding additional information about the effectiveness of an eHealth technology based on alternative forms of randomization.
Serious Games	Games specifically designed to teach skills or promote real-world behaviour change.
Service model	A graphical overview of how an end-user will receive and use a technology in the context of use.

Single-case experimental design (SCED)	A group of high-quality experimental research methods in which individuals serve as both the intervention group and their own control group, for whom an intervention is systematically introduced – and dependent on the type of design, withdrawn – across multiple phases, while outcome variables are frequently and repeatedly measured.
Shared care	The joint participation of general practitioners and hospital consultants in the planned delivery of care for patients with a chronic condition, informed by an enhanced information exchange over and above routine discharge and referral letters.
Shared decision making	Patients, their healthcare professionals, and caregivers actively participating in making decisions about a patient's health and care.
Sketch	A freehand drawing on paper that gives a really low-fidelity representation of a design.
SMART goals	A way to formulate goals, ensuring that they are specific, measurable, achievable, realistic, and timely.
Social marketing	An approach with a focus on marketing principles and compliance strategies to influence a target audience to voluntarily accept, reject, modify, or abandon a behaviour for the benefit of individuals, groups, or society as a whole.
Social media	User generation and sharing of content on social platforms using desktop computers, Internet websites, and mobile applications.
Social support	Social support features motivate users by leveraging social influence of other people. Users can compare themselves with others, such as relatives or unknown people, or share information with those who have the same goal to achieve desired behaviours.
Societal health technologies	Societal health focuses on broad health-related issues that might affect individuals, however, not these individuals, but governments play a vital role in creating policies and regulations. In turn, healthcare inspectorates must implement and maintain these policies and regulations.
Spiral design model	The spiral design model is a traditional software development model that argues for an iterative cycle of prototyping and evaluation, gradually converging to a design via sequential phases.
Stakeholder analysis	The analysis of the interdependencies, responsibilities, and stakes of involved stakeholders.
Stakeholder identification	The systematic, iterative process of finding out who stakeholders are within a specific project.
Stakeholders	People or groups of people who affect or are affected by an eHealth technology.
Storyboard	A series of roughly drawn comic-book style frames that visualize key moments in (the use of) a design and can be used to build a short narrative.
Summative evaluation phase	A phase of the CeHRes Roadmap in the impact, uptake, and working mechanisms of an eHealth technology. Health, the context, behaviour, and stakeholders are assessed.
Supported intervention	A technological intervention provided along with regular human support. This 'supporter' can be a therapist, coach, paraprofessional, or peer.

Supportive care technologies	These types of technologies are characterized by involvement of (multiple) healthcare professionals and, ideally, healthcare professionals and patients work together to manage or improve the health of the patient or client.
System credibility support	System credibility support refers to the trustworthiness and reliability of the system. With the use of the persuasive features, transparency can be given to the background of the system (expertise, authority, etc.). Users need that information, particularly to decide the verifiability of it.
Tailoring	The adapting of an eHealth intervention to the characteristics of a group of individuals.
Technical investigations	A term in Value Sensitive Design; investigations of specific features of technologies and how their properties and mechanisms support human values.
Technology Acceptance Model (TAM)	A well-known model that aims to understand why technologies are used, or not.
Telemedicine	Telemedicine is the use of telecommunication and information technology to provide clinical health care from a distance.
Tertiary prevention	Tertiary prevention is the prevention of further invalidation or deterioration of already diagnosed diseases.
Theory of Planned Behaviour (TPB)	The TPB is a theory that proposes that volitional human behaviour is a function of the intention to perform the behaviour. Intention is hypothesized to be a function of attitudes towards the behaviour, subjective norm, and perceived behavioural control.
Think-aloud method	A type of usability testing in which members of the target group use a prototype to complete tasks/scenarios provided by the researcher, during which they have to think aloud, i.e., verbalize their thoughts and experiences.
Transdisciplinarity	An approach towards problem-solving that goes beyond multi- or interdisciplinary approaches, in which boundaries between disciplines are blurred and knowledge is seamlessly integrated.
uHealth	Technology, such as sensors, that can be used independently from time and place and can seamlessly be incorporated into people's lives.
Unsupported intervention	A technological intervention that either makes use of automated support provided by a computer, or offers no support at all.
Uptake evaluation	Evaluation of the way in which an eHealth technology is used in practice by people and organizations.
Usability	The quality of a product or service which allows users to use it effectively and without effort, immediately learning its use and easily remembering it when returning to usage after a certain amount of time.
Usability testing	The evaluation of a product by testing it with people such as potential users or experts to identify usability problems, flaws, gather overall opinions, or collect recommendations.
User	The person who (is intended to) actively interact with the system.
User engagement	The situation when a full overlap exists between user's intentions and the characteristics of the technology.
User-based usability testing	A form of usability testing in which evaluation is performed with (potential) end-users.

User experience	Perceptions, feelings, and responses by an individual towards the actual or the anticipated use of a product, system, or service.
Unified Theory of Acceptance and Use of Technology (UTAUT)	A model to assess technology acceptance and use, consisting of four key elements explaining behavioural intention and use: Performance expectancy, effort expectancy, social influence, and facilitating conditions.
Value	A broad concept that can refer to what is important to people in their personal lives and what they find important in relation to an eHealth technology.
Value map	A part of the Value Proposition Canvas that describes products and services that support the customers in achieving their goals, taking away their pains, and creating their gains.
Value proposition	An element of business modelling that refers to the offering from the organization to its customer (another organization or an individual) that can be used to create value by means of these offerings.
Value Proposition Canvas	A model that can be used to further aid the development of Value Propositions and Customer Segments elements of the Business Model Canvas.
Value sensitive design	A theoretically grounded approach that accounts for human values throughout the design process.
Value Specification phase	A development phase of the CeHRes Roadmap in which the objectives, values, and requirements for a to-be-developed eHealth technology are formulated.
Virtual reality	Technologies that use software to create sensations (images, sounds, etc.) that replicate the real-world environment. VR is an advanced form of a human-computer interface that enables the user to interact with and be immersed in a computer-generated environment.
Waterfall model	A traditional software development model consisting of sequential phases.
Wearable technologies	Technologies that are small enough to take with you, that are embedded into clothing or accessories, that measure information from your body and lifestyle.
Web 2.0	Web 2.0 allows users not only to read (or consume) information like in Web 1.0, but also interact and collaborate with others to create and share content.
Web-based interventions	Digital platforms that deliver health-related content, tools, and support via the Internet.
Well-being	According to the dictionary, well-being is the state of feeling healthy and happy. Other definitions see well-being as positive mental health, consisting of emotional, psychological, and social well-being.
Wireframe	A representation of the skeleton or basic structure of a design, often used to describe its main functionalities.
Working mechanism	Underlying processes that explain why and how a behaviour change intervention influences individuals to change their behaviour.

Index